HORIZONS IN CANCER RESEARCH

HORIZONS IN CANCER RESEARCH

VOLUME 61

Horizons in Cancer Research

Additional books in this series can be found on Nova's website
under the Series tab.

Additional e-books in this series can be found on Nova's website
under the e-book tab.

HORIZONS IN CANCER RESEARCH

VOLUME 61

HIROTO S. WATANABE
EDITOR

NOVA BIOMEDICAL
New York

Library of Congress Cataloging-in-Publication Data

ISSN: 2159-1326

ISBN: 978-1-63484-503-8

Published by Nova Science Publishers, Inc. † New York

CONTENTS

PREFACE

This book presents original results on the leading edge of cancer research. Chapter One explains unanswered questions of contemporary oncology from the standpoint of karyogamic theory of carcinogenesis. Chapter Two focuses on the molecular players of the human papillomaviruses (HPVs) infection leading to chronic inflammation and cancer. Chapter Three describes Multiple Myeloma (MM), and Monoclonal Gammopathy of Undetermined Significance (MGUS). Chapter Four reviews the role of choline metabolites as second messengers in cellular pathways leading to enhanced cell survival, migration, and proliferation to explore the possibility that *in-vivo* imaging of choline metabolism can be used to obtain readouts of cell signal transduction in cancer. Chapter Five investigates the possible correlation between anatomic melanoma distribution on the specific back area and lack of sunscreen application. Chapter Six describes the known molecular mechanisms of epigallocatechin (EGC) and epigallocatechin-3-gallate (EGCG) in malignant neuroblastoma that can help find new directions for future research. Chapter Seven discusses the burdens of childhood cancer survivorship and the consequences of different treatment therapies on the incidence of CVD and explores potential monitoring methods and the need for consistent cardiovascular monitoring of childhood cancer survivors regarding their cardiovascular health. Finally, Chapter Eight considers a model for implementing recommendations pertaining to Lynch syndrome, and also looks at what is happening in the field now to support Lynch syndrome genetic testing and surveillance, and how a deliberative conference can point the way to changes that need to take place to deliver screening to those at risk.

In: Horizons in Cancer Research. Volume 61
Editor: Hiroto S. Watanabe

ISBN: 978-1-63484-503-8

Chapter 1

SEARCHING FOR A MAGIC KEY IN ONCOLOGY CONTINUES

G. K. Gogichadze*
Tbilisi State Medical University,
Department of Microbiology and Immunology, Tbilisi, Georgia

ABSTRACT

The major criteria of any common (integrative, unitary) theory of carcinogenesis are: systematization and reasonable explanation of the unanswered questions and the mutually exclusive on the face of it facts that have been sufficiently accumulated in modern oncology. In addition, the common theory of carcinogenesis should incorporate major postulates of the theories and hypotheses most accepted in this sphere. Proceeding from the above-mentioned facts, recognition of karyogamic theory as common theory of carcinogenesis acquire a real contoure. Lower we shall try to briefly explain of some unanswered questions of contemporary oncology from the standpoint of karyogamic theory of carcinogenesis.

The origin of malignant tumors, their essence still constitutes one of the great and obscure mysteries of nature. It is thought that the complexity of this problem is still incomprehensible by the human mind, or the cancer problem exceeds the intellectual possibilities of man.

In the history of cancer nature research, scientists repeatedly created an illusion that this century-old problem had been presumably solved, that scientists had found the magic key that would finally open all the doors of the place, where nature has so deeply and skillfully hided a solution to the problem. Unfortunately, in all the cases scientists had to be confronted with a bitter disillusionment. The so hardly found key would, at best, unlock one or two doors, but failed to fit to other doors. As a result, the secret remained and is, regrettably, still unanswered.

* E-mail: gogi_gogichadze@yahoo.com.

The major criteria of any common (integrative, unitary) theory of carcinogenesis are: to systemize and reasonable explain the unanswered questions and the mutually exclusive on the face of it facts (including biological nonsenses!) that have been sufficiently accumulated in modern oncology. In addition, the common theory should incorporate the major postulates of the currently most accepted theories and hypotheses of carcinogenesis.

For example, karyogamic theory of carcinogenesis [1] includes polyetiological, virus, and virus-genetic theories of malignant tumors origin. The etiological factors of tumors according to the last theory may be chemical, physical and biological agents as well, viruses in particular; in other words, all chemical, physical and biological agents with fusogenic abilities [2-7].

Karyogamic theory also include chromosomal theory of malignant tumors genesis, because one of the conditions in formation of both precancerous and tumorous cells are quantitative (tetraploid, subtetraploid, hyperdiploid and other types of quantitative aberrations of chromosomes) and then structural aberrations (translocations, duplications, deletions) of these organoids. After spontaneous or induced arising of tetraploid precancerous synkaryon, in such cells, there exist a number of structural alterations on subcellular and molecular degrees, which assist in malignant transformation. Moreover, in tetraploid cells, there is marked more expressed tendency to arising of chromosomal abberations than in diploid cells.

The most popular and well-ground oncogenes theory of carcinogenesis is presented in karyogamic theory at the stage of promotion, during arising of true cancerous cell. At the stage of promotion, activation of non-expressive sites of parent cells genotype take place, i.e., co-expression and amplification of oncogenes responsible for cells proliferation occur. Thus, activation of oncogenes by the karyogamic theory may be considered as the second stage of cells malignant transformation.

Above-mentioned allows us to consider the karyogamic theory as common (general, integrate, unitary) theory of carcinogenesis. It includes all principal postulated of the most popular and acceptable today theories and hypotheses, devoted to this problem.

Besides, karyogamic (two synkaryons) theory is capable to explain in full volume many aspects of carcinogenesis, insufficiently interpreted by the other hypotheses and theories, such as: formation of first cancerous cell or what is the essence of cancer cell; common mechanism of influence of diametrically different carcinogens on target cells; reason of normal cells spontaneous malignization in tissue culture; reason of arising of tumors in transplantation of allogenic internal organs, in AIDS, in hemolytic anemias; mechanism of arising of malignant neoplasms after inoculation in laboratory animals of some non-carcinogenic, indifferent substances (saline, distilled water, fatty acids, carbohydrates) and so on.

Further we shall try to briefly explain of some unanswered questions of contemporary oncology from the standpoint of karyogamic theory of carcinogenesis.

1. What Is the Essence of the Cancer Cell?

Cancer cell may arise spontaneously, and after the action on normal somatic cells of different agents and factors of chemical, physical and biological nature. Initial target for carcinogenic and non-carcinogenic agents are determinants of cellular membranes, but not the cell's DNA [8, 9].

At the first stage of carcinogenesis, i.e., at the stage of initiation, two normal somatic cells at some favorable conditions may create dikaryons (hetero- or homokaryons). Presumably, during the perforation of cellular membranes induced by different carcinogenic and non-carcinogenic agents, the total negative charge of plasma membranes decrease, and the cells acquire the capability of closely approaching (adhesion), which frequently, especially upon coincidence of the perforated parts, may serve as a prerequisite to fusion process.

As a result of karyogamy, i.e., after synchronous mitosis or simple mechanical assembly of dikaryons nuclei, mononuclear hybrid precancerous cells develop, with tetraploid set of chromosomes on initial stage of hybridization. Received as a result of somatic hybridization, the hybrid synkaryon is a precancerous (initiated, immortal) cell, which exists in a macro organism indefinitely for a long time.

On the promotion stage, after the influence of complete (full) carcinogens or promoters on tissue, where precancerous synkaryons pre-exist, in these cells, the chromosomal aberrations of different types and genes amplifications may arise. From the chromosomal aberrations, the most dangerous in carcinogenic respect are imbalanced translocations, and also duplications, expressed in "complementation" of chromosomes' identical sites, having the same function. This event usually leads to genes' amplification, in consequence of which expression of genes (oncogenes), responsible for the control under the cellular proliferation, ultimately may originate. After this, so-called "over-expressed gene" arose. After above-marked conversion on sub-cellular and molecular levels, there may originate a true tumorous synkaryon, malignant cell with the ability of uncontrolled proliferation. On other words, cancer cell is a hybrid cell, arising after hybridization of two normal somatic cells.

2. Presumptive Common Trigger Mechanism of Action of Different Carcinogens

What are the common signs of all carcinogenic agents and substances, so different by their nature, as, for example, chemical substances, viruses, radiation of different kinds and so on? Is the mechanism of the cells' malignant transformation adequate for carcinogenic and non-carcinogenic factors?

From the position of karyogamic theory, the action of any carcinogen is not associated directly with gene apparatus of cells. Alteration of the cell's genome is induced indirectly; that is, after the somatic cell's fusion and arising of precancerous, tetraploid cell in initial stage of their development [10].

By our opinion the common mechanism of action of diametrically different carcinogens on target-cells is the destruction of the plasma membrane (induction of the perforations of different size) and consequently development of fusogeny - fusion of somatic cells and then development of karyogamy.

It seems that pores in the plasma membrane on the somatic cells formed by the action of different physical, chemical and biological agents, substantially decrease the negative charge of the plasma membrane. In different terms, perforation leads to the weakening on the electrostatic forces and enhancement of the Van der Vaals forces helping somatic cells to overcome intercellular forces and enter into contact with each other. In the case of prolonged contact adhesion process will start to develop.

Thus, influence of carcinogenic agents of different nature on cells is adequate. Adhesion in many cases may be a premise for fusion process.

3. Different Steps of Tumorous Progression Stage

Any combinations of cancer cell with other differentiated and non-differentiated normal somatic cells are possible. A population of tumorous cells, as morphologically, as cytogenetically (and on other signs) in spite of clonal origin of tumors, is highly heterogeneous. Cellular subpopulations are constantly formed in tumors without any obvious regularity, and in any other tumor phenotypically and genotypically different cells can co-exist.

The progression stage, as it seems, should be conditioned by two radically different from one another properties of tumor cells, which is being manifested in the ability to develop invasion process, in the one case, and the metastatic process, on the other case. These two processes significantly differ from one another by their development, cellular mechanisms, etc.

3a. Invasion

It may be supposed that a possible mechanism of invasion process is the hybridization of somatic cells, i.e., the already formed tumorous cells can often be hybridized both with the neighbor same cells or with normal cells [11]. After this formation of dikaryons may take place, in which one nucleus can be represented by tumorous cells, and the second, by normal cells (in case of fusion of tumor and normal cells). After synchronous mitosis or mechanical assembly of nuclei in such cells, a hybrid cell-synkaryon can be formed. This cellular type is represented with new genotypic (and in some cases phenotypic, as well) signs.

What can be said of the invasive growth of cancer cell? It is the known fact that cancer cells, as compared with normal analogs, much easier enter the hybridization process with other cancer and normal cells. If we ratiocinate, in the presence of a high negative charge, cancer cells should not have the ability to effect somatic hybridization with other cells. Apparently, invasion should occur only in the case when cancer cells have a relatively low negative, neutral or even a positive charge. Concurrently, the prerequisite for fusing of cells are perforations of the plasma membrane of both cellular partners (cancer cell and other cancer cell, cancer cell and precancerous cell or normal cell). In case when the plasma membranes of these cells lack pores, these cells will contact with each other but without fusing. The same result is expected in the case of availability of pores in the plasma membrane of one cellular partner only.

On the other hand, the active cell metabolism has been found to condition the suppression of pH towards the acid medium. In its turn, the acid medium contributes to the formation of pores in the plasma membranes of cells, this being accompanied with the negative electric charge suppression on the cell surface. This circumstance is contributory to cell-to-cell contacts, further adhesion and fusing. Moreover that the possibility of the formation of dikaryons and symplast-like structures during low pH is a long-established fact.

Thus, in the case of low pH it is quite possible that the formation of pores on plasma membranes of both partner cells, adhesion, the formation of dikaryons, then karyogamy and, as a result, the process of invasion can take place. In the case of invasion, cancer cells with genetic and phenotypic changes are taking place.

3b. Metastasis

To understand the mechanisms responsible for metastasis is one of the priority goals of cancer research. This process remains one of the most enigmatic aspects of this fatal disease.

Only some cells of the primary cancer are able to metastize (the ability of breaking off from the main focus, migration and attachment to a new place). Once the cancer cell is detached from the primary tumor, it will penetrate blood vessels (or lymphatic channels), retaining viability under the damaging and lethal to it influence, such as blood turbulence and contacts with the immune system cells. Further, by passing the basement membrane, it will go from the blood-vessel endothelium to the target organ. Thus, in order to initiate the process of metastasis, the cancer cell must get detached from the primary tumor seat and penetrate the basement membrane twice in two different directions – from the tumor seat to blood vessels (capillary) and then from the blood vessels to the target organ's tissue. In order to perform such a complex migration, it is necessary that essential alterations of electric potential on the plasma membrane of the cancer cell take place, which should be associated with the hydrogenous index (pH) changes.

The membrane potential of a cancer cell plasmalemma should be connected with the changes of physical and chemical nature occurring in the macro organism, as well as with the metabolic activity of this type of cells proper. The cancer cell metabolism has been found to differ from the normal cell metabolism. Cancer cells can switch on and activated alternative biochemical processes, enhancing thus the metabolism of these cells. As a result, the environmental pH is suppressed, as a result of which cancer cells acquire a relatively low negative, neutral or even a positive charge on their surface. Should a metastatic cell change its high negative charge for a relatively low negative, neutral or even a positive charge, its attachment to a new place and the formation of new cancer cell populations will be quite real [12]. In the case of a relatively suppressed metabolism of cancer cells, the environmental pH increases. In the case of high pH, a cancer cell may develop a high negative charge, which suppresses its adhesion with the tumor bulk and can lead to its detachment and migration in the macro organism.

4. Cells Spontaneous Malignization in Tissue Culture

It is known that in cultures of normal cells *in vitro* not infrequently during 5-8 months a spontaneous malignant transformation takes place without any well-known carcinogenic factors' influences [13].

We concluded that the so-called "spontaneous malignization" of cultivated normal cells is possibly associated with fusion of different (heterokaryons) and homogenous (homokaryons) cellular types, but the possible primary reason of this process may be local damages of plasma membranes under conditions of low pH [14].

After reunion of hetero- and homokaryons' nuclei, a mononuclear hybrid cells – synkaryon (or precancerous cell) is possibly formed there; however, as a result of an additional effect of certain carcinogenic and even non-carcinogenic factors (in our case – low pH exponents), this precancerous cell possibly may transform into a true tumor synkaryon. It is necessary to emphasize that already in 1916 Macklin observed binuclear and multinuclear cells in tissue culture [15]. In 1964, Roberts and Cole reported on some mechanisms of formation of polyploid and heteroploid cells in a murine ascites tumor *in vitro* [16].

It is possible that the cause of cellular cultures' "spontaneous malignization" may be low pH of the environment, which assists local disintegration (damages) of plasma membranes and the follow-up fusion process, following which suitable conditions for tumor cells formation may be created.

Thus, cultures of normal cells *in vitro* are subjects of spontaneous malignant conversion without the effect of any well-known carcinogenic agents and factors. In our opinion, the etiologic factor (initiator) of this state may be low pH. In the basis of experiments, we came to the conclusion that low pH turns out to be a sufficiently strong fusogenic agent, inducing in cultivated somatic cells plasma membranes perforations of different size.

An increased risk of malignization of cultivated normal cells may be induced by trypsin, which usually is applied to long-term, replacement cultures. In our opinion, trypsin in this concrete case (spontaneous malignization *in vitro*) may be promoter of true cancer cell formation.

5. Arising of Tumors in Transplantation of Allogenic Internal Organs

Some clinics dealing with problems of transplantology report that recipients with transplanted internal organs (kidneys, skin, bone marrow, etc.) show a significant rise in the incidence of malignant tumor of certain localization and histogenesis [17, 18]. At the same time, many investigators reported that whole blood and hematopoietic stem cell transplantation was associated with a higher risk of malignant process initiation and relapse.

Until recently, the theory of immunological surveillance of F. Burnet (1957) seemed to be the most justified one [19]. However, based on a number of investigation, it may be supposed that immune deficiency is not the necessary condition for the development of malignant tumors and that immune deficiency is the consequence rather than the reason for malignant processes. Old (1981) made the same conclusion on the basis of careful analysis of his own and literature data [20].

Concretely, what is the mechanism of tumor conversion on allotranstransplantations? In our opinion, tumorous cell represent the hybrid, the so-called tumorous synkaryon, emerging as a result of the fusion of two normal somatic cells. Stem cells, fibroblasts, macrophages, lymphoid cells, undifferentiated cells of various tissues and others show an increased capability to create viable hybrids. During the perforation of cellular membranes induced by some carcinogenic and non-carcinogenic substances and influences, the total negative charge of plasma membranes decrease, and the cells acquire the capability of closely approaching (adhesion). In result of this, may form dikaryons _ heterokaryons or homokaryons. Then, in case of synchronous mitosis or mechanical reunification of nuclei, they may form synkaryons (mononuclear hybrid cells), with tetraploid or hypotetraploid sets of chromosomes on initial stage of hybridization.

Experience in transplantology tentatively testifies that even in cases of maximal antigen compatibility of donors and recipients, immune conflict is unavoidable. As we believe, in immunological conflict between recipient and donor cells, the process of cells' destruction in some cases may be accompanied by damages of plasma membranes and somatic hybridization between immunocompetent cells of the recipient and any cell of transplanted donor's tissue (graft), which may lead to the emergence of a tumorous cell.

As it is shown, the recipients react to the allotransplantant by development of humoral and cellular immune responses (immune cytolysis). In the development of transplantation immunity the most important roles are played by specific antibodies and T-killer cells (immune effectors). 1. Antibody molecules have 2 main functions: they bind to the immunogenic antigens (in this case they are represented by superficial antigens of the allotransplantant cells) and after interaction with the antigen initiates involvement of different cells and molecules. The constant region (C region) of the antibodies defines the type of the response after the antibody-antigen interaction, whether this is complement-mediated lysis, cellular cytotoxicity, enhanced phagocytosis, etc. 2. Cellular immune response is conducted by T-cytotoxic cells: after the sensitization of the recipient by the donor antigens the killer cells are migrating to the transplant tissue and are having inducing the cytotoxic effect. Killers perform their functions either from a distance or when in contact with the target cell. The cytotoxic effect of killers is realized in the target cell plasmalemma by special proteins – perforines, granzymes, etc., which lead to the formation in this organoid of perforations (pores, holes). In the presence of calcium, perforines interact with the plasma membrane of the target cells and after the polymerization they are forming the transmembrane channels (pores). So both antibodies and cytotoxic cells can induce damages (perforations) of different degree on somatic cells plasma membranes, which can represent firstly the precancerous and later the true cancerous cells formation.

Besides, since lymphoid tissue cells as a well as macrophages are the morphological substrate ensuring the formation of the immune response to antigenic stimulation, cells of this type may be one of the essential objects in fusion during organ allotransplantation, especially as the process of contact and penetration of lymphocytes to other cells in immunological conflict ("peripolesis" and "emperipolesis," respectively), as well as facts of fusion of macrophages with other cells are well known. Thus, in the fusion process, the highest activity may be shown by recipient's macrophages and T-lymphocytes, which are effector cells against tissue incompatibility antigens. On the basis of the above and taking into consideration the fact that lymphocytes and macrophages are dominant cells also with respect to phenotypic properties, in the most cases of tumors, malignant cells, which develop during allogenic organ transplantations, may have lymphoid (T- or B-cell), macrophagal or the so-called "intermediate" morphology.

6. Reason of Arising of Tumors in AIDS

Interrelation of oncological diseases and AIDS for certain is more complex than as interpreted by some theories and hypotheses of carcinogenesis.

Besides, as was shown in last years, immune deficit is rather consequence of malignant process development that the cause of cancer cells' formation [20]. In particular, suppression of immune system is not a cause of formation of Kaposi's sarcoma, as this pathology frequently rises already in early stages of HIV-infection, i.e., before essential suppression of organism's immune status.

We attempt to explain the formation of malignant tumors in AIDS from the position of karyogamic theory of carcinogenesis.

As well-known, there are communications about the appearance of the giant, multinuclear formations – polykaryocytes, which were formed by cells' fusion in different tissues and organs of patients with HIV-induced immunodeficiency [21].

In our opinion, along with formation of polykaryocytes the formation of dikaryons is possible as well. Cells, containing two heterotypes (heterokaryons) or same types (homokaryons) of nuclei, possess of high oncogenic potency. As polykaryocytes usually contain lymphoid and macrophagal cellular elements, it is quite possible that exactly these cells participate in formation of dikaryons.

In immunodeficiency of any genesis in the first place, it is necessary to explain formation of malignant tumors, consisting of lymphoid and macrophagal cellular elements (Kaposi's sarcoma, malignant lymphomas, Burkitt's lymphoma, etc.).

Proceeding from this, also taking into consideration that lymphocytes and macrophages are dominant ones in respect of phenotypic properties, the cellular substrate of malignant tumors formed in AIDS have in most cases a lymphoid, macrophagal or so-called "intermediate" morphology.

It is well known that in virus-induced AIDS, the most common manifestation is Kaposi's sarcoma, affecting, first of all, skin and the subcutaneous fat layer, as well as practically all internal organs. It has been also established that so-called spindle-like cells, the origin of which is still uncertain, are the cellular substrate of this malignancy.

It is also well known that the HIV, together with immunocompetent cells, may affect epithelial cells of the skin and the Langerhans cells, localized in this organ.

Therefore, frequent development of Kaposi's sarcoma in AIDS may be due to the fusion of T-lymphocytes and macrophages with epidermocytes or the Langerhans cells with the formation of spindle-like cells. Incidentally, these spindle-like cells resemble macrophages by some of their morpho-functional properties. Specifically, they often reveal signs of phagocytic activity, in particular, in their cytoplasm, there are often present erythrocytes or hemosiderin's granules, etc. [22].

We believe also that the emergence of lymphomas in AIDS maybe caused by the fusion of different immunocompetent cells (lymphocytes), being at different stages of maturation, both between themselves and with cells of other histogenesis.

7. Possible Correlation between Bacterial Membranotoxins and Malignant Neoplasms

The idea that bacteria cause cancer was discarded a hundred years ago, and is still regarded as scientific heresy. At present, an overwhelming body of evidence has determined that relationships among certain bacteria and cancer exist [23-26].

It needs to be noted here that the cellular or molecular mechanisms of this phenomenon are still unknown. Therefore, many questions on this sphere remain.

As it has been found, toxins of different origin, like different carcinogenic chemical substances, irradiations and viruses can, at different doses, show *in vitro* diametrically opposite cytopathogenic effects (cytodestruction, fusogenicity), which will be correspondingly reflected in the clinical picture – beginning at general intoxication and ending with tumor growth. It has not been finally determined but gives a serious cause to expect the same ability and action on the part of some toxins of hemolytic action and generally of membranotoxins of different tropism.

Based on the above, infectious and carcinogenic processes can, irrespective of the principal differences between them (cytodestruction in one case and cytoproliferation in the other), be induced by the same agent: a bacterial membranotoxins, mycotoxins, any infectious or oncogenic viruses, etc.

Such double, diametrically opposed cytopathogenic processes developed in somatic cells by membranotoxins of different tropism (including hemolysins) must be apparently conditioned by: 1) different toxic doses; 2) different rigidity of plasma membranes of target cells proper (e.g., erythrocytes, leucocytes, etc.), and, most important, 3) the so-called perforation degree, or pores (holes) of different size and number formed on the plasma membrane.

At the same time, based on the karyogamic theory of carcinogenesis, the initial target for any carcinogens are determinants of cellular membranes, whereas any agent or effect inducing fusogenicity shall be regarded as a potential carcinogen – or fusogenicity of somatic cells might lead to the formation of first a precancerous and then a tumorous cell.

As rigidity of leucocytes' membranes is higher, it is possible that during destruction of erythrocytes (or immature cells of erythroid line) by hemolytic membranotoxins, reversible damages of plasma membranes (pores of definite size and number) can be formed in leucocytes (or in other type of cells), which can promote the process of adhesion of somatic cells, leading further to the process of fusion in somatic cells and the formation of first precancerous and then cancer cells [27].

Also of importance we consider the circumstance that exotoxins of definite bacteria (e.g., toxins of *Clostridium perfringens* (0-perfringolysin), *Cl. septicum, Cl. histolyticum* and *Cl. novyi,* tetanolysin of *Cl. tetani*, toxins of *Cl. botulinum*, alpha-, beta-, and other toxins of *Staphylococcus aureus*, 0 and S streptolysins of *Streptococcus pyogenes,* etc., are really capable of rendering a strong membranotoxic (hemolytic, cytotoxic, neurotoxic, enterotoxic, etc.) effect on target cells of different types. It has been also found that the perforation of the plasmalemma by membranotoxins (pore-forming toxins) causes an influx of Ca (2+) and an efflux of cytoplasmic proteins.

Membranotoxins affect primarily determinants of plasma membranes of cells that are tropic to them: they link to specific receptors of plasma membranes, provoke their lysis and, correspondingly, the development of perforations of different size and number in these organoids which can, in some cases, become a precondition for fusogenicity.

To all appearance, a decisive importance in the development of different type, often diametrically opposed pathologies (infections, tumors, etc.) acquires the so-called perforation degree, or the volume or quantity of pores formed in the target-cell plasma membrane by some toxins (and other agents). Based on the above, the following 3 options are considered below:

1. In the case of large-size pores (supposing approximately 8-10 nm and larger), irreversible changes and cytolysis occur. The target cells fail to complete reparation processes, what result in cytodestruction (cytolysis). A clinical presentation of pathogenic effect can be an infectious process or a severe intoxication; while in the case of tropism to immunocompetent cells or stem cells, immune deficiencies and teratogenic effects may be induced, accordingly.
2. In some cases, when pores of lesser volume are developed, membranotoxins induce simultaneous arising of nonviable polykaryocytes (in the case of reversible changes in the plasmalemma) or cytolysis in somatic calls (in the case of irreversible changes in this organoids), and can provoke immune deficiency of different degrees (in the case of immunocompetent cells tropism) or teratogenic effects (in the case a stem cells of any organ is damaged). Most multinuclear cells (polykaryocytes) formed as a result of fusion are not likely to proliferate. They are nonviable, nonfunctional formations that tend to quickly break down and perish.
3. In the case of formation of even lesser pores, when reversible changes of the plasmalemma occur, the total negative charge of this organoids decrease and the cells develop an ability to come closer to each other (adhesion). This last process frequently, especially on coincidence of the perforated parts, will likely become a prerequisite to fusion process. Thus, at this stage, together with multinuclear cellular structures (polykaryocytes), the binuclear cells, carriers of high carcinogenic potency, are formed. As a result of karyogamy, i.e., after synchronous mitosis or simple mechanical assembly of heterokaryons (or homokaryons) nuclei, mononuclear hybrid precancerous cells develop with a tetraploid set of chromosomes in the initial stage of hybridization [28]. Toxins (and other pathogenic agents, e.g., viruses) strongly stimulate the occurrence of chromosomal abnormalities in these cells. The hybrid synkaryon produced as a result of somatic hybridization is a precancerous (initiated, immortal) cell, which can exist in a macro organism indefinitely for a long time.

On the promotion stage, after the effect of complete (full) carcinogens or promoters or the same toxin on tissue, where precancerous cells pre-exist, the chromosomal aberrations of different types and gene amplifications may arise in these cells. After above-marked conversion on sub-cellular and molecular levels, there may arise true tumorous synkaryon, cancer cell with the ability of uncontrolled proliferation. This last cell represents a clone, from which the formation of malignant tumor substrate at the early stage of carcinogenesis commences.

Thus, some bacterial membranotoxins of different tropism are capable, as a result of damages of the plasma membrane of the target cell of various degrees (perforation, lysis), of inducing both infectious processes as well as the formation of first precancerous and then cancer cells.

8. Reason of Arising of Tumors in Hemolytic Anemias

Hemolytic anemias may be induced by means of some exogenic hemolytic factors: by different organic and inorganic hemolytic toxins (phosphorus, phenylhydrazin, saponins, arsenic, lead) and biotoxins (snake venom, mushrooms poisons, mycotoxins, etc.), some medical preparations, radiations, some infectious agents and heavy burns. Besides, in some cases, hemolytic anemias are induced by antibodies and immunocompetent cells against own tissue (autoimmune hemolytic anemia). A strong relationship exists between autoimmunity and B-cell oncogenesis [29, 30]. According to clinical studies, malignant tumors in autoimmune hemolytic anemias appear in 45-47%.

At the same time in the opinion of some scientists, some toxins, even different infectious viruses (for instance, viruses of influenza, rubella, HIV) and carcinogenic agents may induce both fusion process and cytolytic (destructive) effects on somatic cells. Such different effects possibly depend on the size of plasma membranes' pores induced by them. In the case of large pores irreversible changes and cytolysis take place. For instance, high doses of carcinogenic agents lead to partial increasing of quantity of giant polynuclear cells, but further increase of this dose induces massive cellular lysis. In a case of these agents tropism to immunocompetent cells (HIV), immune deficit of different degree may be induced. In lesser doses of carcinogenic agents, dikaryons are observed most frequently. Thus, in hemolytic anemias of different genesis side by side with hemolysis, process of somatic cells fusion may take place. For instance, after a bite of venom with hemolytic action, together with massive destruction of erythrocytes (hemolysis), there may be induced a fusion process of other cellular types with more rigid plasma membranes (for instance, leucocytes of different maturity, and probably of cells of other type), with the possible development of precancerous, and then true cancerous cell [31]. In autoimmune hemolytic anemias, there are 2 possibilities of inducing a malignant process: 1) the destructive action of autoimmune antibodies and immunocompetent cells (for example, T-killers) on erythrocytes and their fusogenic effect on these cells and cells of other types, with the possible development of cancerous cells (in more detail see chapter about the allotransplantation); 2) some immunosuppressive drugs used in autoimmune states increase considerably the risk of malignant tumors arising, in particular, on lymphomas, in resemblance of cancer of other kind. Besides, the immunosuppressive drugs, strongly increase the occurrence of chromosomal abnormalities in patients with connective tissue diseases. It is possible that these substances, together with cytolysis of immunocompetent cells, may induce the process of fusion with the possible formation of a cancer cell. Thus, cell fusion may in some cases of autoimmune process produce cells with tumor properties. Carcinogenic agents or some other reasons may create the autoimmunization background in a macro organism, which may lead to multiple intercellular contacts between immunocompetent cells and cells with aberrant antigens. In case of cells fusion, initiation of malignant neoplasms of lymphoid or macrophagal histogenesis is expected to take place.

9. Arising of Malignant Neoplasms by Some Non-Carcinogenic Substances

In experimental oncology, examples are known on induction of malignant neoplasms in experimental animals after inoculation with indifferent at first sight substance, such as some fatty acids, carbohydrates, physiological solution (saline), even distilled water, etc. The similar result was obtained after an epidemiological analysis of some of these agents, e.g., respect of dietary fats and carbohydrates.

The explanation of these strange facts by means of the already existing different hypotheses and theories of carcinogenesis (as polyetiological, virus-genetic, oncogenes and so on) is impossible.

In this chapter we make an attempt to explain the essence of these occurrences by means of karyogamic theory of carcinogenesis.

9a. Fatty Acids

In experiments in mice and rats etiologic role of dietary fats in producing malignant tumors of different histogenesis and localization, in particular, breast, colon and prostate cancers were confirmed [32]. It was demonstrated that polyunsaturated fatty acids increase process of carcinogenesis more intensively, than saturated fatty acids [33].

At the same time, some scientists report on the fusogenic effect of different (but not all!) fatty acids in tissue culture *in vitro* [34]. These scientists concluded that the fusion process proceeds most easily in the case of unsaturated fatty acids. Various degrees of cells' fusion were seen with linoleic, undecylenic, myristoleic, palmitoleic acids and glyceryl monooleate. In this connection, of interest is to mention the already confirmed fact that although glyceryl monooleate induced intensive fusogeny process, the glyceryl dioleate induces only agglutination (nor fusion), whereas glyceryl trioleate induces neither fusion nor agglutination. Ahkong et al. explain the fusogeny process by an increase in the permeability of plasma membranes of the target cells [34]. In our opinion, the permeability increase of the plasma membranes is associated with the plasmalemma structure changes. In other words, the permeability growth should be in direct bond with the development of perforations in this organoid. A perforation may, in turn, precondition fusogeny only on condition that pores are not of very large size (which will necessarily lead to the destruction of cells) and most important, the coincidence of the perforated sections of the neighbor cells' plasmalemma takes place. In case the pores of large volume (size) are produced, the abnormally high permeability might occur in the plasma membranes, because of which the cells deteriorate.

Parallelism between carcinogenicity and fusogeny processes of these substances, allow us to consider this phenomenon as confirmation of karyogamic theory of carcinogenesis [35].

Our experiments established that polyunsaturated (linoleic) and monounsaturated (oleic) fatty acids differ from saturated acids by a high intensity of interaction with cellular membranes. Especially high fusogenic activity was revealed by the oleic acid. However, the epidemiological analysis failed to detect the carcinogenic activity of this fatty acid. What is the reason of this strange occurrence? A reverse correlation between fusogenic and carcinogenic abilities has been revealed: the higher is the fusogenic activity of this or that substance or agent, the lower is its carcinogenic activity and vice versa. In particular, in the case of high fusogenic ability of an oleic acid the formation of unviable giant polykaryocytes is induced and carcinogenic effect is less manifested; and vice versa, the carcinogenic effect is higher in the presence of low fusogenic ability of the linoleic acid because of the formation of mainly dikaryons with high oncogenic potency.

9b. Carbohydrates

In experiments in mice and rats etiological role of carbohydrates in producing malignant tumors were confirmed [36]. The mechanism of influence of carbohydrates (glucose, fructose, galactose, et al.) on the experimental conditions is yet unknown.

In scientific literature there are only few data on the possible fusogenic action of several sugars. In 1917 Kalashnikov studied the action of glucose solution on spawn of perch [37]. Author observed giant syncytiums with many nuclei in resting phase or dividing by means of amitosis. Author assumed that in some cases fusion of several nuclei into one does occur. It was shown also that hybridization of somatic cells promoted by sucrose. Recently Smeland and Funderud have reported about the possible interrelation of the cellular adhesion by sugar molecules and the tumor arising [38]. In the last years some authors have reported about the fusogenic activity of glucose, lactose, fructose, with the exception of starch.

The above-mentioned correlations between the fusogenic and carcinogenic properties of several carbohydrates may indicate that following the effect of some carbohydrates in experimental conditions, malignant tumors may arise by means of somatic cells fusion and further hybridization. The effect of some carbohydrates on the target cells plasma membranes may induce perforations or modifications of these organoid. This may be a reason of the cell's further fusion and the formation of dikaryons, then precancerous cells and then true tumor synkaryon.

9c. Distilled Water

As was shown after experimental works of Warabioka, Watanabe and his co-authors the daily inoculation of distilled water into intraperitoneal cavity of rats, in some cases development of sarcomas in particular, fibrosarcomas, maybe induced [39, 40].

At the first sight it is complicated to explain these events from the position of karyogamic theory too, such as the fusogenic properties of distilled water are unknown yet.

On the other hand it is known, that in some conditions distilled water has the capability to induce destruction of somatic cells, in particular, erythrocytes, what is followed by the intensive hemolysis. Distilled water in cells with more rigid plasma membranes (leucocytes, fibroblasts and so on) may induce smaller, reparable perforations in neighboring cells, which frequently, especially upon coincidence of the perforated parts of plasma membranes, may serve as a prerequisite to fusion process.

As has been noted above, any fusogenic agent or factors may induce perforations of definite size or modifications of cells' plasma membranes with the follow-up fusion of cellular membranes. Perforations of big size induce a considerable destruction of cytoplasmic membranes, cytolysis and perishing of the cells. Based on the above, we may assume that daily injections of distilled water into the intraperitoneal cavity (or subcutaneously) of experimental animals may in some cases induce the perforations of different size of neighboring cells' plasma membranes, which sometimes assist their approaching and follow-up fusion process.

One may think that in sites of inoculation (or near them) distilled water may induce in cellular plasma membranes perforations of big size, which from the oncological point of view are nor dangerous. And only in the tissues localized little far from the site of inoculation, the condition favorable for cells' approaching, their fusion and follow-up somatic hybridization with arising of precancerous cell are formed.

9d. Saline

Some data of scientific literature testify the carcinogenic action of a physiological solution under experimental conditions. In 1940 a Japanese scientist Tokoro reported on the development of reticulosarcoma and spindle-cell sarcoma in the site of daily subcutaneous injection of 5-20% physiological solution in two rats [41]. The said report is so far the only one and this strange fact cannot be explained by the existing theories and hypotheses of carcinogenesis.

The explaining of this phenomenon by the karyogamic theory of carcinogenesis is also difficult because in scientific literature there is extremely little data on fusogenic properties of this substance. However, in 1917 Kalashnikov observed giant syncytium with many nuclei in the rest phase and during division when he acted on spawn of perch by physiological solution [37].

As has been shown by the some researchers in the last years, saline may under some conditions modify the properties of cytoplasmic membranes' lipid bilayer. This may ultimately induce alterations of the negative charge of cells' surface, which may assist to the approaching of somatic cells and as a result - their fusion (in case of coincidence of plasma membranes perforated sites). Thus, this strange fact we may explain by means of karyogamic theory of carcinogenesis.

CONCLUSION

In our opinion, the above-mentioned facts rather convincingly evidence the karyogamic theory's pretensions to the unitary (general) role of carcinogenesis. The principal merit of this theory consists in its ability to integrate the earlier scientific theories and hypotheses dedicated to this problem. In other words, it encompasses the major postulates of leading theories of carcinogenesis and answers rather convincingly the questions unanswered before in the experimental and clinical oncology.

The karyogamic theory is based on several key theses of modern oncology (which are not fully shared by all the scientists engaged in this sphere), namely:

1) cancer is concurrently a polyetiological and monopathogenic process;
2) cancer cell represents hybrid formed as a result of fusion of 2 normal somatic cells;

3) cancer cells are devoid of antigens foreign to the macro organism;
4) the mechanism of action of carcinogenic agents and factors (viruses, irradiations, chemical agents, etc.) of diametrically different nature on target cells is adequate;
5) The initial target of carcinogenic agents and factors is the plasma membrane of somatic cells rather than the genetic apparatus;
6) Immunologic alterations are a result of tumor transformation rather than its cause, etc.

The initiation stage of carcinogenesis should be seemingly begin from the perforations of the plasma membrane of target cells induced by different agents and factors. One of the evidences in corroboration of the above is the fact that all carcinogenic agents (viruses, irradiations, aromatic hydrocarbons, toxins, fatty acids, low pH, etc.) are characterized of exactly the same effect (or formation of pores) on plasma membranes. In addition, much importance is given to the quantity of formed pores (PQ) and their volume (PV).

As will be seen, this at the first sight insignificant process – perforation, may, in a number of cases, become a direct cause of rather dramatic processes ongoing in the macro organism at the cellular, sub-cellular and molecular levels (or the formation of a cancer cell).

As has already been mentioned, initiation stage consists of the following 4 steps:

Step I – perforations of the plasma membranes of the target cells. As has been established, any carcinogenic or non-carcinogenic agents have a common mechanism of action on the target cells: they all induce perforations or the production of pores (holes) in the plasmalemma of the cell. This process may become a prerequisite for reduction of the summary negative charge on the cell's surface and approach of the cells. As it seems, the degree of perforations (quantity, volume) should be of decisive importance in the realization of any clinical state (infection, tumor process, teratogeny, etc.):

a) In the case of development of comparatively big size pores or upon their massive formation – rapid repair of the plasma membrane by the cells becomes impossible and the cells undergoes irreversible changes (destruction, cytolysis). The clinical manifestation of the above may be the development of any infectious process;
b) In the case of development of lesser size pores – the transformation of the target cells into giant, nonviable polykaryocytes. The letter represents the so-called genetic impasse, for they fail to enter the S-phase of the cell cycle, subsequent mitosis and tend to be soon destroyed. The clinical manifestation of the above may be an infectious process, immune deficiency, teratogeny;
c) In the case of development of still lesser size pores – the formation of a precancerous cell, the direct cause of which might be a reduction of the summary negative charge on the surface of the plasma membrane of 2 neighbor normal somatic cells.

Step II – approach of two normal somatic cells, their contact and follow-up adhesion.

Step III – fusogeny. In the case of coincidence of the perforated parts of the plasmalemma of 2 neighbor somatic cells, a binucleate cell of high oncogenic potency – dikary on (hetero- or homokaryon) may be formed.

Step IV – karyogamy and then tetraploidy (at the early stage of a precancerous cell formation). As a result of synchronous mitosis or mechanical reunion of nuclei of the dikaryons, a mononuclear hybrid cell – synkaryon, with a tetraploid set of chromosomes, may be formed. At this stage, this cell may be called a precancerous cell. Thereafter, the phenomenon of chromosomes segregation will take place.

For promotion stage (i.e., formation of a cancer cell) the necessary precondition is active proliferation (hyperplasia) of the corresponding tissue. Under the effect of complete carcinogens, promoters, non-specific influences or some extreme situations, precancerous synkaryon can transform into a tumor one. The pre-existence in the corresponding tissue and organs of precancerous cells has been described elsewhere. The mechanism of malignant transformation of the precancerous cell into a tumorous one probably has the molecular and sub-cellular foundation. In terms of oncology, particular dangerous are: chromosomal translocations (especially of non-balanced type), duplications, deletions and gene amplifications.

Progression stage should seemingly be initiated in two processes - invasive and metastatic. Invasive process is developed by involvement of new, intact cells and tissues into carcinogenesis, where a great role should be again given to somatic hybridization. At this time, malignant cells of a new type are being formed. As it is well-known, the genotypic and phenotypic instability is the primary manifestation in cancer. In the second manifestation of the progression – upon metastasis or arising of secondary tumor loci, the key role should be given to the variable electric potentials arising on the surface of cancer cells.

REFERENCES

[1] Hallion, L. Sur la pathogenie du cancer; theorie karyogamique. *Press Med. Par.* 1907; XV:10-11.

[2] Mekler, LB. Mechanisms of tumor induction in light of general theory of oncogenesis. *Usp. Sovr. Biol.* 1978; 85:134-151.

[3] Elkort, RJ; Handler, AH; Kobrick S. et al. The relationship of somatic cell hybridization to carcinogenesis. *Europ. J. Cancer* 1972; 8 :259-261.

[4] Kuppers, G; Zimmerman, U. Cell fusion by spark discharge and its relevance for evolutionary process. *FEBS lett.* 1983; 164 :323-329.

[5] Gogichadze, GK. Karyogamic theory of malignant neoplasms in the light of biological approach. *Proc. Acad. Sciences of Georgia (seria biol.).* 1988, 14:166-173.

[6] Qian, LW. A hypothesis on the pathogenesis of cancer: cancer might arise following an event of normal somatic cell fusing. Med. Hypotheses 1993; 46:521-524.

[7] Lu, X; Kang, Y. Cell fusion hypothesis of the cancer stem cell. *Adv. Exp. Med. Biol.* 2011, 714:129-140.

[8] Gogichadze, GK; Gogichadze, TG. *Karyogamic theory of cancer cell formation from the view of the XXI century.* Nova Biomedical Books, New York. 2010.

[9] Gogichadze, GK; Gogichadze, TG. *Somatic hybridization as a primary reason of malignization.* Lambert Academic Publisher, Saarbruken. 2013.

[10] Gogichadze. GK; Gogichadze, T; Kamkamidze, G. Presumably common trigger mechanism of action of diametrically different carcinogens on target cells. *Cancer and Oncology Research* 2013, 1 (2):65-68.

[11] De Baetselier, P. *Neoplastic progression by somatic cell fusion.* Influence Tumor Dev. Host.-Dodrecht, etc. 1989.

[12] Gogichadze, G; Gogichadze, T; Kamkamidze, G. Possible effect of variable membrane potential of a cancer cell on different carcinogenic processes. *Georgian Medical News* 2014, 9 (234):116-120.

[13] Le Boeuf, RF; Lin, P; Kerckaert, GA. et al. Ultracellular acidification is associated with enhanced morphological transformation in Sirian hamster embryo cells. *Cancer Res.* 1992, 52:144-148.

[14] Arvinte, T; Cudd, A; Schulz, B. et al. Low-pH associated of proteins with the membranes of intact red blood cells. II. Studies of the mechanism. *Bioch. Et. Bioph. Acts* 1989, 98:61- 68.

[15] Macklin, CC. Binucleate and multinucleate cells in tissues cultures. *Anat. Res.* 1916, 10:225.

[16] Roberts, DC; Cole, C. Some mechanisms of formation of polyploid and heteroploid cells in a murine ascites tumor *in vitro*. *J. Natl. Cancer Inst.* 1964, 32:1023-1030.

[17] Penn, I. De novo malignancy in pediatric organ transplant recipients. *J. Pediatr. Surg.* 1994, 29:221-226.

[18] Fiedor, P; Wierbicki, Z; Pawelec, K. et al. Human papillomavirus as a risk factor for development of cancer in allograft recipients. *Ann. Transplantology. Index Copernicus J. abstract.* 2009, 14 (Suppl.1):24.

[19] Burnet, FM. Cancer - a biological approach. *Brit. Med. J.* 1957, 17:779-793.

[20] Old, LJ. Cancer immunology: the search for specifity – G.H.A. Clowes memorial lecture. *Cancer Res.* 1981, 41:361-375.

[21] Lifson, JD; Reyes, G; Mc Grath, MS. et al. AIDS retrovirus induced cytopathology: giant cell formation and involvement of CD4 antigen. *Science* 1986, 232:1123-1127.

[22] Gogichadze, GK; Dolidze, TG. Hypothesis explaining simultaneous development of acquired immunodeficiency syndrome and malignant tumors. *Med. Hypotheses* 1995, 44:307-308.

[23] Parsonnet, J. Bacterial infection as a cause of cancer. *Environ. Health Perspect.* 1995, 103, Suppl. 8:263-268.

[24] Lax, AJ. Opinion: bacterial toxins and cancer – a case to answer? *Nat. Rev. Microbiol.* 2005, 3 (4):343-349.

[25] Chang, AH; Parsonnet, J. Role of bacteria in oncogenesis. *Clin. Micr. Reviews* 2010, 23:837-857.

[26] Caygill, CRJ; Gatenby, PA. *Epidemiology of the association between bacterial infections and cancer.* Springer Science + Business media B.V. 2012:1-24.

[27] Gogichadze, GK; Misabishvili, EV; Gogichadze, TG. Tumor cells formation by normal somatic cells' fusion and cancer prevention prospects. *Med. Hypotheses* 2006, 66, 1:133- 136.

[28] Gogichadze, T; Gogichadze, G. On a possible mechanism of tumor conversion induced by bacterial membranotoxins. Proc. 4th World Congress on Cancer Science and Therapy, Chicago, 2014. doi:10.4/72/1948-5956. S1.035.

[29] Batailler, ER; Klein, B; Durie, BGM. et al. Interrelationship between autoimmunity and B-lymphoid cell oncogenesis in humans. *Clin. Exp. Rheumatol.* 1989, 7:319-328.

[30] Lechner, K; Obermeier, HL. Cancer-related microangiopathic hemolytic anemia: clinical and laboratory features in 168 reported cases. *Medicine (Baltimore)* 2012, 91:195-205.

[31] Gogichadze, GK. *Common characteristics of a cancer cell and logical corroborations of its hybrid essence.* Advances in Genetic Research. Ed. Kevin V. Urbano. 2011, 46:161-178.

[32] Gross, L. Inhibition of the development of tumors or leukemia in mice and rats after reduction of food intake. *Cancer Res.* 1988; 62:1463-1465.

[33] Freedman, LS; Clifford, C; Messina, M. Analysis of dietary fat, calories, body weight, and the development of mammary tumors in rats and mice: a review. *Cancer Res.* 1990; 50: 5710- 5719.

[34] Ahkong, QF; Cramp, FC; Fischer, D. et al. Studies on chemically induced cell fusion. *J. Cell Sci.* 1972; 10: 769-787.

[35] Gogichadze, GK; Gogichadze, TG. Cancer as a result of somatic cells fusion caused by some dietary fats and carbohydrates. *Med. Hypotheses* 2005; 65:622- 623.

[36] Nishiyama, Y. Experimentalle erzeugung des sarkoms bei ratten durch wiered-holte injectionen von glucoselosung [Experimental production of sarcoma in rats by wired took injections of glucose solution]. *Gann* 1938; 32: 85-98.

[37] Kalashnikov, PP. Observations over development of eggs of Persa fluviatillis in artificial solutions. Works of Soc. *Natural Scientists of Petrograd* 1917: XLV-LII.

[38] Smeland, EB; Funderud, S. Sugar molecules, cell adhesion and cancer etiology. *Tidsskrift. Nor Laegeforen* 1992; 112:2834.

[39] Warabioka, K. On the induction of sarcoma in rats injected with aqua distillata gelida. Second report. *Gann* 1957; 48: 577-578.

[40] Watanabe, T; Ibata, H; Sugikoto, T. et al. Production and inhibition of hepatic sarcomata in rats by injections of trypan blue. *Gann* 1957; 48: 576-577.

[41] Tokoro, Y. Uber die artificielle erzeugung des sarkoms bei den weissen ratten mittels konzen trierte kochsalzlosun [About the artificial generation of sarcoma in white rats by concentrated kochsalzlosun]. *Gann* 1940; 34:149-155.

In: Horizons in Cancer Research. Volume 61
Editor: Hiroto S. Watanabe

ISBN: 978-1-63484-503-8

Chapter 2

MECHANISMS OF CANCER FORMATION UNDER INTERPLAY BETWEEN HOST IMMUNITY AND HUMAN PAPILLOMAVIRUS (HPV) INFECTION

Masachika Senba[1] and Naoki Mori[2]
[1]Department of Pathology, Institute of Tropical Medicine, Nagasaki University, Nagasaki, Japan
[2]Department of Molecular Virology and Oncology, Gradual School of Medicine, University of the Ryukyus, Okinawa, Japan

ABSTRACT

The cervical, penil, anal, and oropharyngeal cancers are caused by high-risk human papillomaviruses (HPVs). HPVs have developed strategies to escape host defense by innate and adaptive immunity. HPVs can induce immune evasion of the infected cells, which enable the virus to be undetectable for long time. Immune response evasion has been considered significant aspect of HPVs persistence, which is the principal contributing factor leading to HPV associated with cancers. HPVs have evolved in a different way of evading immune system. The macrophages and natural killer (NK) cells are classified as innate immune cells, and dendritic cells (DCs), cluster of differentiation $CD4^+/CD8^+$ T-cells and regulatory T-cells are classified as adaptive immune cells. HPV associated with cancers expressing viral oncogenes E6 and E7 are potentially recognized by the immune system. The major histocompatibility complex (MHC) class I molecules are patrolled by NK cells and $CD8^+$ cytotoxic T lymphocytes. This recognition system is a main target for the strategies of immune evasion deployed by viruses. The long latency period from initial infection to persistence signifies that HPV evolves mechanisms to escape the immune response. The integration of the viral genome into the host cells results in induced cellular immortalization, transformation, and carcinogenesis, due to their interference with cell cycle and apoptosis control. Most importantly, high-risk HPV E6 and E7 oncoproteins are able to bind and degrade tumor suppressor p53 and pRb genes, respectively. Therefore, interaction of p53 and pRb proteins can give rise to an increased genomic instability following induced immortalization, transformation, and carcinogenesis. Toll-like receptors (TLRs) are specific pattern recognition molecules that bind to HPV components to trigger innate and adaptive immunity. HPVs modulate TLRs expression and interfere with TLRs signaling pathways, lead to persist viral infection and oncogenesis. Overexpression of NF-κB in HPVs associated with cancers suggests that NF-κB activation is a key modulator in driving chronic inflammation to cancer. HPVs oncogene-mediated suppression of NF-κB activity contributes to HPV escape from the immune system. This review focuses on the molecular players of the HPVs infection lead to chronic inflammation and cancer.

INTRODUCTION

Papillomaviruses have been discovered in a large number of vertebrate species. More than 300 papillomaviruses have been identified, including 200 human papillomaviruses (HPVs) (Egawa, 2015). The link between genital HPV infection and cervical cancer was first reported in the early 1970s by Harold zur Hausen (2009). His laboratory was the first to demonstrate that genital warts (condyloma) contain HPV genes, and also discovered the relationship between HPV infection and cervical cancer (Gissmann, & zur Hausen, 1980; de Villiers, Gissmann, & zur Hausen, 1981). He was awarded the Nobel Prize for Medicine in 2008 for the detection and isolation of HPV types 16 and 18 DNA from cervical cancer (Dürst, Gissmann, Ikenberg, & zur Hausen H, 1983; Boshart et al., 1984). HPV infection is associated with a broad spectrum of benign and malignant neoplastic epithelial changes. Epidemiological, clinical, and pathological studies have indicated that the virus causes sexually transmitted infections. The sexually active men and women are susceptible to genital HPV infection. Incidence and prevalence peak are at young age because young people are exposed to HPV infection for their sexual behavior. Cervical cancer is a major cause of morbidity and mortality in women worldwide. More than 500,000 new cases of cervical cancer and 275,000 deaths are reported each year worldwide (Tay, 2012). HPV persistent infections and precancer are established typically within 5 to 10 years (Schiffman et al., 2007). The worldwide HPV prevalence in cervical cancer is estimated to be 99.7% (Walboomers et al., 1999). HPV infection is commonly found in the genital organs of both men and women. More than 40 HPV genotypes are able to infect the genital organs of females and males, including the vulva, vagina, cervix and penis. HPV-DNA has also been identified in the head and neck cancers, in the oral cavity (the oropharynx and the larynx) cancers in both sexes. The association of HPV with neoplastic transformation has been reported in the lesions of the uterine cervix. The role of HPV in malignant transformation of penile cancer may be a similar way in cervical cancer. However, its association with penile cancer is not clearly understood (Senba et al., 2006; 2009a; 2010a; 2010b; 2011a).

The causal relationship between chronic inflammation and cancer is widely accepted. Specifically, there is a strong association between tumor viruses and the development of human cancers. Approximately 12% of human cancers are caused by oncoviruses, and more than 80% of cases occurred in the developing countries. (Bouvard et al., 2009; de Martel et al., 2012; Mesri, Feitelson, & Munger, 2014). The mechanisms of oncogenesis associated with infection and inflammation have been proposed. Effective host immune responses are essential for the control of HPV infection and persistence of HPV. However, failure to eliminate HPV infected cells increases the risk of developing chronic inflammation and cancers. Therefore, HPV associated with cancers are the most common outcome of high-risk

HPV infection, which are preceded by a phase of persistent HPV infection due to host immune system failure to eradicate HPV. Innate (cellular) and adaptive (humoral, antibody, and acquired) immune responses are induced in most individuals infected with HPV but are insufficient to eradicate the virus. The prevalence of overall HPV in women with normal cytology was estimated at 10.4-12%. Worldwide HPV prevalence was Africa 22.1-24%, Central America and Mexico 20.4%, North America 11.3%, Europe 8.1%, and Asia 8.0% (de Sanjosé et al., 2007). 90% of the HPV infections are cleared within 2 years mainly as a result of innate immune responses directed against early HPV proteins (Bulkmans et al., 2007; Forman et al., 2012). The majority of HPV infections are cleared before the occurrence of cancer formation. However, if the host immune system fails to eliminate the virus, persistent HPV infection occurs. The persistent HPV infection occurs due to the HPV avoiding immune surveillance and control. HPV prolonged persistence leads to genomic instability resulting in formation of cancer. HPV oncoproteins E7 and E6 are essential factors for HPV oncogenesis. E7 and E6 react with the tumor suppressor gene products pRb (retinoblastoma tumor suppress protein) and p53 in host cell proteins, respectively. E7 and E6 induced genetic instability leading to the activation of oncogenesis as well as inactivation of tumor suppressor genes (Münger et al., 2004; Senba et al., 2009b; 2009c; 2011b; 2012).

Although many investigators have proposed oncogenesis due to inflammation associated with cancer development, the mechanisms underlying the relationship between chronic inflammation and cancer still remain unresolved (Martin, & Gutkind, 2008; White, Pagano, & Khalili, 2014; Mesri, Feitelson, & Munger, 2014). Cancer formation due to the host immune response to high-risk HPV infection needs to be understood. This review focuses on the recent advances in the understanding of the molecular mechanisms of HPV infection and cancer formation.

HPV Types

Molecular epidemiologic evidence clearly indicates that certain types of HPV are the principal cause of cervical cancer, but the risk associated with the various HPV types has not been adequately assessed (Muñoz et al., 2003). At present, about 200 HPV genotypes have been identified and classified according to the sequence of the gene encoding the major capsid protein L1 (Haedicke, & Iftner, 2013). Approximately 40 genotypes infect the genital mucosa. A new HPV type is defined as showing less than 90% homology to any of the known on the basis of the L1 region. Subtype or variants of the same genotype correspond to a nucleotide identity of between 90% and 98%, respectively (Lazarczyk et al., 2009). Genital HPV types have been classified into low-risk groups, which are found mainly in benign tumors, and high-risk groups, which are frequently associated with malignant tumors. Low-risk HPV types typically induce benign tumors and are rarely associated with malignant tumors. In contrast, persistent high-risk HPVs induce malignancy. Thus, HPV is classified into low-risk types (6, 11, 30, 34, 40, 42, 43, 44, 54, 55, 57, 61, 62, 64, 67, 70, 71, 72, 74, 79, 81, 83, and 84); only 15 HPV types (16, 18, 31, 33, 35, 39, 45, 51, 52, 56, 58, 59, 68, 73, and 82) are consistently classified as entailing high-risk; and three (26, 53, and 66) are classified as probable high-risk types (Table 1) (Muñoz et al., 2003).

The high-risk types are associated with more than 90% of cervical cancers. Moreover, three main groups of HPV are classified depending on their localization, as follows; skin HPV types (1, 2, 3, 4, 5, 7, 8, and 10), skin and mucosal HPV types (2 and 7), and mucosal HPV types (2, 6, 7, 11, 16, 18, 31, 32, 33, 40, 42, 44, 51, 52, 54, 61, 72, 81, and 89) (Table 2) (Muñoz et al., 2003; Gross, & Pfister, 2004; de Villiers et al., 2004; Cogliano et al., 2005). The most frequently associated with particular diseases of HPV are localized three lesions, as follows; skin HPV types (1, 2, 3, 4, 5, 7, 8, and 10), anogenital HPV types (6, 11, 16, 18, 31, 33, 40, 42, 43, 44, 45, 51, 52, 54, 61, 72, 81, and 89), and oropharyngeal HPV types (2, 6, 7, 11, 16, 18, 32, and 57) (Table 2) (Cubie, 2013).

Table 1. Classification of low and high-risk HPV types

	HPV types
Low-risk	6, 11, 30, 34, 40, 42, 43, 44, 54, 55, 57, 61, 62, 64, 67, 70, 71, 72, 74, 79, 81, 83, 84
Probably high-risk	26, 53, 66
High-risk	16, 18, 31, 33, 35, 39, 45, 51, 52, 56, 59, 68, 73, 82

Table 2. HPV types associated with diseases

Diseases		Most frequently associated HPV types
Skin benign tumors	Warts	HPV 1, 2, 3, 4, 7, 10
Skin malignant tumors	Carcinomas	HPV 5, 8
Anogenital benign tumor	Warts	HPV 6, 11, 40, 42, 43, 44, 54, 61, 72, 81, 89
Anogenital malignant tumor	Carcinomas	HPV 16, 18, 31, 33, 45, 51, 52
Oropharyngeal benign tumor	Papillomas	HPV 2, 6, 7, 11, 16, 18, 32, 57
Oropharyngeal malignant tumor	Carcinomas	HPV16

The most important players are HPV-16, found in 50 to 70% of cases, and HPV-18, found in 7 to 20% of cases (Senba et al., 2006; Muñoz, Castellsagué, de González, & Gissmann, 2006; Parkin, & Bray, 2006; Koutsky, 2009). Therefore, the high-risk strains, HPV-16 and HPV-18 are the most closely associated with cervical and penile cancers. HPV-6 and HPV-11 are typically found in genital warts and condyloma acuminata of the genital organs (zur Hausen, 1996; Wallin et al., 1999; Walboomers, et al., 1999; Khan et al., 2005; Bernard, 2005; Stanley, 2010). In cervical cancer, HPV-33, HPV-45, and HPV-31 are the next most frequently detected HPV, except for Asia where HPV-58, HPV-33, and HPV-52 are the next most prevalent types (Bosch et al., 2008). In penile cancer, HPV-16 (60.23%), HPV-18 (13.35%), HPV-6/11 (8.13%), HPV-31 (1.16%), HPV-45 (1.16%), HPV-33 (0.97%), HPV-52 (0.585), and other HPV types (2.47%) are reported (Laimins, 1993; zur Hausen, & de Villiers, 1994; Miralles-Guri et al., 2009).

HPV Genome

HPV is members of the *Papovaviridae* family. HPV is a small nonenveloped DNA tumor virus, with a diameter of 50-55 nm. HPV induces hyperproliferative lesions in cutaneous and mucosal epithelia. The genome of HPV is a long circular double-stranded DNA molecule of approximately 8,000 base pairs (de Villiers, 2013) (Figure 1). The HPV genomes are organized into three regions; the HPV genomes contain one regulatory region designated as the URR (upstream regulatory region) or LCR (long control region), which contains transcription factor-binding sites and the replication origin, and two groups of ORFs (open reading frames). These ORFs are designated the late (L) gene (L1 and L2), the early (E) gene (E1, E2, E3, E4, E5, E6, E7, and E8) (Delius et al., 1994; Terai, & Burk, 2002). Viral genes are divided into early and late categories dependent on the time of expression.

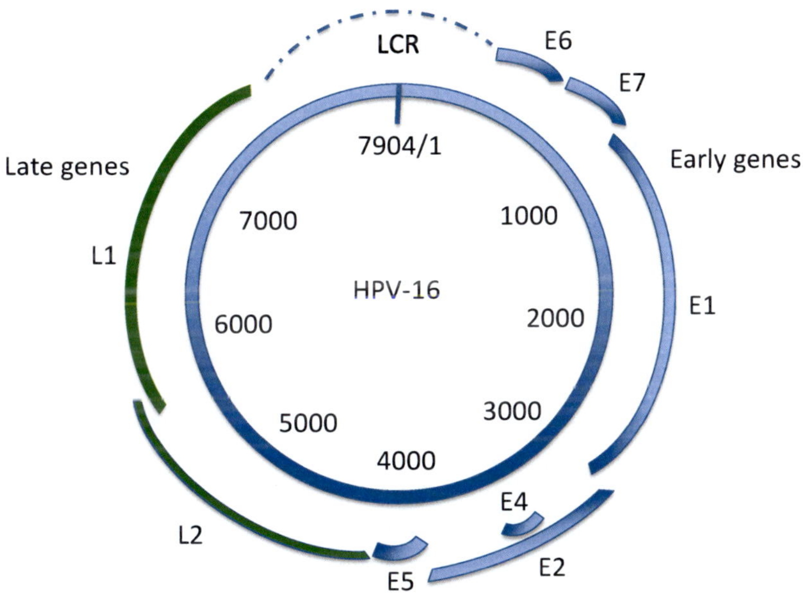

Figure 1. Typical genome organization of the high-risk type is illustrated by the genome of HPV-16. HPV genome is a circular double-stranded DNA molecule of approximately 8,000 base pairs. The six early ORFs (E1, E2, E4, E5, E6, and E7) are expressed from the different promoters during epithelial cell differentiation. The two late ORFs (L1 and L2) are expressed from promoter in the upper epithelial layers. L1 is the major capsid protein and L2 is the minor capsid protein. E1, E2, L1, and L2 are core proteins that are present early during HPV evolution. E4 protein may also be a core protein. In general, these proteins are involved in virus cell cycle. The LCR/URR contains the replication and post-transcriptional control that contributes to HPV genotype expression.

These core genes include the E1 and E2 proteins necessary for viral replication and control of gene transcription (Bergvall, Melendy, & Archambault, 2013; McBride, 2013), and the late proteins L1 and L2 (Buck, Day, & Trus, 2013; Wang, & Roden, 2013). E1 encodes a virus-specific DNA helicase, and E2 functions in viral transcription, replication, and genome partitioning. The E4 protein is expressed in the later stages of infection when complete virions are assembled. The E4 protein is considered to play an important role in the maturation and replication of HPV, and it is involved in the induction of the release of virions from infected cells (Doorbar et al., 1991). The E4 also carries out its common function at different anatomical sites where epithelial structure differs. These remaining viral E5, E6, and E7 genes may be considered as accessory genes that have developed to easily replication in stratified epithelium (Egawa et al., 2015). The E5 protein has weak activity in maintaining the malignant transformation of the host cells (Leptak et al., 1991). The oncogenic HPV E6 and E7 proteins promote cellular proliferation, delay cellular differentiation, and promote immune evasion (McLaughlin-Drubin, Meyers, & Munger, 2012). Proteins E6 and E7 have been shown to induce immortalization and transformation of the host cells. Therefore, E6 and E7 oncogene proteins have been shown to be the main contributors to the development of HPV-induced cancers and overexpression in cancer tissues (Phelps et al., 1988; Münger et al., 1989; Scheffner et al., 1990; Werness, Levine, & Howley, 1990; Klaes et al., 1999). Functions of E3 and E8 proteins are not clear.

The late gene regions, L1 (major capsid protein) and L2 (minor capsid protein) encode for viral capsid proteins during the late stages of virion assembly. The protein encoded by L1 is highly conserved among different HPV species (Table 3).

The minor capsid protein encoded by L2 has more sequence variations than those of the L1 protein (Ozbun, & Meyers, 1997). Early viral transcription is regulated by an element located in the non-encoding region proximal to the open reading frames called the LCR or the URR. The HPV LCR is located between the end of L1 and the start of the early region and contains promoter elements, transcription factor binding sites, and the viral origin of replication (Doorbar et al., 2015). The HPV LCR has numerous binding sites for many repressors and activators of transcription. It has been suggested that the LCR plays a part in determining the characteristics of HPV types (Morris, Dent, Ring, & Latchman, 1993; Tan, Leong, Walker, & Bernard, 1994; Kanaya, Kyo, & Laimins, 1997). Eighty-six complete genomes of HPV have been characterized and about 120 are partially characterized (de Villiers, 2013). The replication origin located in the LCR of the viral genome, and the LCR contains binding sites for both E1 and E2 proteins (Ustav, Ustav, Szymanski, & Stenlund, 1991). E1 and E2 are required for initial amplication and establishment of viral DNA and late vegetative replication, but E1 is dispensable for maintenance replication (Kim, & Lambert, 2002; Egawa et al., 2012).

Table 3. Human papullomavirus gene functions

Gene category	Gene		Function
Early genes	E1	Core proten	Viral DNA replication and control of gene transcription
	E2	Core protein	Modulation of replication and transcription
	E3		Unknown
	E4	Core protein	Viral assembly, and contribute to virus release and transmission
	E5	Accessory protein	Growth stimulation
	E6	Accessory protein	Oncoprotein due to interaction with p53 protein, telomerase activation, anti-apoptosis effect, induction of genemic instability, and drives cell cycle entry to allow genone
	E7	Accessory protein	Oncoprotein due to interaction with pRb protein, transformation of E2F-dependent promoters, induction of genomic instability, and drives cell cycle entry to allow genone
	E8		Unknown
Late genes	L1	Core protein	Major capsid protein, assembles into pentomeric capsomeres
	L2	Core protein	Minor capsid protein, virus entry and trafficking to the nucleas

E: early, L: late.

HPV LIFE CYCLE

HPV is the etiologic agents of cervical and other cancers. Persistence of infections by high-risk HPV types is the greatest risk factor for malignant progression. The life cycle of genital HPV is tightly adapted to their host tissue in the differentiating epithelial cells of skin or mucosa. HPV virions migrate to the nucleus as episomes and early HPV promoter is activated. The early (E) genes consist of E6 and E7 are oncoproteins in high-risk HPV. These factors act to alter the function of cell cycle regulators to allow for persistence of episomal genomes in undifferentiated cells, and replication of genomes or amplification in differentiated cells (Münger et al., 2004).

Latent infection. The organization of the life cycle is a major factor contributing to the HPV persistence infection. Viral early proteins are produced in undifferentiated keratinocytes in the basal layers of stratified epithelium. Normal squamous epithelial cells grow as stratified epithelium. Amplifying stem cells in the basal layer differentiate, and one of the daughter cells migrates upward and begins to undergo terminal differentiation. The other daughter cells remain in the basal layers of the epithelia, where HPV binds to and enter into cells through small wounds (Kines et al., 2009). The mechanism by which HPV actively invades cells involves the interaction with a heparin sulfate proteoglycans (HSPG) receptor. The replication cycle within the epithelium can be divided into the latent and the lytic infections. In the latent infection, the HPV genome is replicated to low copy numbers, approximately 10 to 200 genomes per cell within the nucleus of initially infected keratinocytes, subsequently basal cells (Doorbar, 2005; Moody, & Laimins, 2010). In basal epithelial cells, HPV self-renewal can ensure long-term maintenance of the viral genome. Maintenance of the viral episome in basal cells is the basic function of the early phase of the viral life cycle. E1, E2, E6, and E7 are each necessary for continued episomal maintenance of genomes (Stubenrauch et al., 1998; Thomas, Hubert, Ruesch, & Laimins, 1999; Park, & Androphy, 2002). The early HPV genes E1 and E2 are essential for DNA replication in the basal cells, whereas E6 and E7 modulate cell cycle regulators to maintain long period replication (Frattini, & Laimins, 1994; Sedman, & Stenlund, 1995). HPV DNA is replicated coordinately with host cell chromosomes, and HPV genomes are segregated into the two daughter cells. At the viral persistence state, the immune system may confine the infection to these basal cells.

Lytic infection. When infected daughter cells migrate to the upper layers of the epithelium, viral late gene products are produced to initiate the vegetative phase of the HPV life cycle, resulting in high-level amplification of the viral genome. The HPV virions are synthesized at the upper layers of stratified squamous epithelia. Activation of the late viral promoter in response to host cell differentiation occurs in the upper epithelial layer. For high levels of viral protein expression, the transcript levels of the E1, E2, E1^E4 (a fusion of the first amino acids of E1 to the E4 ORF), and E5 genes increase dramatically, resulting in virus copy number amplifies from 50 to 200 copies per cell (Bodily, & Laimins, 2011). For multiplication of viral DNA, the early genes E5, E6, and E7 are thought to coordinate a suitable environment in the host cells. The late promoter activates the late gene products, resulting in the vegetative phase of the HPV life cycle leading to high-level amplification of the viral genome. The HPV virions replicate in the superficial layers of the epithelium, and consequently the progeny HPV virions are released from the cell to re-initiate infection (Fehrmann, & Laimins, 2003; Doorbar, 2005). Following genome amplication, the virus capsid proteins L1 and L2 are produced in the late phase and virions are assembled. For a better understanding, the life cycle of HPV was divided into four parts; HPV genome maintenance, HPV genome amplification, HPV virion assembly, and virus release (Figure 2).

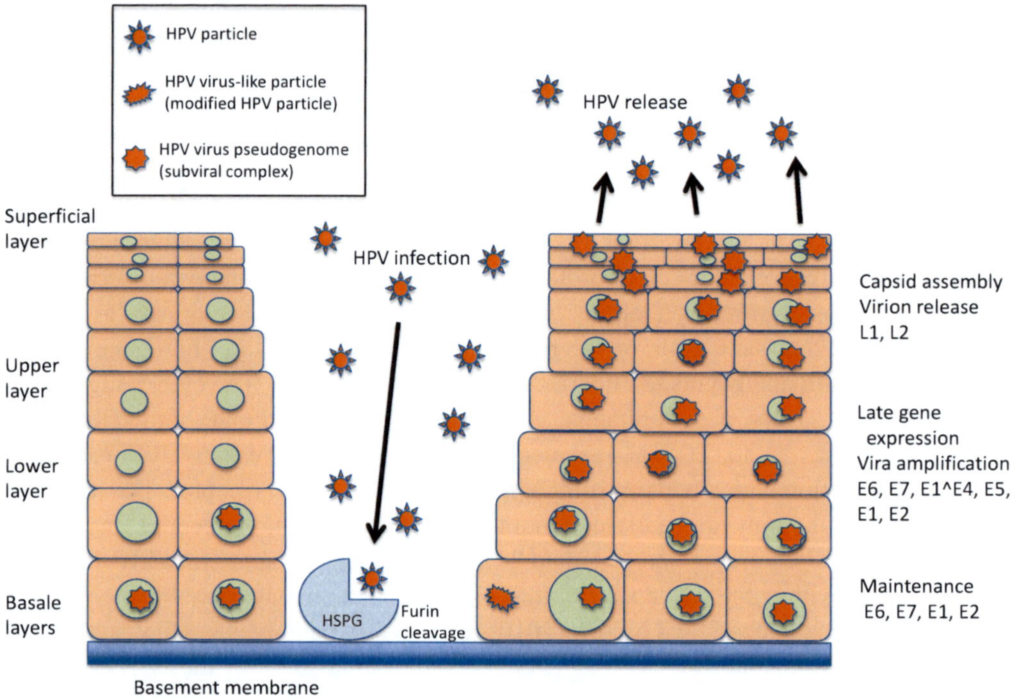

Figure 2. Model of life cycle of HPV. HPV infects keratinocytes and basal cells in the basal layer of stratified epithelium. HPV binds to and enter into cells through small wounds. HPV actively invades cells through the interaction with a heparin sulfate proteoglycans (HSPG) receptor. The replication cycle within the epithelium can be divided into the latent and the lytic infections. As the basal epithelial cells differentiation, the life cycle of HPV was divided into four parts; HPV genome maintenance (latent infection), HPV genome amplification (lytic infection), HP virion assembly (lytic infection), and virus release (lytic infection). The HPV proteins increase with differentiation of basal cells. Replication of HPV virion particles is released from superficial layer cells.

Mechanisms of HPV Entry

The early events of infection are viral replication and viral production functions. HPV is entry in host cell, which is initiated by binding of the virus particle to cell surface receptors. It has been suggested that virus particle binds initially to the basal keratinocyte cell surface (Roberts et al., 2007; Sapp, & Bienkowska-Haba, 2009a). Following step is HPV entering basal cells of stratified epithelia. The keratinocytes are main targets of HPV and entry in these cells for the productive infection. HPV virus-like particles are also able to enter dendritic cells (DCs) and Langerhans cells (LCs). An anti-HPV immune response is avoiding immune evasion for HPV using DCs and LCs presentation (Fausch, Da Silva, & Kast, 2003; Horvath et al., 2010). The identity of the receptors and the mechanism of internalization are known for many viruses. (Roden et al., 1994; Müller et al., 1995; Volpers et al., 1995; Sapp, & Day,

2009b). Glycosaminoglycans (GAGs) chains, especially HSPG, were suggested as initial attachment receptors for HPV particles (Joyce et al., 1999; Giroglou et al., 2001; Combita et al., 2001; Drobni, Mistry, McMillan, & Evander, 2003). HSPG are found on the surface of most cells and frequently in the extracellular matrix (Spillman, 2001; Liu, & Thorp, 2002). Cell surface HSPG has been shown to be the key attachment factor for HPV prticles. A few studies suggest that certain HPV particles or HPV virus-like paricles preparations may infect cells independent of HSPG (Buck et al., 2006; Cruz, & Meyers, 2013; Johnson, et al., 2009; Patterson, Smith, & Ozbun, 2005). HPV particles or HPV virus-like paricles can bind to the extracellular matrix though interactions with HSPG and lamini-332 (Joyce et al., 1999; Cerqueira, et al., 2013; Culp, Budgeon, & Christensen, 2006a; Culp et al., 2006b; Selinka, et al., 2007). This primary attachment is dependent only on L1 and does not require L2 (Horvath et al., 2010).

L2 proteins of all sequenced HPV virus-like particles contain at their N-termini a consensus cleavage motif for furin. Exposue of the L2 N-terminus allows access to a highly conserved consensus furin convertase recognition site and subsequent cleavage by furin on the cell surface, rendering the cross-neutralization epitopes accessible to antibody binding (Day, Lowy, & Schiller, 2008; Richards, Lowy, Schiller, & Day, 2006). The primary function of HSPG binding is to enable cell surface furin cleavage of the minor capsid protein L2, and furin cleavage is necessary for successful infection (Day, Lowy, & Schiller, 2008). HPV virus-like particles are internalized rapidly, within minutes after the initial receptor encounter and engagement (Williams, & Fuki, 1997). Significantly, HSPG-dependent events have been shown to occur on the extracellular basement membrane (Kines et al., 2009). The interaction with the putative secondary non-HSPG receptor may trigger infectious uptake. The identity of the putative secondary non-HSPG receptor has remained elusive despite extensive efforts to identify HPV (Selinka et al., 2003; Day, Lowy, & Schiller, 2008). However, HPV virus-like particles interaction with the cell surface during the initial stage of infection is not completely understood.

Interaction with secondary receptor and HPV viral-like particles must be internalized into the cell to establish an infection. Productive entry of HPV virus-like particles are involved in internalization by endocytosis. The dynamics of HPV virus-like particles interaction with the cell surface during the initial stages of infection are not completely understood and the entry mechanisms are highly controversial. The comprehensive study focused on HPV virus-like particles endocytosis into keratinocyte-derived cells, using HPV-based assays, indicates vesicle formation during HPV virus-like particles endocytosis is actin-dependent, clathrin-independent, caveolin-independent, and lipid raft-independent uptake of HPV virus-like particles, and that implicate tetraspanin-enriched microdomains (TEM) as entry mediators (Spoden et al., 2008). The successful infection requires the low-pH-dependent step of endocytic vesicles. Some endocytic pathways have been described and clathrin-independent caveolin-independent are two main pathways using by non-enveloped viruses to infect cells (Pelkmans, & Helenius, 2003; Smith, & Helenius, 2004).

HPV virus-like particles are trafficked through the early endosomal compartment. HPV viral-like particles were found to traffic via caveosomes to early endosomal compartment (Smith, Campos, Wandinger-Ness, & Ozbun, 2008). HPV virus pseudogenome (subviral complex) must pass through the late endosomal compartment. The HPV virus pseudogenome is detected in multivesicular endosomes and late endosomal compartment (Spoden et al., 2008; Schelhaas et al., 2012). The infection did not require functional Rab7. It was suggested that infections genomes exit the endocytic pathway prior to transit into late endosomal compartment (Smith, Campos, Wandinger-Ness, & Ozbun, 2008; Schelhaas et al., 2012; Day et al., 2013). The L1 is retained within late endosomal compartment. The HPV virus pseudogenome is transferred to the trans-Golgi network (Day et al., 2013). The nuclear envelope breakdown is required for establishment of HPV infection (Pyeon et al., 2009). Moreover, the nuclear access most likely occurs in mitotic cells, because nuclear envelope breakdown allows nuclear access rather than entry through a nuclear pore (Aydin et al., 2014). L2 is bound to the HPV virus like particles within the early endosomal compartment, and the HPV virus pseudogenome is processed through the late endosomal compartment, and delivers the HPV virus pseudogenome into the nucleus where it localized to ND 10 bodies (McKinney, Hussmann, & McBride, 2015). However, many controversies remain, especially, regarding the endocytosis, intracellular trafficking, and transport to the nucleus (Sapp, & Bienkowska-Haba, 2009a; Sapp, & Day, 2009b) (Figure 3).

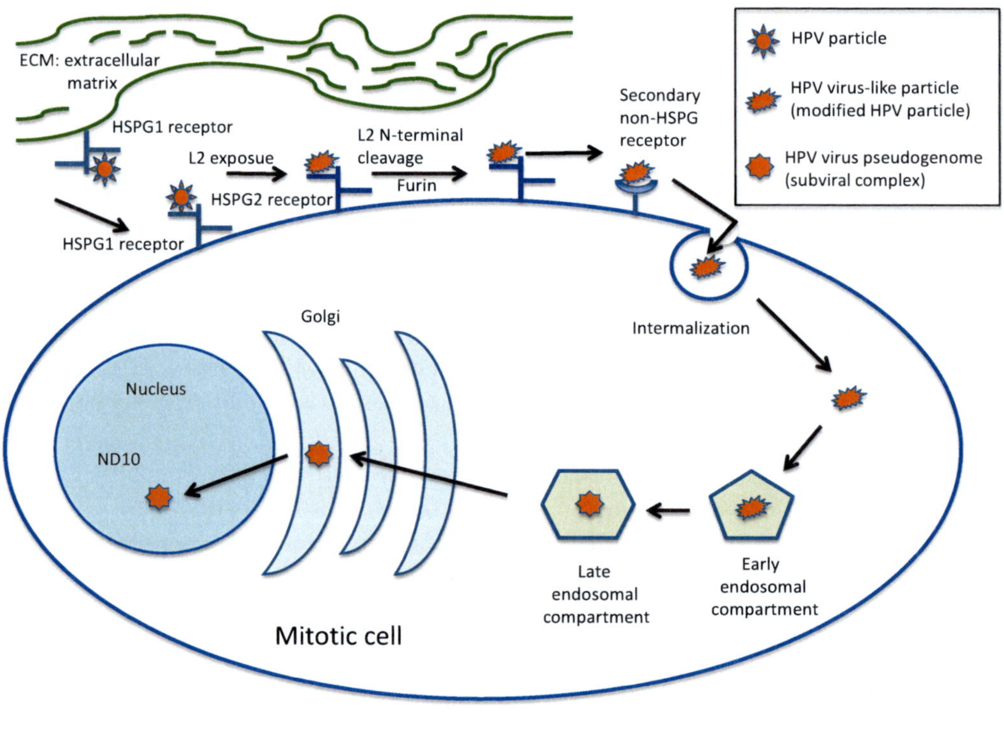

Figure 3. Putative model of HPV entry into cell surface and cell body nucleus. HPV particles bind to primary attachment receptors, HSPG1, appearance in the extracellular matrix (ECM) and cell surface. HPV capsids bind to ECM-resident laminin-332. HPV particles are changed to HPV virus-like particles and bind to HPSG2 receptor on the cell surface. HPV virus-like particles interact with HSPG2 resulting in the exposure of furin cleavage site. HPV virus-like particles are transferred to the secondary non-HSPG receptor on the cell surface. The secondary non-HSPG receptor interacts with HPV virus-like particle, subsequent to enter into the cell body. After intermalization, the structurally modified HPV virus-like particles are delivered to an early and late endosomal compartments, and HPV virus-like particles are changed to HPV virus pseudogenome (subviral complex) particles. After mitotic nucleus penetration, HPV virus pseudogenome locates to ND10 in the nucleus. However, many controversies remain in the endocytosis, intracellular events, and transport to the nucleus.

MHC CLASS I AND HPV IMMUNE EVASION

Both innate and adaptive immune responses are essential for the clearance of HPV, however, HPV has evolved mechanisms to avoid immune attack. HPV enters permissive cells and leaves the infected cells, resulting in hijack cellular metabolic pathways to generate progeny viruses. Hosts have developed innate and adaptive immune system and designed to recognize and eliminate these invaders. However, viruses have also evolved strategies to the host defense response. The most of the DNA viruses alter the host immune response for their life-long persistent infections. HPV infection is not accompanied by cell injury and cell death and inflammation. HPV reduces a little or no release of proinflammatory cytokines, resulting in weak-activation or non-activation for migration antigen presenting cells (APCs) (Stanley, 2006). HPV is an exclusively intraepithelial pathogen, and there is no viremic phase of the life cycle, thus, minimal amounts of virus are exposed to immune defenses. HPV in keratinocytes and basal cells is far from sites of immune surveillance, which is invisible to the host defenses. Therefore, HPV can remain in the host cells for long time, resulting in persistence and chronic infection. High-risk HPV persistence is required neoplasm formation due to avoidance of immune attack from the host.

The immune evasion target is the major histocompatibility complex (MHC) class I antigen presentation pathway. The cells are under constant control from $CD8^+$ cytotoxic T lymphocytes (CTLs) that continuously scaning the somatic cell surface for MHC class I molecules presenting non-self-peptides are recognized by the T-cell receptor, such as viral particles, and also $CD8^+$ CTLs are able to eliminate the infected cells through recognition of pathogen-derived peptides presented by MHC class I molecules at the cell surface. The MHC class I antigen presentation pathway enables infected cells with intracellular pathogens to signal the presence of the invader to the immune system. It has been suggested that HPV and HPV-infected cells have evolved mechanisms to avoid immune attack. T-cell mediated immune responses against oncogenic HPV are believed to play a central role in cervical oncogenesis. The MHC class I molecules are present on almost all the nucleated cells, and protect against invading HPV. MHC class I molecules at the cell surface consist of a transmembrane heavy (H) chain (45,000 MW), the soluble β_2-microglobulin (β_2m) light (L) chain (12,000 MW) subunit, and an eight or ten residue peptides in length (Tindle, 2002). The assembly of MHC class I molecules is regulated by series of interactions with endoplasmic reticulum (ER) resident chaperones and accessory molecules. The viral peptides result from proteosome degradation of proteins in the cytosol, which are translocated by the transporter associated with antigen processing 1 (TAP1) in the ER. They are loaded into newly synthesized MHC class I molecules. This stage of assembly is characterized by the formation of the peptide loading complex (PLC) and the acquisition of optimal peptides (Antonios, Powis, & Elliott, 2003). The PLC retains MHC class I molecules within the ER until they are loaded with high affinity peptides. Once loaded high affinity peptides have been bound, MHC class I molecules exit the ER, and transit through the Golgi apparatus to the cell surface to present their cargo to $CD8^+$ CTLs. This extra level of quality control is performed by the PLC distinguishes MHC class I molecules from many other proteins that assemble within the ER. MHC class I molecules can sample both the intracellular and extracellular milieus for defective and foreign proteins by presenting peptide fragments to immune effector cells. The MHC class I peptide complexes are patrolled by cells of both the innate and adaptive immune systems, namely natural killer (NK) cells and $CD8^+$ CTLs, respectively. Decreased MHC class I expression on infected cells renders the cells susceptible to NK cells mediated killing. Immune evasions selectively target the MHC class I molecules that preferentially present viral peptides (HLA-A and HLA-B) and spare the MHC class I alleles that act as dominant ligands of NK cells inhibitory receptors (HLA-C and HLA-E) (Kloover et al., 2002; van de Weijer, Luteijn, & Wiertz, 2015).

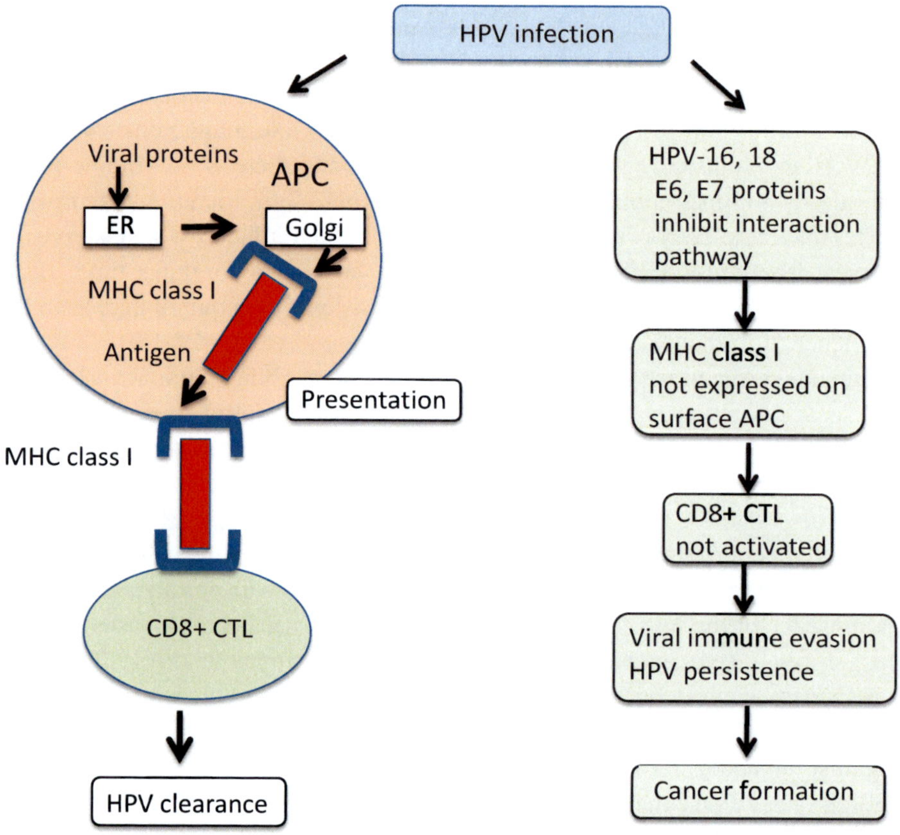

Figure 4. There is a strong association between HPV infection and the development of cancer formation due to viral immune evasion. The primary mechanism of viral immune evasion for HPV is avoidance of antigen presentation. HPV-16, and HPV-18, E6 and E7 interfere with the interferon pathways, therefore, the amount of major histocompatibility complex (MHC) class I molecules is reduced on the cell surface. CD8+ cytotoxic T lymphocytes (CTLs) play an important role in the elimination of viral-infected cells. However, MHC class I is not expressed on the cell surface of antigen presenting cells (APCs), resulting in inactivation of CD8+ CTLs. Continuous viral immune evasion leads to viral persistence and cancer formation in the long term. ER: endoplasmic reticulum.

The HPV-16 E6 and E7 oncoproteins are expressed constitutively in the majority of precancer and cancer lesion. HPV specific memory CTLs from cancer patients are recognized in the HPV-16 E6 and E7 oncoproteins presented by MHC class I molecules (Nimako et al., 1997). NK cells clearly respond to the viral infection through cytolysis and secreting proinflammatory cytokines, as well as the downregulation of surface MHC class I molecules in order to avoid recognition by $CD8^+$ T-cells, and molecules induced by viral invasion of cells. Ligands for NK cells receptors are primary for viral immune evasion. NK cells are important components of the innate immune system directly involved in the anti-viral immune response. NK cells inhibitory receptors monitor the normal levels of MHC class I molecules, whose expression is frequently altered by virus infection. Therefore, HPV infected associated with altered self-MHC class I molecules are protected HPV infected cells from NK cells, but lack of those are eliminated. E7 has been reported to downregulate the TAP1. Thereby interfering with presentation of antigens via the MHC class I pathway (Ghittoni et al., 2010). Moreover, NK cells are being considered for cancer treatment in antitumor activity (Cerwenka, & Lanier, 2001; Yokoyama, 2005; Pyzik, Kielczewska, & Vidal, 2008; Jonjić, Babić, Polić, & Krmpotić; 2008; Shastri, Nagarajan, Lind, & Kanaseki, 2014) (Figure 4).

HPV infections are predominantly controlled by MHC class I restricted CTLs. High-risk HPV-16 and HPV-18 E7 proteins have been shown to repress the MHC class I heavy chain gene promoter, which might lead to a loss of recognition of virus infected cells for MHC class I restricted CTLs (Georgopoulos, Proffitt, & Blair, 2000). The ability of HPV-18 E7 to avoid MHC class I might confer an increased oncogenic potential. The mechanism of MHC class I downergulation might be pertinent to a link with transformation. Downregulation of transcription of the MHC class I heavy chain gene by high-risk E7 proteins is associated with transformation. HPV immune evasion mechanisms lead to a loss of MHC class I expression, and loss of TAP1 function, resulting in increase the risk of malignancy, but not all MHC class I downregulatory mechanisms are associated with oncogenesis (O'Brien, & Campo, 2003). E7 can suppress cytotoxic response through the downergulation of the TAP1. E7 reduces the expression of TAP1, which is a key molecule of the antigen processing pathway for peptide transportation and loading. TAP1 inhibition subsequently reduces MHC class I dependent antigen presentation dramatically impairing the CTLs response (Cromme et al., 1993; Vambutas, Bonagura, & Steinberg, 2000; Vambutas et al., 2001; Senba, & Mori, 2012; van de Weijer, Luteijn, & Wiertz, 2015).

IMMUNE RESPONCES IN HPV INFECTION

The immune system plays a central roe in determining the outcome of HPV infection and immune response essential for the clearance of HPV. Defense mechanisms include components of both the innate and adaptive immune systems. The innate immune response has an important role in antiviral defense. The components of the innate immune response are activated complement components destroying virus infected cells and virus itself. The innate immune system responds early after exposure to a broad range of pathogens. HPV infects keratinocytes of the basal layer of the mucosal epithelium (Sterling, Skepper, & Stanley, 1993; Stanley MA, 1994) and also infects the basal layer cells (Maglennon, McIntosh, & Doorbar, 2011; Gravitt, 2012). The keratinocytes play an important role during the initiation of the HPV infection and are part of the innate immune defense system. The immune response plays an important role in clearing most of HPV infection, however, some HPV infections cannot be eliminated and persist for several years (zur Hausen, 1996). During the early stages of HPV infection, the host innate immune response becomes the first line of defense against the infection.

HPV must be detected by pattern-recognition receptors (PRRs) before innate immune responses. PRRs are specifically recognition of microbe-specific pathogen-associated molecular patterns (PAMPs). PRRs activate specific signaling cascades to induce the gene expression of targets, including the activation of type 1 interferons (IFNs) and proinflammatory cytokines. DNA viruses including HPV have mechanisms for inhibiting interferon synthesis and signaling. HPV infected keratinocytes are activated the antiviral defense due to the type 1 IFNs secretion. Type 1 IFNs, such as IFN-α and IFN-β, have antiviral, and immunostimulatory properties, that act as a bridge between innate and adaptive immunity (Le Bon, & Tough, 2002; Theofilopoulos, Baccala, Beutler, & Kono, 2005; Coccia, & Battistini, 2015). Type 1 IFNs play a critical role in anti-viral innate immunity to eradicate viruses and are secreted by macrophages or DCs. IFNs regulate the activation of immunity, such as the maturation of DCs, activation of NK cells and differentiation of CTLs. Thus, type 1 IFNs play an important role in the overall regulation of anti-viral immune response and anti-proliferative functions. HPV E6 and E7 can cooperatively inhibit the type I IFNs pathway, and contribute to establishment of persistent infection. High-risk HPV-16 E6 binds to interferon regulatory factor-3 (IRF-3), and inactivates the function of the transcription factor IRF-3 (Ronco, Karpova, Vidal, & Howley, 1998), a member of the interferon regulatory factor (IRF) family that has a crucial role in regulating IFN-α and IFN–β genes. On the other hand, E7 interacts with IRF-1, and represses its transcriptional activity for the IFN-β promoter (Park et al., 2000). E6 and E7 can block anti-viral and anti-proliferative functions of IFN-α (Li et al., 1999; Barnard, Payne, & McMillan, 2000). This interaction does not occur with low-risk HPV-6 E6 associated with benign tumor (O'Brien, & Campo, 2003). High-risk HPV-16 and low-risk HPV-11 E7 have shown to avoid the IFN-α and IFN–β responses (Park et al., 2000; Barnard, Payne, & McMillan, 2000). Thus, E7 inhibits IFN-α mediated signal transduction due to binding to p48/IRF-9. Stimulation of the cells of the innate immune system leads to the proliferation and differentiation of cells that participate in the adaptive immune response. This process is essential for anti-viral $CD4^+$ T-cells because they are integral components for successful innate and adaptive immune defenses. $CD4^+$ T-cell activity has a direct influence on the function and predominance of both T-cell and B-cell effector responses. Most DNA viruses have evolved mechanisms for inhibiting IFN synthesis and signaling. High-risk HPV downregulates IFN-α inducible gene expression (Chang, & Lamins, 2000; Nees et al., 2001), and HPV-16 E6 and E7 oncoproteins directly interact with components of the IFNs signaling pathway (Ronco, Karpova, Vidal, & Howley, 1998; Barnard, & McMillan, 1999). The keratinocytes can function as non-professional antigen presenting cells and are able to induce the expression of $CD4^+$ helper T-cell (Th), Th1 and Th2 type cytokines and cytotoxic responses in $CD4^+$ and $CD8^+$ memory T cells, respectively (Black et al., 2007; Nestle, di Meglio, Qin, & Nickloff, 2009). Keratinocytes constitutively express low levels of several cytokines. Pro-inflammatory cytokines, including several interleukins (ILs) and tumor necrosis factor (TNF) are important mediators of skin and mucosal inflammation. One of these cytokines, TNF is a major regulator of inflammation response in injury and infection (Locksley et al., 2001; Hehlgams et al., 2005). This cytokine activate multiple signaling pathways involved an antiviral activities, growth arrest, cell proliferation, differentiation, apoptosis, and growth factor availability (Locksley et al., 2001). Transforming growth factor (TGF)-β is other pro-inflammatory cytokines in HPV related diseases. For instance, HPV-16 E6 and E7 oncoproteins can inhibit the expression of TGF-β2 isoform, and TGF-β1 isoform may promote chromosomal instability (Deng, et al., 2008). Importantly, local concentration of pro-inflammatory cytokines may have an impact on the adaptive immune response to HPV (Boccardo, Lepique, & Villa, 2010). HPV positive keratinocytes show significantly reduced expression of a wide range of inflammatory cytokines including IL-1, IL-6, TNF-α, and TGF-β (Arany, & Tyring, 1996; Castrilli et al., 1997; Fichorova, & Anderson, 1999; Alcocer-Gonzalez et al., 2006), and expression of the anti-inflammatory IL-10 is increased (Alcocer-Gonzalez, et al., 2006; Ghittoni et al., 2010). A role of IL-6 in cervical oncogenesis is supported by the detection of higher levels of this protein in cervical cancer as compared with precursor and normal tissues (Castrilli et al., 1997). Interestingly, IL-6 production and macrophage chemoattractant protein-1 silencing might contribute to local immunosuppression allowing HPV infected cells to escape the immune system (Boccardo, Lepique, & Villa, 2010). Keratinocytes also constitutively express low levels of INF-α, IFN-β, and IFN-κ. Expression of IFN-κ is suppressed in HPV positive cells. This could contribute to inhibition of expression of interferon inducible genes (Rincon-Orozco et al., 2009). Importantly, IFN-κ was downregulated in cervical cancer tissues when compared with normal cervical tissues (Rincon-Orozco et al., 2009). Therefore, HPVs have evolved different ways of targeting cytokine and chemokine signaling as well as antigen presenting pathways to impair both HPV infected cells and immune effector cells (Boccardo, Lepique, & Villa, 2010). One of the functions of IFN production by HPV infected cells induced an antiviral state in surrounding cells. The importance of IFN response in controlling HPV infection is clear. Moreover, very effective immune evasion mechanism is inhibition of IFNs expression due to HPV infection.

The expressions of $CD4^+$ Th1-type and Th2-type cytokines are present in the subepithelial cervical tissue (al-Saleh et al., 1998). Importantly, lower percentages of Th1 cells with higher proportion of IL-4+ and IL-6+ cells were observed in high-grade squamous cell tissues compared to normal tissues. Predominant Th2 type cytokines in $CD4^+$ T-cells were also found in high-grade cervical lesions. IFNs induce an antiviral state in infected cells (Ronco, Karpova, Vidal, & Howley, 1998; Li et al., 1999; Perea, Massimi, & Banks, 2000; Park et al., 2000; Nees et al., 2001; Paradkar et al., 2014). Healthy women had lower concentrations of IFN γ (Th1 cytokine) and IL-5 (Th2 cytokine), which are important proinflammatory proteins in the blood. This suggests that both cell-mediated (Th1 cytokine) and antibody-mediated (Th2 cytokine) response may be negatively affected by oncogenic HPV infection (Deligeoroglou et al., 2013). $CD4^+$ T-cells are important for launching an efficient immune response against HPV. Anti-viral $CD4^+$ T-cell responses in healthy individuals presumed to have transient HPV-16 infections have been reported, while no response in some individuals with pre-cancer or cancerous lesions has been observed (de Jong, 2004). If $CD4^+$ T-cells are not activated, clearance of the offending pathogen will be hampered. For inhibitory signals, the cytolytic functions of $CD8^+$ T-cells are inhibited by the up-regulated expression of NK cell receptors on tumor infiltrating lymphocytes (TILs) derived from cervical cancer. These cells promote cell-mediated and antibody-mediated immune responses. Further studies are needed to determine whether HPV actively in vaccine-induced protection against primary HPV infection (Sheu et al., 2007).

The innate immune system consists of the epithelial barrier, phagocytosis, the complement cascade, some APCs, effector cells, such as, macrophages, neutrophils, and NK cells. DCs and LCs are highly specialized local APCs. DCs, LCs, NK cells, and keratinocytes are important cells involved in promoting a good immune response against HPV infection. LCs are the principal DC population in the epidermis of the skin. Moreover, NK cells are able to directly recognize and eliminate HPV infected cells (Renoux et al., 2011). However, NK cell activity is reduced in HPV infection (O'Brien, & Campo, 2002). Immature DCs take residence primarily in the dermis, whereas LCs found mostly within the epidermis and the superficial epithelial layers of the mucosa (Banchereau et al., 2000). DCs are key regulatory cells in the immune system, which are bridge between the innate and adaptive immune system. The intraepithelial of HPV has evolved to evade immune recognition at DCs and LCs. One prominent evasion mechanism is the ability to replicate without inducing cell death. This mechanism can possibly result in unactivated or partially activated DCs with a limited ability to migrate to the lymph node (Stanley, 2006). DCs are clearly the most potent APCs for stimulating an effective CTLs response. Generally, DCs both capture and process antigens, express lymphocyte co-stimulatory molecules, migrate to lymphoid organs, and secrete cytokines to initiate immune responses. T- and B-lymphocytes are the key mediators of cellular immunity under the control due to the activation of HPV specific T-cells. DCs bound to MHC class I or class II molecules interact with $CD4^+$ T-cells and $CD8^+$ T-cells, respectively. $CD8^+$ CTLs facilitate the destruction of cells with $CD4^+$ T-cells providing cytokines such as IL-2. Local APCs are probably recruited and secrete mediators that enhance the inflammatory response.

Antibodies specific for viral surface antigen block binding and/or fusion of virus to host cells. The coat of the virus particles facilitate receptor-mediated phaogocytosis and/or complemented mediated lysis of the virus. The infection is established, in a case, CTLs are the major component of cell-mediated immunity, and play a more important role in the defense against viral infections. CTLs are a major effector component of Th1 immune responses and are capable of killing virally infected cells. Most HPV therapeutic vaccines are targeted to the induction of CTLs to HPV E6 and E7, because these proteins have an important role in HPV infection and tumor progression. T-cell mediated immune responses against high-risk HPV are believed to play a central role in cancer formation (Sheu et al., 2007). CTLs targeted against E6 and E7 should be able to kill even HPV-infected basal cells in which only the early phase of viral replication. Conversely, CTLs targeted against L1 and L2 would not kill these cells, because these viral proteins are only detected later in the HPV life cycle at cervical squamous cells. CD8+ CTLs responses specific to HPV E6 or E7 have been detected only in a low percentage of cervical cancer cases, and a few responses are found in high-grade cervical intra-epithelial neoplasia (CIN) cases (de Gruijl et al., 1996; de Jong et al, 2004; Steele et al., 2005; Einstein et al., 2009; Mizuuchi et al., 2012; Di Bonito et al., 2015).

Interestingly, HPV may suppress CTLs responses via downregulation of the TAP1. For instance, TAP1 is necessary to load MHC class I with the processed viral protein before the complex is shuttled to the membrane. This interaction could explain the reduction in MHC class I presentation of HPV peptides by MHC class I molecules could inhibit both the induction of HPV-specific CTLs and the recognition of infected cells by effector CTLs. Moreover, specific T-cells have been confirmed that cervical cancer associated with keratinocytes expressing high levels of E6 and E7 could escape the attack from CTLs (Einstein et al., 2009; Kin, Kwon, & Sin, 2013; Song, Li, Li, & Dai, 2015), and also HPV-specific CTLs exist predominantly in cervical cancer (Bontkes et al., 2000).

HPV-specific CTLs infiltrating cervical cancer may play an important role in restricting disease progression. Cell mediated immunity is though to be important in the control of HPV infection. High-risk HPV specific CTLs have been demonstrated in the peripheral blood of cervical cancer patients. HPV infections initiate and progress to genital cancers after more than decades without any effective immune response to resolve the initial HPV infection. The regional immune escape may play an important role in cancer formation arising from the HPV infected area (Evans, Man, Evans, & Borysiewicz, 1997; Sheu et al, 1999). $CD8^+$ CTLs play an important role in the elimination of HPV infected cells. $CD8^+$ CTLs detect viral antigen peptides presented by MHC class I molecule on the cell surface. This pathway is designed to sample the intracellular milieu and present the information to the CTLs trafficking the area. DNA viruses with large genome coding capacity have been proven to be particularly adept at preventing CTLs recognition through the action of dedicated immune evasion proteins. In addition, viral immune evasion proteins contribute to viral defense and replication (Wagner et al., 2002; Antoniou, Powis, & Elliott, 2003; Ambagala, Solheim, Srikumaran, 2005; Antoniou, & Powis, 2008). The abnormal immune responses are leading to HPV persistence. The viral immune evasion leads to the development from chronic inflammation to cancer associated with HPV infection.

Basal kerachinocytes express PRRs, such as Toll-like receptors (TLRs), NOD-like receptors, and DNA receptors (Medzhitow, & Janeway, 1997; Medzhitow, 2007). TLRs are perhaps the best studied of PRRs, and ligation of host signaling pathways mediated via Mal/Myd88 or TRIM/TRIF adaptor molecules and in the initiation of both innate and adaptive immune responses (Akira, & Hemmi, 2003; Stanley 2012). TLRs are a family of immunological receptors that PAMPs with infectious agents. TLRs recognize various PAMPs derived from viruses, bacteria, fungus, and protozoa. Ligand specificity has been presented for TLRs. They are activation initiates signaling pathways that result in innate and adaptive immune responses in the face of immunological danger. TRLs have been established to play an essential role in sensing and initiating antiviral immune responses. The binding of viral PAMPs to host evolutionarily conserved pattern recognition receptors such as TLRs activates signaling pathways associated with multiple immune responses. These involved in activation of DCs, LCs, macrophages, NK cells, NF-κB, mitogen activated protein kinases (MAPKs), expression of proinflammatory cytokines, and induction of adaptive immunity (Beutler, 2004; Medzhitov, 2007; Zhou, Zhu, & Cheng, 2013). E6 and E7 have the ability to directly interfere with immune response related pathways favouring viral persistence. HPV E6 and E7 modulate innate immune responses mediated by a family of TLRs that are key sensors of evading HPVs. Keratinocytes in cervical tissues have been shown to express TLR1, TLR2, TLR3, TLR4, TLR5, TLR6, and TLR9, and also keratinocytes response firstly against pathogenic microbe (Miller, 2008; Nasu, & Narahara, 2010; Tummers, & Burg, 2015). TLRs play an important role in combating viral infections and in the recognition of viral nucleic acids. The activation of TLRs promotes the production of cytokines including type 1 IFN (Hasan, 2014). Specifically, activation of TLR-9 in keratinocytes produces TNF-α, IL-8, CCL2, CCL20, CXCL9 and type 1 IFN (Lebre et al., 2007; Miller, & Modlin, 2007; Amador-Molina et al., 2013). HPV is able to modify cytokine levels as an immune evasion mechanism (Stanley, 2012). Expression of TLR5 and TLR9 were undetectable or weak in normal squamous cell. However, the expression gradually increases from low-grade CIN to high-grade CIN, and squamous cell carcinoma (Lee et al., 2007; Kim et al., 2008). HPV-16 E6 and E7 oncogenes are able to block TLR9 induced cytokine secretion by keratinocytes (Hasan et al., 2007). The impaired TLR9 function might contribute to reduce host immune responses during persistent HPV infection (Hasan et al., 2007). This immune evasion strategy could promote establishment of persistent HPV infection and subsequent cancer formation. The effect of high-risk HPV on the innate immune system is not clear, however, avoidance of stimulation of the innate immune system permits persistence in the mucosal epithelium due to high-risk HPV using an immune evasion strategy (Amador-Molina et al., 2013; Zhou, Zhu, & Cheng, 2013). Moreover, HPV modulates TLRs expression and interferes with TLRs signaling pathways, leading to persistent viral infection and oncogenesis. Immunotherapeutic strategies based on TLRs agonists have emerged to be one of the novel drugs in treatment of HPV associated with diseases in the future (Zhou, Zhu, & Cheng, 2013).

The immune system plays a pivotal role in determining the outcome of HPV infection. The important role of host innate and adaptive immune responses protects from established HPV infections. Defense mechanisms against HPV infections are regulated in concert with innate and adaptive immunity. The main players of adaptive immune responses to HPV infections are production of neutralizing antibodies and induction of NK cells (Nakagawa et al., 2000; de Jong et al., 2004; Sheu et al., 2007; Pichlmair, & Reis e Sousa, 2007; Woo et al., 2010). Antibody specific for viral surface antigens block binding and/or fusion of virus, and coat the viral particles to facilitate receptor mediated phagocytosis and/or complement mediated lysis of virus. Antibodies production from the mucosal tissues prevents HPV infection in the mucosal surface. Cervical anti-HPV immunoglobulin (Ig), IgA and IgG are strongly associated with HPV-DNA and cervical diseases (Hagensee et al., 2000; Bierl et al., 2005). It is suggested that mucosal antibodies protect against HPV infection (Sheu et al., 2007).

Basic Functions of E6 and E7 in Oncogenesis

HPV oncoproteins high-risk E6 and E7 play a key role for HPV oncogenesis because of the immune response and cellular transformation. HPV-16 E6 and E7 oncoproteins are constitutively expressed in cancer lesions as putative targets for the immune response against HPV (Kadish et al., 1997). The overexpression of both E6 and E7 genes are most virulent for causing cervical cancer. E7 and E6 react with the tumor suppressor gene products pRb and p53 in host cell proteins, respectively, resulting in induced cellular immortalization, transformation, and carcinogenesis, due to their interference with cell cycle and apoptosis control (Münger et al., 2004; Duensing, & Münger, 2004). E7 and E6 induced genetic instability leads to the activation of oncogenes and inactivation of tumor suppressor genes (Jabbar et al., 2010; Moody, & Laimins, 2010).

The HPV oncogenes, E7 and E6, have been shown to be the main contributors to the development of HPV induced cancers, probably due to integration of the viral genes in the host cell genome. Inactivation of tumor suppressors p53 and pRb is a common event in the carcinogenesis of human cells. In HPV infection, the significant interactions are both p53 and pRb proteins, which are important molecules in the cell cycle and apoptosis control. Remarkably, p53 and pRb proteins are mutated in many human cancers. Both E7 and E6 oncogenes interact with pRb and p53, which inhibit the activities of these tumor suppressors. S phase progression of the cell cycle would normally lead to apoptosis by the action of p53. However, in HPV infected cells, this process is counteracted by the viral E6 protein, which targets p53 for proteolytic degradation. High-risk HPV causes persistent infections, which induce the initiation and progression of malignant tumor formation. As an aberration of virus infection, the constant activity of the viral proteins E7 and E6 leads to increasing genomic instability, and accumulation of oncogene mutations, resulting in cancer formation. Specifically, those involving tumor suppressor genes can give rise to an immortalization associated with activation of telomerase. Extensive studies have linked the efficiency of mucosal HPV types in promoting cancer development to the viral E6 and E7 proteins. The E6 and E7 genes are thought to play causative roles, since E6 promotes the degradation of p53 through its interaction with E6 associated protein (E6-AP), an E3 ubiquitin ligase, whereas E7 binds to pRb and disrupts its complex formation with E2F transcription factors (Huibregtse, Scheffner, & Howley, 1993; Scheffner, Huibregtse, Vierstra, & Howley, 1993). In addition, E6 and E7 cause degradation of the cellular genes controlling G2/M phase transition and progression (Walboomers et al., 1999; Patel, Incassati, Wang, & McCance, 2004).

E6 and E7 proteins may immortalize various types of human cells independently, however, their cooperative interaction leads to substantially enhanced immortalization efficiency. E7 binds to cyclin-kinase complexes and cyclin-dependent kinase (CDK) inhibitors. E7 directly binds to cyclin A/CDK2 as well as indirectly interacts with the cyclin E/CDK2 complexes via p107 protein of the pRb family, which acts to increase cyclins A and E in the epithelial cells. E7 also binds to the CDK inhibitors, p27 and p21 (Tommasino et al., 1993; McIntyre, Ruesch, & Lamins, 1996; Zerfass-Thome et al., 1996; Funk et al., 1997; Ruesch, & Laimins, 1998).

The E7 is an oncogene that mediates the initiation of DNA synthesis and transform cells into continuously growing cells. It hereby induces genetic abnormalities that enhance the likelihood of malignant progression. The E7 protein can interact with pRb, an important negative regulator of entry into S phase of the cell division cycle. It is thought that the high-risk HPVs have a unique ability to induce the proteolytic degradation of pRb. In the hypophosphorylated state, combined E7 and pRb activates the E2F transcription factor, which triggers the expression of proteins necessary for DNA replication and cell cycle progression. Phosphorylation of pRb by G1 cyclin-dependent kinases releases E2F leading to cell cycle progression into S phase. Because E7 is able to bind to unphosphorylated pRb, it may prematurely induce cells to enter S phase by disrupting pRb-E2F complexes (Boyer, Wazer, & Band, 1996; Jones, Thompson, & Münger, 1997: Berezutskaya et al., 1997; zur Hausen, 2000; 2002; Nguyen, Wesbroook, & McCance, 2002).

In addition to the inactivation of pRb family members, numerous functions of E7 have been reported. Histone deacetylases and transcriptional co-repressors have been reported to associate with E7 via Mi2 to promote cell growth. The interaction of E7 with cyclin E/CDK2 has also been reported. These cyclin-kinase complexes can phosphorylate the pRb proteins. Furthermore, E7 binds to the CDK-inhibitors, p27 and p21, confirming the abrogation of cell-cycle inhibition. Despite these multifunctional properties of the E7 protein, however, the expression of a mutant form of pRb that is selective for binding E7 revealed that the effects of E7 on epidermal differentiation are indeed due to pRb inactivation (zur Hausen, 2000; Nguyen, Wesbroook, & McCance, 2002).

The most manifest function of the E6 protein is to promote the degradation of p53 under E6 protein associated with E6AP protein, an E3 ubiquitin ligase. The affinity of E6AP for p53 is likely to be modified by the association with E6. The p53 is a tumor suppressor gene involved in apoptosis after DNA damage, and regulation of both G1/S and G2/M cell cycles. HPV-infected cells induce inhibition of apoptosis by E6 inactivation of p53. In addition, E6 interferes with other proapoptotic proteins, such as Bak, flavin adenine dinucleotide (FADD) and procaspase 8 (Thomas, Pim, & Banks, 1999; Garnett, Filppova, & Duerksen-Hughes, 2006) (Figure 5).

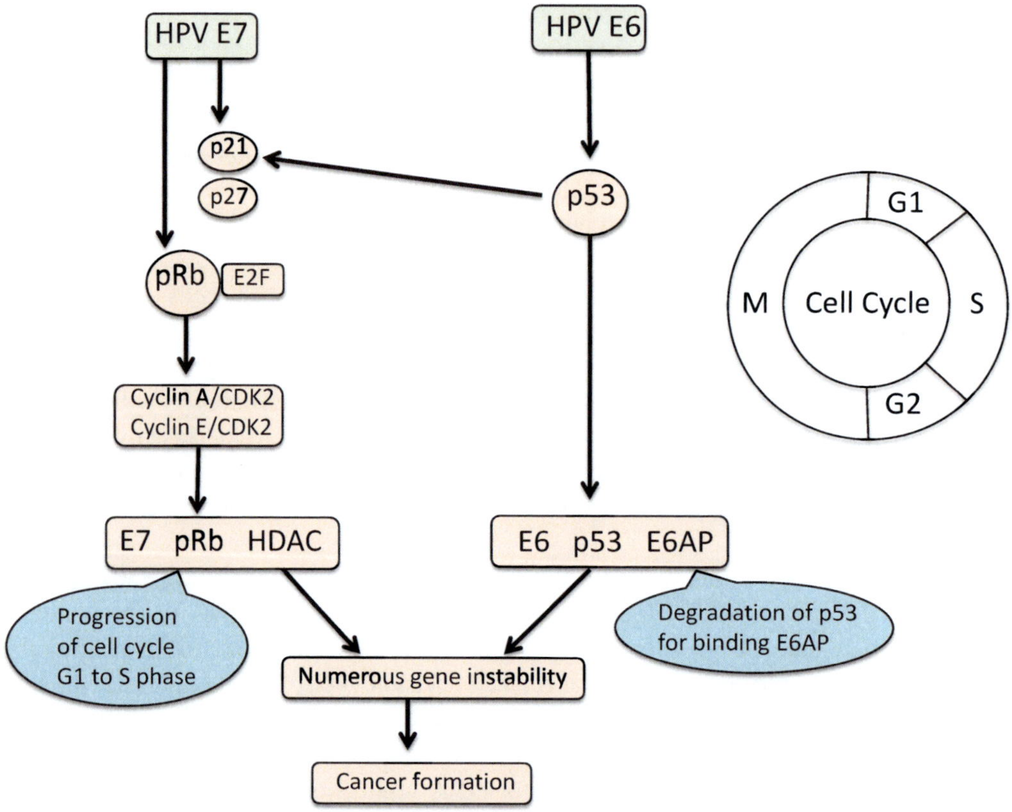

Figure 5. Essential mechanisms for the interaction of HPV E7 oncoprotein bind to retinoblastoma tumor suppressor protein (pRb), and the related pRb family members p107 and p130. E7 binds to pRb leading to E2F mediated gene transcription and activation of cyclin/CDK2 complexes. HPV E6 oncoprotein binds to p53. HPV E6 oncoprotein progresses cell cycle G to S, most likely by abrogating G2 to M checkpoint control.

The high-level expression of E6 and E7 in cancer tissue is often observed, and high-risk HPV DNA is frequently found to integrate into the host genome (Woodman, Collins, & Young, 2007; Pett, & Coleman, 2007). The integration sites are no evidence for insertion mutagenesis (Ziegert et al., 2003; Wentzensen, Vinokurova, & von Knebel Doeberitz, 2004). However, common fragile sites are suggested to be preferential targets for HPV DNA integration, and FRA8C at chromosome 8q24 near the c-Myc locus has been reported (Ferber et al., 2003). The c-Myc gene is observed in multiple cervical cancer cell lines, and it is suggested that HPV gene insertion at a signal integration site near the c-Myc locus (Macville et al., 1999; Herrick et al., 2005; Peter, et al., 2006). HPV gene integration sites are usually found at a single or a few chromosomal loci in clonal cell populations of cervical cancers. The molecular mechanism of integration is not clear.

Furthermore, E2 has been reported to inhibit E6 and E7 activity through direct protein interactions, repress the hTERT promoter, and induce apoptosis independent of the repression of E6 and E7 transcription (Webster et al., 2000; Lee et al., 2002; Demeret, Garcia-Carranca,

& Thierry, 2003). Therefore, HPV E6 and E7 integrate associated with chromosomal abnormalities leading to activation of oncogenesis and/or inactivation of tumor suppressor genes, resulting in inducing genomic instability and malignant progression (zur Hausen, 2002; Woodman, Collins, & Young, 2007). E6 and E7 induced genomic instability leading to cervical cancer development. HPV E6 and E7 integration in host cells is the most significant risk factor driving malignant progression after HPV infection (Yugawa, & Kiyono, 2009).

TRANSFORMING FUNCTIONS OF E7 IN ONCOGENESIS

Among the early proteins, E7 appears to be one of the most efficient cell cycle deregulator. HPV-16 E7 is an acidic phosphoprotein of 98 amino acids. E7 is an oncogene that mediates the initiation of DNA synthesis and transforms cells into continuously growing cells. It thereby induces genetic abnormalities that enhance the likelihood of malignant progression. It is thought that the high-risk HPVs have a unique ability to induce the proteolytic degradation of pRb. In the hypophosphorylated state, 2 combined E7 and pRb activate the E2F transcription factor, which triggers the expression of proteins necessary for DNA replication and cell cycle progression. HPV E7 interacts with many proteins, most of which are important regulators of cell growth, especially the phosphorylation of pRb by G1 cyclin-dependent kinases, and releases E2F leading to cell cycle progression from the G1 to S phase of mitosis. Because E7 is able to bind to unphosphorylated pRb, which induces cells to enter the S phase for disrupting pRb-E2F complexes (Boyer, Wazer, & Band, 1996; Jones, Thompson, & Munger, 1997; Berezutskaya, Yu, Morozov, Raychaudhuri, & Bagchi, 1997; Nguyen, Westbrook, & McCance, 2002). These interactions are the likely ways in E7 deregulates cell cycle, and leads to increased cell proliferation, immortalization, and transformation. The pRb family members play a pivotal role in cell cycle regulation. The other two members of the pocket protein family, p107 and p130, are associated with E2F4 or E2F5, respectively. These are involved in controlling additional cell cycle checkpoints p130 exerts its transcriptional regulatory function during the G0/G1 transition, while p107 is active in the G1/S transition and in the G2 phase (Cobrinik, 2005; Dimova, & Dyson, 2005).

The $p16^{INK4a}$ is the principal member of the Ink4 family of CDK inhibitors, which prevents the phosphorylation of pRb family members. The $p16^{INK4a}$ contributes to the regulation of cell cycle progression by inhibiting the S phase. The $p16^{INK4a}$ binds to CDK4/6, inhibiting cyclin D-CDK4/6 complex formation and CDK4/6 mediated phosphorylation of Rb family members in hypophosphorylated state, which promotes binding to E2F and leads to G1 cell cycle arrest (Serrano, Hannon, & Beach, 1993; Koh, Enders, Dynlacht, & Harlow, 1995; Khleif et al., 1996; Serrano, 1997). Therefore, overexpression of $p16^{INK4a}$ results in inhibition of E2F dependent transcription and inhibition of cell cycle progression at the G1 to S checkpoint (Zhang, Postigo, & Dean, 1999). The repression of $p16^{INK4a}$ gene expression by hypermethylation or mutation is a common occurrence in cancers. The $p16^{INK4a}$ phosphorylation induces formation of the $p16^{INK4a}$/CDK4 complex, preventing cyclin D binding and subsequenent kinase function. Cytoplasmic location of $p16^{INK4a}$ due to CDK4a sequestration has been suggested to occur in neoplastic cells as an indirect phenomenon of an alteration in the Rb pathway (Zhao, Mao, & Talbot, 2006). The $p16^{INK4a}$ protein is involved in regulation of the cell cycle. The $p16^{INK4a}$ is negatively controlled associated with the pRb gene product. Usually, $p16^{INK4a}$ is expressed at very low concentrations in healthy cells, whereas it is strongly over expressed in cervical cancer cell lines in which pRb has been functionally inactivated by the high-risk HPV E7 oncoprotein (Khleif et al., 1996; Nakao et al., 1997). The $p16^{INK4a}$ and $p19^{ARF}$ proteins have antiproliferative biological activity, and are involved in the pRb and p53 pathways, respectively (Weber, at al., 2000; Pei, & Xiong, 2005). These protein interactions are crucial for understanding the key points of tumor suppression. The $p16^{INK4a}$ is considered a tumor suppressor protein because of its physiological role and downregulated expression in the tumors (Romagosa et al., 2011).

The $p16^{INK4a}$ overexpression in HPV-related cancers is used as a diagnostic tool and has been directly associated with high-risk genotypes of HPV (Klaes et al., 2001; Cuschieri, & Wentzensen, 2008; Mulvany et al., 2008). The presence of E7 and E6 HPV oncoproteins is the molecular mechanism that explains $p16^{INK4a}$ overexpression in high-risk genotypes of HPV. The $p16^{INK4a}$ could be a prognostic tool in HPV associated with cancers. Malignant transformation is sometimes associated with $p16^{INK4a}$ overexpression due to pRb failure (Romagosa et al. 2011). The overexpression frequency of $p16^{INK4a}$ was reported to be 55 to 97% in cervical squamous cell carcinoma (Sano et al., 1998; Klaes et al. 2001), and 48 to 80% in cervical adenocarcinoma (Milde-Langosch et al., 2001; Zielinski et al., 2003). The overexpression frequency of $p16^{INK4a}$ was reported to be 29 to 53% in penile squamous cell carcinoma (Ferreux et al., 2003; Prowse et al., 2008; Senba et al., 2009a; 2010b). There is a close association between $p16^{INK4a}$ overexpression and high-risk HPV infection. Therefore, overexpression of $p16^{INK4a}$ is suggested to be a useful marker for evaluating HPV activity in cancer lesions (Sano et al., 1998; Ferreux et al., 2003; Carozzi et al., 2008).

E7 protein function enables HPV replication in the upper layers of the epithelium. HPV-16 E7 oncoprotein contains 98 amino acids and has casein kinase II phosphorylation sites at serine residues 31 and 32. E7 is a small nuclear phosphoprotein divided into three domains as CR1, CR2, and CR3 (Barbosa, et al., 1990; Dyson, Guida, Münger, & Harlow, 1992), and E7 is known to bind to pRb, pRb family members (p107, p130), histone deacetylases (HDAC), AP-1 transcription factors, TATA box binding protein (TBP), cyclins, CDKs and CDK inhibitors, and M_2 pyruvate kinase (M2-PK) via a LXCXE motif necessary for pRb binding in the CR2 region of E7 (Chellappan et al., 1992; Gonzalez, Stremlau, He, Basile, & Münger, 2001; Münger et al., 2001). E7 in the CR1 domain leads to cellular immortalization and transformation (Ruesch, & Laimins, 1998; Schulze et al., 1998).

In addition to the inactivation of pRb family members, numerous functions of E7 have been reported. HDAC and transcriptional co-repressors have been reported to associate with E7 via Mi2 to promote cell growth. Cyclin E-CDK 2 is essential for DNA synthesis (Ohtsubo et al., 1995). E7 contained keratinocytes express increased levels of cyclin E-CDK 2 activity (Funk et al., 1997; Ruesch, & Laimins, 1997, 1998). In proliferating cells, the G1/S phase cyclins and CDKs (cyclin D-CDK 4, cyclin E-CDK 2, cyclin A-CDK 2) are the key regulators of DNA synthesis, and cell cycle progression. The interaction of E7 with CDK2/cyclin A, as well as CDK2/cyclin E, has also been reported. These cyclin-kinase complexes exhibit kinase activities that can phosphorylate and inactivate of pRb proteins. Cyclin A-CDK 2 interacts with and phosphorylates E2F (Tommasino et al., 1993). E7 binds to cyclin A-CDK 2 in a cell cycle dependent manner and also contributes the S and G2 phases. Furthermore, E7 binds the CDK-inhibitors (CKIs), $p27^{KIP1}$ and $p21^{WAF/CIP1}$, confirming the abrogation of cell-cycle inhibition. Cells co-expressing HPV-16 E7 and $p21^{WAF/CIP1}$ or $p27^{KIP1}$ are still able to enter S phase, while in the absence of E7 are arrested in

G1 phase (Funk et al., 1997; Jones, Thompson, & Munger, 1997). For evasion of the immune system, E7 also interacts with p48, as well as IRF1. Recently, p600 has been identified as a cellular target of E7 that contributes to anchorage-independent growth and cellular transformation. Because knockdown of p600 sensitized cells to apoptosis induced by cell detachment irrespective of the presence of E7, and it has been suggested as a novel target of cancer treatment (Huh, 2005; White, 2012). Binding of E7 with both the 35-kDa catatytic and 65-kDa structural subunits of PP2A has been reported, resulting in the sequestration of these subunits and inhibition of their interaction with PKB/Akt, thereby maintaining its signaling by blocking its dephosphorylation. CR2 contains a LXCXE (amino acids 22-26) domain involved in binding to the tumor suppressor protein pRb and its related protein p107 and p130, also termed pocket proteins. Despite these multifunctional properties of the E7 protein, however, the expression of a mutant from of pRb (Delta LXCXE) that is selectively defective for binding E7 revealed that most the effects of E7 on epidermal differentiation are indeed due to pRb inactivation (zur Hausen, 2000; 2002).

TRANSFORMING FUNCTIONS OF E6 IN ONCOGENESIS

HPV-16 E6 is a 151 amino acid protein. The major structural characteristic of E6 is the presence of two atypical zinc fingers. The base of fingers is two motifs containing two cysteines, which are conserved in all E6 HPV types. E6 is one of the primary oncogenes of the virus, and its causes immortalization and transformation of cells. E6 binds to p53, CBP/p300, E6-AP, E6 binding protein (E6-BP), paxillin, mammalian homologue of disc large (hDLG), Bak, Tyk2, E6 targeting protein 1 (E6TP1), protein kinase N (PKN), Gps2, and IRF-3. E6 also alters the rate of transcription of human telomerase catalytic subunit (hTERT) and vascular endothelial growth factor (VEGF) genes. The most manifest function of the E6 protein is to promote the degradation of p53 under E6 protein associated with E6AP protein and an ubiquitin ligase. The affinity of E6AP for p53 is likely to be modified by the association with E6. E6-AP is also essential for p53 degradation in an infected cell. The p53 is a tumor suppressor gene involved in apoptosis after DNA damage, and regulation of both the G1/S and G2/M cell cycles. HPV-infected cells induce inhibition of apoptosis by E6 inactivation of p53. In addition, E6 interferes with other pro-apoptotic proteins, such as Bak, FADD and procaspase 8 (Thomas, Pim, & Banks, 1999; Garnett, Filppova, & Duerksen-Hughes, 2006).

The tumor suppressor p53 has been implicated in many important cellular processes, including in stimulation of the repair processes and protective mechanism, or the cessation of cell division and the induction of acquired cell death. The tumor suppressor p53 plays a central role in response to DNA damage. The p53 gene function is not an oncogene but a tumor suppressor that is very frequently genetic alterations in approximately 50% of human solid cancer cases worldwide. On the other hand, mutant p53 protein is basically undetectable in normal cells, however, rapidly increases in response to a variety of stress signals (Yoshida, & Miki, 2010). As a transcription factor, p53 mediates changes in gene expression that promote apoptosis, senescence or a reversible and protective cell cycle arrest. These mechanisms eliminate the damaged cells and suppress oncogenesis. Overexpression of the mutant p53 protein product was reported to be 41 to 89% in penile cancer cases (Lam and

Chan. 1999; Lopes et al., 2002; Humbey et al., 2003; Senba et al., 2009a; 2010b). New functions of this protein were revealed including the regulation of metabolic pathways and cytokines that are required for embryo implantation (Levine, & Oren, 2009). A frequent anticancer therapeutic strategy is to reactivate the p53 pathway in order to induce tumor clearance, but its induction by chemotherapy may paradoxically limit the effectiveness of the treatment (Goh et al., 2011). The recent research may see new p53-based drugs to treat cancer (Brown et al., 2009). The primary transforming activity of high-risk HPV is provided by the E7 and E6 oncoproteins. The efficient binding of Rb and E7 can lead to inhibition of cell growth and apoptosis through a p53 dependent pathway. As a result, high-risk E6 proteins have evolved to target the tumor suppressor p53 for degradation, and preventing cell growth inhibition in both undifferentiated and differentiated cells (Moody, & Laimins, 2010).

E6 has the ability to alter keratinocyte differentiation via targeting the Notch signaling pathway. The Notch1 gene family encodes for conserved trans-membrane receptors, which play a key role in cell-fate determination and differentiation. Notch activity increased in primary epithelial cells, resulting in cell cycle exit. Notch1 function has been observed as an oncogene in the development of human T-cell acute lymphoblastic leukemia, and breast cancers, but also acts as a determinant of keratinocyte differentiation and tumor suppressor in the epidermis. Notch1 expression also leads to squamous cell carcinoma of cervix (Zagouras et al., 1995). Moreover, Notch1 gene can induce growth suppression of cervical cancer cell lines through suppression of both E6 and E7 (Talora et al., 2002). Notch1 gene has been identified as a novel target of p53 and can be downregulated by E6 through p53 degradation (Lefort et al., 2007; Yugawa et al., 2007). Downregulation of Notch1 by E6 may lead to inhibition of cancer development. Induction of Noch1 through p53 occurs in response to genotoxic stress. HPV-16 E6 binds to the conserved LXXLL motif of a 100 kDa cellular protein, termed E6-AP, which functions as an ubiquitin protein. Therefore, its down regulation through p53 with E6/E6AP has been revealed as a novel tumor suppressor mechanism that blocks the development of HPV induced oncogenesis which leads to HPV related cancers (Lefort et al., 2007; Yugawa et al., 2007).

Telomerase is active in more than 90% of immortal and cancer cells, but it is absent in normal cells (Kim et al., 1994). Lack of telomerase activity in normal cells leads to the progressive breakdown of the telomerase DNA at the end of chromosomes due to incomplete end DNA replication, resulting in chromosomal instability and aging (Harley, Futcher, & Greider, 1990). Activation of telomerase is commonly observed in human cancers along with inactivation of pRb and p53 pathways. Inactivation of the pRb pathway and activation of telomerase are also required for immortalization of human epithelial cells. HPV E7 inactivates the pRb pathway and E6 induces hTERT expression and activation of telomerase for cellular immortalization associated with HPV infection. An important function of the E6 protein is the activation of telomerase in infected cells. Target proteins of E6 might contribute to cellular transformation with telomerase. Human telomerase is a ribbonucleoprotein complex composed of at least the hTERT and RNA component (hTR). The hTERT is expressed in specific germ-line cells, proliferative stem cells of renewal tissues, and cancer cells. In normal cells, the expression of hTERT reconstitutes telomerase activity and suppresses senescence.

High telomerase activity is observed in the most human cancer cells, which strongly suggests an important role in oncogenesis. Telomerase shortening is an important factor for limits the lifespan of normal cells. However, E6 induces telomerase activity, resulting in a contribution to the immortalization of epithelial cells by maintaining telomerase length. HPV-16 E6 mutant deficient for E6AP binding are still able to stimulate the expression of hTERT. The E6 protein has been shown to increase telomerase activity, and hTERT. Interaction between E6 and Myc has been observed to activate the telomerase reverse transcriptase promoter (Klingelhutz, Foster, & Mc Dougall, 1996; Oh, Kyo, & Lamins, 2001; McMurray, & McCance, 2003; Veldman, Liu, Yuan, & Schlegel, 2003; Gewin, Myers, Kiyono, & Galloway, 2004; Katzenellenbogen et al., 2007). NFX1-91 is an identified novel cellular repressor of the hTERT promoter (Xu et al., 2008), which is targeted by E6 for degradation in an E6AP HECT domain E3 ubiquitin ligase-dependent manner (Gewin et al., 2004). HPV-16 E6 associated with E6AP promote the degradation of the transcriptional repressor NFX-91, and consequently to activate hTERT transcription. E6 can also increase cellular fibronectin gene expression, transactivation of the prothymosin-α, c-Myc, and TGF-1β promoters (Dey et al., 1997; Kinoshita et al., 1997).

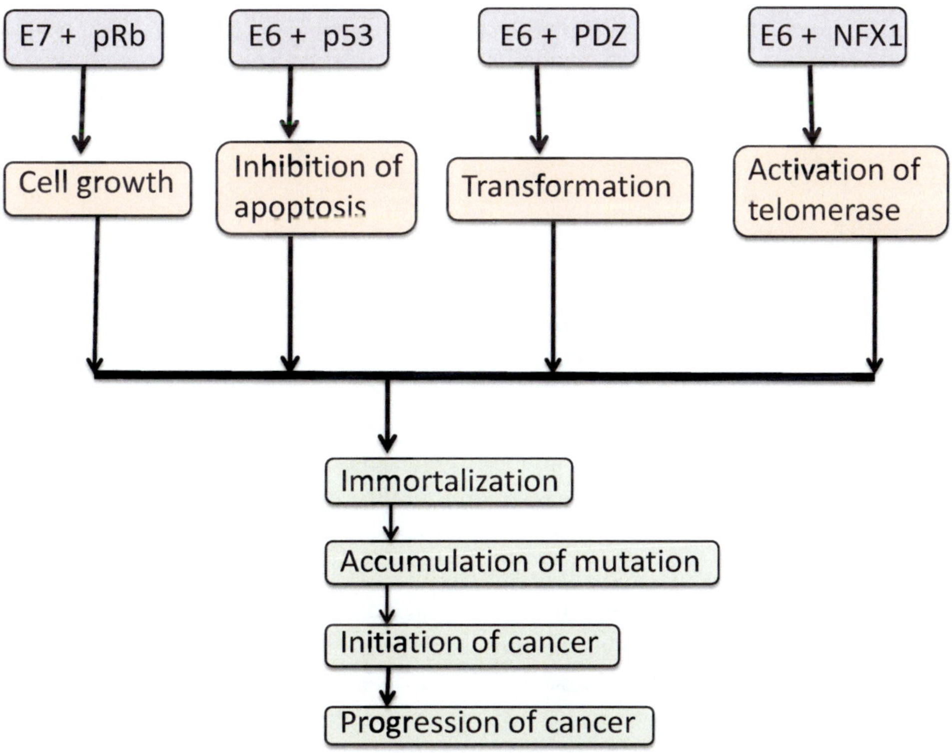

Figure 6. HPV E7 and E6 oncoproteins of the high-risk HPV can inactivate tumor suppressors pRb and p53, respectively. NFX is a recently identified novel cellular receptor of the hTERT promoter. PDZ-domain containing proteins lead to degradation of p53, which is important for cell transformation.

High-risk HPV E6 has been shown to interact with PSD95/Dlg/Zo-1 (PDZ) domain containing proteins leading to their degradation. The PDZ domain itself is composed of 80 to 100 amino acid residues and mediates binding to a C-terminal motif or other PDZ domains within its interaction partners. The majority of these binding partners are transmembrane proteins located at the plasma membrane including transmembrane receptors and channel proteins (Jelen, Oleksy, Smietana, & Otlewski, 2003). E6 targets several other cellular proteins for degradation and possesses the ability to bind and degrade p53. This is important for cell transformation because PDZ-domain-containing proteins are involved in a variety of cellular functions such as cell signaling, cell adhesion, ion exchange, and tight-junction integrity. PDZ proteins have also been found to be target proteins by oncoproteins from other tumor viruses, such as human T-cell lymphoma virus Tax and adenovirus E4 orfl. E6 interacts with several PDZ proteins, including MAGUKs (Dlg, Scribble, MAGI-1, MUPP1), and TIP-1, via a C-terminal PDZ binding motif on the E6 protein. E6 binding to these proteins appears to be particularly important for transformation and oncogenesis in cultured cells and transgenic mice. Recently, several PDZ-domain-containing proteins have been identified as targets of E6 protein. E6-induced degradation of these proteins potentially causes loss of cell-cell contacts mediated by tight junctions. E6 also contributes to the loss of cell polarity in HPV associated cancers. The tumor suppressor properties of these proteins against the development of HPV associated cancer have been reported. HPV E6 transforming properties are strong reduction for loss of PDZ binding domain in *in vitro* and *in vivo* experimental models. The targeting of PDZ domain containing proteins may lead to oncogeneic transformation associated with moleculer changes (Glaunsinger, Lee, Thomas, Banks, & Javier, 2000; Nguyen, Nguyen, Lee, Griep, & Lambert, 2003; Watson, Thomas, Banks, & Roberts, 2003; Lee, & Laimins, 2004; Favre-Bonvin, Reynaud, Kretz-Remy, & Jalinot, 2005; Storrs, & Silverstein, 2007) (Figure 6).

Mechanisms of Inflammation to Cancer Formation

The mechanisms of oncogenesis associated with infection and chronic inflammation have not been elucidated. However, many oncogenic mechanisms have been proposed for infection and chronic inflammation. Host pathogen interactions are usually initiated via recognition of PAMPs by host sensors known as PRRs, such as TLRs, RIG-1-like receptors, NOD-like receptors, and DNA receptors. PAMPs rapidly trigger host immune responses. The complex signaling pathways induce inflammatory responses and the eradication of viruses. NF-κB is a transcription factor composed of homo- or heterodimers of Rel homology domain-containing proteins, including p65 (RelA), RelB, cRel, p105/p50 (NF-κB1), and p100/p52 (NF-κB2). The intranuclear translocation of activated NF-κB signaling pathway induces the expression of numerous genes involved in innate and adaptive immune regulation, inflammatory responses, and anti-apoptosis. The intracellular translocation of activated NF-κB signaling pathway is regulated by a variety of posttranslational modifications, including phosphorylation and multiple ubiquitinations. Activation of the NF-κB and IRF transcription factor pathways is crucial for the immune early step of immune activation. NF-κB is activated by a variety of diverse extracellular or intracellular stimuli, including microbial pathogens and PAMPs. Many oncogenic viruses activate NF-κB to facility transformation of infected cells. Some viruses maintain a delicate balance between activation and suppression of NF-κB in order to maintain long-term persistence. As viral strategies, impairing NF-κB activation is proposed as a means of avoiding the innate immune response of the host. Aberrant NF-κB signaling is implicated in multiple disorders, such as chronic inflammation and cancer (Karin, 2008; 2009; Senba, Mori, & Wada, 2009b; Le Negrate, 2012; Zhao et al., 2015).

The relationship between chronic inflammation and cancer progression has long been known. Persistent infection with high-risk HPVs is the main case of cancer formation. Numerous investigations have identified NF-κB as an important modulator in driving chronic inflammation to cancer. This transcription factor is indispensable for the malignant progression of transformed cells associated with various inflammatory cells and a network of signaling molecules. The expression and the function of numerous cytokines, chemokines, growth factors, and survival factors are NF-κB-dependent. NF-κB activation has been implicated in a variety of processes related to transformation and oncogenesis, including proliferation, migration, angiogenesis, and prevention of apoptosis. NF-κB activity is involved in the regulation of the angiogenesis process for cancer cell growth and invasiveness. VEGF is the main member of angiogenic factors, and is under the transcriptional control of NF-κB (Kiriakidis et al., 2003). TLRs are possible signal initiators for NF-κB activation due to inflammation inducing carcinogenesis. In most cancer cells, the activation of NF-κB plays an important role in cancer initiation, progression, and metastasis. Among the major activators of NF-κB, TLRs are the front line receptors in response to microbial infection. The activation of NF-κB through stimulated TLRs in local chronic inflammation may serve as an initiator. NF-κB is constitutively activated during human cervical cancer progression (Chen, Alvero, Silasi, & Mor, 2007; Chen et al., 2008; El-Omer, Ng, & Hold, 2008; Senba et al., 2011a) and penile cancer progression (Senba et al., 2009a; 2010a; 2010b).

Increased NF-κB activity is associated with many cancers, especially cancers associated with viral infections. NF-κB dependent proliferation and protection from apoptosis are likely to have significant effects on the oncogenesis of HPV associated with cancers. HPV E6 and E7 positive cells have shown that IL-1β induces NF-κB activation and exhibits elevated levels of NF-κB components. E6 rather E7 expression was found to be associated with the nuclear location of these components (Havard et al., 2002). It is frequently reported that HPV encoded E6 and E7 oncoproteins are important regulatory proteins in host cells, which are associated with the transcriptional activity of NF-κB. A fraction of the E7 protein is found to be associated with the IκB kinase (IKK) complex and attenuate induced kinase activity of IKKα and IKKβ, thus resulting in impaired IκBα phosphorylation and degradation. While E7 obviates IKK activation in the cytoplasm, the E6 protein reduces NF-κB p65-dependent transcriptional activity within the nucleus. It is suggested that HPV oncogene-mediated suppression of NF-κB activity contributes to HPV escape from the immune system (Nees et al., 2001; Spitkovsky et al., 2002; Harvard, Rahmouni, Boniver, & Delvenne, 2005; Mishra et al., 2006). HPV E7 and E6 oncogenes are key regulatory proteins inside host cells and are associated with the transcriptional activity of NF-κB. Therefore, overexpression of NF-κB in penile and cervical cancer cases suggested that NF-κB activation is a key modulator in driving chronic inflammation to cancer (Senba et al., 2009a; 2010a; 2010b; 2011a; 2012).

PDZ domain-containing proteins have been identified as binding partners for the oncoprotein E6 of the high-risk type HPV. The PDZ binding motif of E6 is required for activation of NF-κB and the non-PDZ domain mutant from E6 is unable to activate NF-κB (James, Lee, & Kingelhutz, 2006). TNF, other cytokines, and growth factors stimulate the activation of NF-κB and the transcription of antiapoptotic target genes, including the inhibitor of apoptosis proteins XIAP, ciap-1, and ciap-2 (Gaur, & Aggarwal, 2003). NF-κB and TNF are functionally important molecules in inflammation-associated with cancers (Coussens, & Werb, 2002; Pikarsky et al., 2004). Prevention of DNA damage or cytokine induced apoptosis by activation of NF-κB may be a major obstacle in the treatment of HPV associated with cancers. NF-κB activation in HPV infected cells is likely to play a role in the proliferative capacity of the cells in addition to protection from apoptosis, which is reflected in the diminished ability of E6 mutants that are not able to bind PDZ domains or activate NF-κB to promote oncogenesis. Investigation of the potential role of NF-κB activation in the pathogenesis of HPV associated with cancers is significant importance with regard to the treatment and prevention for viral cancers (James, Lee, & Kingelhutz, 2006). NF-κB activity is triggered in response to infective agents and proinflammatory cytokines via the IKK complex. TNF, ILs, chemokines, COX-2, 5-LOX, and MMP-9 are all regulated by the transcription factor NF-κB. NF-κB activation is induced by a wide variety of stimuli of inflammation and formation of cancer, because inflammatory mediators induce oncogenesis (Kanodia, Fahey, & Kast, 2007; Mantovani, Romero, Palucka, & Marincola, 2008). Inflammatory biomarkers can also be exploited to develop new antiinflammatory drugs, which can be used not only for prevention but also for therapy of cancer. Moreover, inhibitors of NF-κB activation can block the cancer transformation response, which is a new approach in cancer treatment (Wang, Cusack Jr, Liu, & Baldwin Jr, 1999; Kim, Hawke, & Maldwin, 2006; Karin, 2008; 2009) (Figure 7).

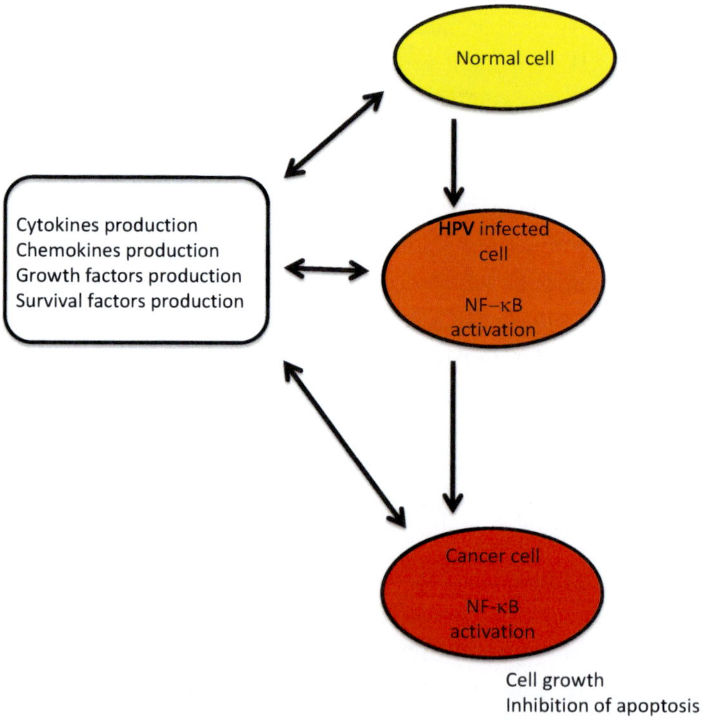

Figure 7. Relationship between chronic inflammation and cancer demonstrated link among Toll-like receptor (TLR), inflammation, and oncogenesis. TLR activated NF-κB, resulting in the production of inflammatory cytokines, growth factors, and survival factors, which could enhance malignant transformation.

Human leukocytes antigen (HLA) molecules are fundamental to the T-cell mediated adaptive immune response due to antigen presentation. HLA-G is a non-classical HLA class I molecule with multiple immune regulatory properties (Carosella, HoWangYin, Favier, & LeMaoult, 2008). It is different from classic HLA class I molecules by its low polymorphisms. HLA-G is a non-classical MHC class I antigen with seven isoforms, including both membrane-bond forms (HLA-G1, -G2, -G3, and -G4), and soluble forms (HLA-G5, -G6, and –G7). HLA-G has been known to suppress the immune system by modulating the release of the Th2 cytokines, which are associated with the anti-cancer immunity. Th2 cytokines are including IL-10, which induces HLA-G expression.

HLA-G and IL-10 expression in cervical cancer tissues are highly expressed locally in biopsies from patients with premalignant and cervical cancer lesions. It is suggested that HPV, HLA-G and IL-10 may play an important role in cervical cancer progression (Wang, Liu, Li, & Li, 2013). High levels of IL-10 may prevent cervical cancer for the elimination of HPV (Farzaneh et al., 2006). IL-10 increases Th1 cytokine production and the cytotoxic potential of HPV-specific $CD8^+$ CTLs. IL-10 associated with IL-12 is using treatment of cervical cancer (Santin et al., 2000). Therefore, HLA-G and IL-10 might be associated with cancer progression of the cervix. The HLA-G expression has been detected in a wide variety of human cancers, however, HLA-G expression in the normal tissues has been found to be restricted to a few tissue types, including trophoblastic cells and thymic epithelium (Rouas-Freiss et al., 2005; Carosella, HoWangYin, Favier, & LeMaoult, 2008). Recent investigations indicate strong immune inhibitory properties in cancer cells that may favor their escape from anti-cancer immune responses. Interestingly, abnormal HLA-G expression has been identified in cervical cancer tissues, and correlated positively with tumor progression (Yoon et al., 2007; Dong et al., 2010; Zheng et al., 2011; Li et al., 2012). It is suggested that HLA-G expression in tumors may contribute to escape from host immune surveillance, and also inhibition of cell mediated immune response. HLA-G molecules are associated with HPV infection, persistence, and cervical cancer development (Simoes et al., 2009; Ferguson et al., 2011, 2012; Silva et al., 2013; Yang et al., 2014). Numerous women are infected with high-risk HPV, but the majority of them never develop cervical cancer. The persistent infection with high-risk HPV is required for cervical cancer. However, the presence of HPV infection alone is not sufficient to induce cancer formation. HLA-G acts as a negative regulator of immune responses and its expression in cervical cancer cells may enable them to avoid immune attack. The role of HLA-G in cervical cancer lesions has not been defined clearly. Moreover, recent studies also detected soluble HLA-G in body fluids of patients with various types of cancers (Gros et al., 2006; Rebmann et al., 2007; Pistoia, Morandi, Wang, & Ferrone, 2007). It is suggested that soluble HLA-G expression is useful for diagnosing HPV associated with cancers and as a tumor marker (Morandi et al., 2007; Yan, 2011). HLA-G molecule acts as a powerful modulator of innate and adaptive immune responses. It plays an important role in the inhibition of the cytotoxic function and proliferation of T and NK cells, and the maturation and function of antigen presenting cells through direct binding to inhibitory receptors expressed on different immune cells (Carosella, HoWangYin, Favier, & LeMaoult, 2008; Loustau, Wiendl, Ferrone, & Carosella, 2012). These finding suggested that HLA-G could contribute to cancer cell immune evasion and cancer progression, and also soluble HLA-G is a diagnostic and prognostic biomarker to identify cancers, as well as a novel therapeutic target in cancers.

ACKNOWLEDGMENT

The authors thank Dr. Mihoko Kikuchi, Department of Immunogenetics, Institute of Tropical Medicine, Nagasaki University, for helpful advice. This work was supported in part by a Grant-in-Aid (No. 24592432) from the Ministry of Education, Culture, Sports, Science and Technology of Japan.

REFERENCES

Akira, S., & Hemmi, H. (2003). Recognition of pathogen-associated molecular patterns by TLR family. *Immunol Lett*, Jan 22; 85 (2): 85-95. Review.

Alcocer-González, J.M., Berumen, J., Taméz-Guerra, R., Bermúdez-Morales, V., Peralta-Zaragoza, O., Hernández-Pando, R., Moreno, J., Gariglio, P., & Madrid-Marina, V. (2006). *In vivo* expression of immunosuppressive cytokines in human papillomavirus-transformed cervical cancer cells. *Viral Immunol, Summer*, 19 (3): 481-491.

Al-Saleh, W., Giannini, S.L., Jacobs, N., Moutschen, M., Doyen, J., Boniver., J., & Delvenne, P. (1998). Correlation of T-helper secretory differentiation and types of antigen-presenting cells in squamous intraepithelial lesions of the uterine cervix. *J Pathol*, Mar; 184 (3): 283-290.

Amador-Molina, A., Hernández-Valencia, J.F., Lamoyi, E., Contreras-Paredes, A., & Lizano, M. (2013). Role of innate immunity against human papillomavirus (HPV) infections and effect of adjuvants in promoting specific immune response. *Viruses*, Oct 28; 5(11): 2624-2642. doi: 10.3390/v5112624. Review.

Ambagala, A.P., Solheim, J.C., & Srikumaran, S. (2005). Viral interference with MHC class I antigen presentation pathway: the battle continues. *Vet Immunol Immunopathol*, Aug 15; 107 (1-2): 1-15.

Antoniou, A.N., Powis, S.J., & Elliott, T. (2003). Assembly and export of MHC class I peptide ligands. *Curr Opin Immunol*, Feb; 15(1): 75-81. Review. No abstract available.

Antoniou, A.N., & Powis, S.J. (2008). Pathogen evasion strategies for the major histocompatibility complex class I assembly pathway. *Immunology*, May; 124 (1): 1-12. doi: 10.1111/j.1365-2567.2008.02804.x. Epub 2008 Feb 18. Review.

Arany, I., & Tyring, S.K. (1996). Status of local cellular immunity in interferon-responsive and -nonresponsive human papillomavirus-associated lesions. *Sex Transm Dis*, Nov-Dec; 23(6): 475-480.

Aydin, I., Weber, S., Snijder, B., Samperio Ventayol, P., Kühbacher, A., Becker, M., Day, P.M., Schiller, J.T., Kann, M., Pelkmans, L., Helenius, A., & Schelhaas, M. (2014). Large scale RNAi reveals the requirement of nuclear envelope breakdown for nuclear import of human papillomaviruses. *PLoS Pathog*, May 29; 10 (5): e1004162. doi: 10.1371/journal.ppat.1004162. eCollection 2014.

Banchereau, J., Briere, F., Caux, C., Davoust, J., Lebecque, S., Liu, Y.J., Pulendran, B., & Palucka, K. (2000). Immunobiology of dendritic cells. *Annu Rev Immunol*, 18: 767-811. Review.

Barnard, P., & McMillan, N.A. (1999). The human papillomavirus E7 oncoprotein abrogates signaling mediated by interferon-alpha. *Virology*, Jul 5; 259 (2): 305-313.

Barnard, P., Payne, E., & McMillan, N.A. (2000). The human papillomavirus E7 protein is able to inhibit the antiviral and anti-growth functions of interferon-alpha. *Virology*, Nov 25; 277 (2): 411-419.

Barbosa, M.S., Edmonds, C., Fisher, C., Schiller, J.T., Lowy, D.R., & Vousden, K.H. (1990). The region of the HPV E7 oncoprotein homologous to adenovirus E1a and Sv40 large T antigen contains separate domains for Rb binding and casein kinase II phosphorylation. *EMBO J*, Jan; 9 (1): 153-160.

Berezutskaya, E., Yu, B., Morozov, A., Raychaudhuri, P., & Bagchi, S. (1997). Differential regulation of the pocket domains of the retinoblastoma family proteins by the HPV16 E7 oncoprotein. *Cell Growth Differ*, Dec; 8 (12): 1277-1286.

Bergvall, M., Melendy, T., & Archambault, J. (2013). The E1 proteins. *Virology*, Oct; 445 (1-2): 35-56. doi: 10.1016/j.virol.2013.07.020. Epub 2013 Sep 10. Review.

Bernard, H.U. (2005). The clinical importance of the nomenclature, evolution and taxonomy of human papillomaviruses. *J Clin Virol*, Mar; 32 Suppl 1: S1-6. Review.

Beutler, B. (2004). Inferences, questions and possibilities in Toll-like receptor signalling. *Nature*, Jul 8; 430 (6996): 257-263. Review.

Bierl, C., Karem, K., Poon, A.C., Swan, D., Tortolero-Luna, G., Follen, M., Wideroff, L., Unger, E.R., & Reeves, W.C. (2005). Correlates of cervical mucosal antibodies to human papillomavirus 16: results from a case control study. *Gynecol Oncol*, Dec; 99 (3 Suppl 1): S262-268. Epub 2005 Oct 17.

Black, A.P., Ardern-Jones, M.R., Kasprowicz, V., Bowness, P., Jones, L., Bailey, A.S., & Ogg, G.S. (2007). Human keratinocyte induction of rapid effector function in antigen-specific memory CD4+ and CD8+ T cells. *Eur J Immunol*, Jun; 37 (6): 1485-1493.

Boccardo, E., Lepique, A.P., & Villa, L.L. (2010). The role of inflammation in HPV carcinogenesis. *Carcinogenesis*, Nov; 31 (11): 1905-1912. doi: 10.1093/carcin/bgq176. Epub 2010 Sep 5. Review.

Bodily, J., & Laimins, L.A. (2011). Persistence of human papillomavirus infection: keys to malignant progression. *Trends Microbiol*, Jan; 19 (1): 33-39. doi: 10.1016/j.tim.2010.10.002. Epub 2010 Nov 1. Review.

Bontkes, H.J., de Gruijl, T.D., van den Muysenberg, A.J., Verheijen, R.H., Stukart, M.J., Meijer, C.J., Scheper, R.J., Stacey, S.N., Duggan-Keen, M.F., Stern, P.L., Man, S., Borysiewicz, L.K., & Walboomers, J.M. (2000). Human papillomavirus type 16 E6/E7-specific cytotoxic T lymphocytes in women with cervical neoplasia. *Int J Cancer*, Oct 1; 88 (1): 92-98.

Bosch, F.X., Burchell, A.N., Schiffman, M., Giuliano, A.R., de Sanjose, S., Bruni, L., Tortolero-Luna, G., Kjaer, S.K., & Muñoz, N. (2008). Epidemiology and natural history of human papillomavirus infections and type-specific implications in cervical neoplasia. *Vaccine*, Aug 19; 26 Suppl 10: K1-16. doi: 10.1016/j.vaccine.2008.05.064. Review.

Boshart, M., Gissmann, L., Ikenberg, H., Kleinheinz, A., Scheurlen, W., & zur Hausen, H. (1984). A new type of papillomavirus DNA, its presence in genital cancer biopsies and in cell lines derived from cervical cancer. *EMBO J*, May; 3 (5): 1151-1157.

Bouvard, V., Baan, R., Straif, K., Grosse, Y., Secretan, B., Ghissassi, F., Benbrahim-Tallaa, L., Guha, N., Freeman, C., Galichet, L., & Cogliano, V.; WHO International Agency for Research on Cancer Monograph Working Group. (2009). A review of human carcinogens--Part B: biological agents. *Lancet Oncol*, Apr; 10 (4): 321-322. No abstract available.

Buck, C.B., Thompson, C.D., Roberts, J.N., Müller, M., Lowy, D.R., & Schiller, J.T. (2006). Carrageenan is a potent inhibitor of papillomavirus infection. *PLoS Pathog*, Jul; 2(7): e69.

Boyer, S.N., Wazer, D.E., & Band, V. (1996). E7 protein of human papilloma virus-16 induces degradation of retinoblastoma protein through the ubiquitin-proteasome pathway. *Cancer Res*, Oct 15; 56 (20): 4620-4624.

Brown, C.J., Lain, S., Verma, C.S., Fersht, A.R., & Lane, D.P. (2009). Awakening guardian angels: drugging the p53 pathway. *Nat Rev Cancer*, Dec; 9 (12): 862-873. doi: 10.1038/nrc2763. Review.

Buck, C.B., Day, P.M., & Trus, B.L. (2013). The papillomavirus major capsid protein L1. *Virology*, Oct; 445 (1-2): 169-174. doi: 10.1016/j.virol.2013.05.038. Epub 2013 Jun 22. Review.

Bulkmans, N.W., Berkhof, J., Bulk, S., Bleeker, M.C., van Kemenade, F.J., Rozendaal, L., Snijders, P.J., & Meijer, C.J.; POBASCAM Study Group. (2007). High-risk HPV type-specific clearance rates in cervical screening. *Br J Cancer*, May 7; 96 (9): 1419-1424. Epub 2007 Mar 6.

Carosella, E.D., HoWangYin, K.Y., Favier, B., & LeMaoult, J. (2008). HLA-G-dependent suppressor cells: Diverse by nature, function, and significance. *Hum Immunol*, Nov; 69 (11): 700-707. doi: 10.1016/j.humimm.2008.08.280. Epub 2008 Sep 24. Review.

Carozzi, F., Confortini, M., Dalla Palma, P., Del Mistro, A., Gillio-Tos, A., De Marco, L., Giorgi-Rossi, P., Pontenani, G., Rosso, S., Sani. C., Sintoni, C., Segnan, N., Zorzi, M., Cuzick, J., Rizzolo, R., & Ronco, G.; New Technologies for Cervival Cancer Screening (NTCC) Working Group. (2008). Use of p16-INK4A overexpression to increase the specificity of human papillomavirus testing: a nested substudy of the NTCC randomised controlled trial. *Lancet Oncol*, Oct; 9 (10): 937-945. doi: 10.1016/S1470-2045(08)70208-0. Epub 2008 Sep 8.

Castrilli, G., Tatone, D., Diodoro, M.G., Rosini, S., Piantelli, M., & Musiani, P. (1997). Interleukin 1alpha and interleukin 6 promote the *in vitro* growth of both normal and neoplastic human cervical epithelial cells. *Br J Cancer*, 75 (6): 855-859.

Cerqueira, C., Liu, Y., Kühling, L., Chai, W., Hafezi, W., van Kuppevelt, T.H., Kühn, J.E., Feizi, T., & Schelhaas, M. (2013). Heparin increases the infectivity of Human Papillomavirus type 16 independent of cell surface proteoglycans and induces L1 epitope exposure. *Cell Microbiol*, Nov; 15 (11): 1818-1836. doi: 10.1111/cmi.12150. Epub 2013 May 6.

Cerwenka, A., & Lanier, L.L. (2001). Natural killer cells, viruses and cancer. *Nat Rev Immunol*, Oct; 1 (1): 41-49. Review.

Chang, Y.E., & Laimins, L.A. (2000). Microarray analysis identifies interferon-inducible genes and Stat-1 as major transcriptional targets of human papillomavirus type 31. *J Virol*, May; 74 (9): 4174-4182.

Chen, R., Alvero, A.B., Silasi, D.A., & Mor, G. (2007). Inflammation, cancer and chemoresistance: taking advantage of the toll-like receptor signaling pathway. *Am J Reprod Immunol*, Feb; 57 (2): 93-107.

Chen, R., Alvero, A.B., Silasi, D.A., Steffensen, K.D., & Mor, G. (2008). Cancers take their Toll--the function and regulation of Toll-like receptors in cancer cells. *Oncogene*, Jan 7; 27 (2): 225-233. doi: 10.1038/sj.onc.1210907. Review.

Chellappan, S., Kraus, V.B., Kroger, B., Munger, K., Howley, P.M., Phelps, W.C., & Nevins, J.R. (1992). Adenovirus E1A, simian virus 40 tumor antigen, and human papillomavirus E7 protein share the capacity to disrupt the interaction between transcription factor E2F and the retinoblastoma gene product. *Proc Natl Acad Sci USA*, May 15; 89 (10): 4549-4553.

Cobrinik, D. (2005). Pocket proteins and cell cycle control. *Oncogene*, Apr 18; 24 (17): 2796-2809.

Coccia, E.M., & Battistini, A. (2015). Early IFN type I response: Larning from microbial evasion strategies. *Semin Immunol*, Mar; 27 (2): 85-101. doi: 10.1016/j.smim.2015.03.005. Epub 2015 Apr 11. Review.

Cogliano, V., Baan, R., Straif, K., Grosse, Y., Secretan, B.E., & Ghissassi, F.; WHO International Agency for Research on Cancer. (2005). Carcinogenicity of human papillomaviruses. *Lancet Oncol*, Apr; 6 (4): 204. No abstract available.

Combita, A.L., Touzé, A., Bousarghin, L., Sizaret, P.Y., Muñoz, N., & Coursaget, P. (2001). Gene transfer using human papillomavirus pseudovirions varies according to virus genotype and requires cell surface heparan sulfate. *FEMS Microbiol Lett*, Oct 16; 204 (1): 183-188.

Coussens, L.M., & Werb, Z. (2002). Inflammation and cancer. *Nature*, Dec 19-26; 420 (6917): 860-867. Review.

Cromme, F.V., Snijders, P.J., van den Brule, A.J., Kenemans, P., Meijer, C.J., & Walboomers, J.M. (1993). MHC class I expression in HPV 16 positive cervical carcinomas is post-transcriptionally controlled and independent from c-myc overexpression. *Oncogene*, Nov; 8 (11): 2969-2975.

Cruz, L.1, & Meyers, C. (2013). Differential dependence on host cell glycosaminoglycans for infection of epithelial cells by high-risk HPV types. *PLoS One*, Jul 4; 8 (7): e68379. doi: 10.1371/journal.pone.0068379. Print 2013.

Cubie, HA. (2013). Diseases associated with human papillomavirus infection. *Virology*, Oct; 445 (1-2): 21-34. doi: 10.1016/j.virol.2013.06.007. Epub 2013 Aug 9.

Culp, T.D., Budgeon, L.R., & Christensen, N.D. (2006a). Human papillomaviruses bind a basal extracellular matrix component secreted by keratinocytes which is distinct from a membrane-associated receptor. *Virology*, Mar 30; 347 (1): 147-159. Epub 2005 Dec 27.

Culp, T.D., Budgeon, L.R., Marinkovich, M.P., Meneguzzi, G., & Christensen, N.D. (2006b). Keratinocyte-secreted laminin 5 can function as a transient receptor for human papillomaviruses by binding virions and transferring them to adjacent cells. *J Virol*, Sep; 80 (18): 8940-8950.

Cuschieri, K., & Wentzensen, N. (2008). Human papillomavirus mRNA and p16 detection as biomarkers for the improved diagnosis of cervical neoplasia. *Cancer Epidemiol Biomarkers Prev*, Oct; 17 (10): 2536-2545. doi: 10.1158/1055-9965.EPI-08-0306. Review.

Day, P.M., Lowy, D.R., & Schiller, J.T. (2008). Heparan sulfate-independent cell binding and infection with furin-precleaved papillomavirus capsids. *J Virol*, Dec; 82 (24): 12565-12568. doi: 10.1128/JVI.01631-08. Epub 2008 Oct 1.

Day, P.M., Thompson, C.D., Schowalter, R.M., Lowy, D.R., & Schiller, J.T. (2013). Identification of a role for the trans-Golgi network in human papillomavirus 16 pseudovirus infection. *J Virol*, Apr; 87 (7): 3862-3870. doi: 10.1128/JVI.03222-12. Epub 2013 Jan 23.

de Gruijl, T.D., Bontkes, H.J., Stukart, M.J., Walboomers, J.M., Remmink, A.J., Verheijen, R.H., Helmerhorst, T.J., Meijer, C.J., & Scheper, R.J. (1996). T cell proliferative responses against human papillomavirus type 16 E7 oncoprotein are most prominent in cervical intraepithelial neoplasia patients with a persistent viral infection. *J Gen Virol*, Sep; 77 (Pt 9): 2183-2191.

de Jong, A., van Poelgeest, M.I., van der Hulst, J.M., Drijfhout, J.W., Fleuren, G.J., Melief, C.J., Kenter, G., Offringa, R., & van der Burg, S.H. (2004). Human papillomavirus type 16-positive cervical cancer is associated with impaired $CD4^+$ T-cell immunity against early antigens E2 and E6. *Cancer Res*, Aug 1; 64 (15): 5449-5455.

Deligeoroglou, E., Giannouli, A., Athanasopoulos, N., Karountzos, V., Vatopoulou, A., Dimopoulos, K., & Creatsas, G. (2013). HPV infection: immunological aspects and their utility in future therapy. *Infect Dis Obstet Gynecol*, 2013: 540850. doi: 10.1155/2013/540850. Epub 2013 Aug 20. Review.

Delius, H., Van Ranst, M.A., Jenson, A.B., zur Hausen, H., & Sundberg, J.P. (1994). Canine oral papillomavirus genomic sequence: a unique 1.5-kb intervening sequence between the E2 and L2 open reading frames. *Virology*, Oct; 204 (1): 447-452.

de Martel, C., Ferlay, J., Franceschi, S., Vignat, J., Bray, F., Forman, D., & Plummer, M. (2012). Global burden of cancers attributable to infections in 2008: a review and synthetic analysis. *Lancet Oncol*, Jun; 13 (6): 607-615. doi: 10.1016/S1470-2045(12)70137-7. Epub 2012 May 9. Review.

Demeret, C., Garcia-Carranca, A., & Thierry, F. (2003). Transcription-independent triggering of the extrinsic pathway of apoptosis by human papillomavirus 18 E2 protein. *Oncogene*, Jan 16; 22 (2): 168-175.

Deng, W., Tsao, S.W., Kwok, Y.K., Wong, E., Huang, X.R., Liu, S., Tsang, C.M., Ngan, H.Y., Cheung, A.N., Lan, H.Y., Guan, X.Y., & Cheung, A.L. (2008). Transforming growth factor beta1 promotes chromosomal instability in human papillomavirus 16 E6E7-infected cervical epithelial cells. *Cancer Res*, Sep 1; 68 (17): 7200-7209. doi: 10.1158/0008-5472.CAN-07-6569.

de Sanjosé, S., Diaz, M., Castellsagué, X., Clifford, G., Bruni, L., Muñoz, N., & Bosch, F.X. (2007). Worldwide prevalence and genotype distribution of cervical human papillomavirus DNA in women with normal cytology: a meta-analysis. *Lancet Infect Dis*, Jul; 7 (7): 453-459. Review.

de Villiers, E.M., Gissmann, L., & zur Hausen, H. (1981). Molecular cloning of viral DNA from human genital warts. *J Virol*, Dec; 40 (3): 932-935.

de Villiers, E.M., Fauquet, C., Broker, T.R., Bernard, H.U., & zur Hausen, H. (2004). Classification of papillomaviruses. *Virology*, Jun 20; 324 (1): 17-27. Review.

de Villiers, E.M. (2013). Cross-roads in the classification of papillomaviruses. *Virology*., Oct; 445 (1-2): 2-10. doi: 10.1016/j.virol.2013.04.023. Epub 2013 May 16. Review.

Dey, A., Atcha, I.A., & Bagchi, S. (1997). HPV16 E6 oncoprotein stimulates the transforming growth factor-beta 1 promoter in fibroblasts through a specific GC-rich sequence. *Virology*, Feb 17; 228 (2): 190-199.

Di Bonito, P., Ridolfi, B., Columba-Cabezas, S., Giovannelli, A., Chiozzini, C., Manfredi, F., Anticoli, S., Arenaccio, C., & Federico, M. (2015). HPV-E7 delivered by engineered exosomes elicits a protective $CD8^+$ T cell-mediated immune response. Viruses, Mar 9; 7 (3): 1079-1099. doi: 10.3390/v7031079.

Dimova, D.K., & Dyson, N.J. (2005). The E2F transcriptional network: old acquaintances with new faces. *Oncogene*, Apr 18; 24 (17): 2810-2826. Review.

Dong, D.D., Yang, H., Li, K., Xu, G., Song, L.H., Fan, X.L., Jiang, X.L., & Yie, S.M. (2010). Human leukocyte antigen-G (HLA-G) expression in cervical lesions: association with cancer progression, HPV 16/18 infection, and host immune response. *Reprod Sci*, Aug; 17 (8): 718-723. doi: 10.1177/1933719110369183. Epub 2010 May 5.

Doorbar, J., Ely, S., Sterling, J., McLean, C., & Crawford, L. (1991). Specific interaction between HPV-16 E1-E4 and cytokeratins results in collapse of the epithelial cell intermediate filament network. *Nature*, Aug 29; 352 (6338): 824-827.

Doorbar, J. (2005). The papillomavirus life cycle. *J Clin Virol*, Mar; 32 Suppl 1: S7-15. Review.

Doorbar, J., Egawa, N., Griffin, H., Kranjec, C., & Murakami, I. (2015). Human papillomavirus molecular biology and disease association. *Rev Med Virol*, Mar; 25 Suppl 1: 2-23. doi: 10.1002/rmv.1822.

Drobni, P., Mistry, N., McMillan, N., & Evander, M. (2003). Carboxy-fluorescein diacetate, succinimidyl ester labeled papillomavirus virus-like particles fluoresce after internalization and interact with heparan sulfate for binding and entry. *Virology*, May 25; 310 (1): 163-172.

Duensing, S., & Münger, K. (2004). Mechanisms of genomic instability in human cancer: insights from studies with human papillomavirus oncoproteins. *Int J Cancer*, Mar 20; 109 (2): 157-162. Review.

Dürst, M., Gissmann, L., Ikenberg, H., & zur Hausen. H. (1983). A papillomavirus DNA from a cervical carcinoma and its prevalence in cancer biopsy samples from different geographic regions. *Proc Natl Acad Sci USA*, Jun; 80 (12): 3812-3815.

Dyson, N., Guida, P., Münger, K., & Harlow, E. (1992). Homologous sequences in adenovirus E1A and human papillomavirus E7 proteins mediate interaction with the same set of cellular proteins. *J Virol*, Dec; 66 (12): 6893-6902.

Egawa, N., Nakahara, T., Ohno, S., Narisawa-Saito, M., Yugawa, T., Fujita, M., Yamato, K., Natori, Y., & Kiyono, T. (2012). The E1 protein of human papillomavirus type 16 is dispensable for maintenance replication of the viral genome. *J Virol*, Mar; 86 (6): 3276-3283. doi: 10.1128/JVI.06450-11. Epub 2012 Jan 11.

Egawa, N., Egawa, K., Griffin, H., & Doorbar, J. (2015). Human Papillomaviruses; Epithelial Tropisms, and the Development of Neoplasia. *Viruses*, Jul 16; 7 (7): 3863-3890. doi: 10.3390/v7072802. Review.

Einstein, M.H., Schiller, J.T., Viscidi, R.P., Strickler, H.D., Coursaget, P., Tan, T., Halsey, N., & Jenkins, D. (2009). Clinician's guide to human papillomavirus immunology: knowns and unknowns. *Lancet Infect Dis*, Jun; 9 (6): 347-356. doi: 10.1016/S1473-3099(09)70108-2. Review.

El-Omar, E.M., Ng, M.T., & Hold, G.L. (2008). Polymorphisms in Toll-like receptor genes and risk of cancer. *Oncogene*, Jan 7; 27(2): 244-252. doi: 10.1038/sj.onc.1210912. Review.

Evans, E.M., Man, S., Evans, A.S., & Borysiewicz, L.K. (1997). Infiltration of cervical cancer tissue with human papillomavirus-specific cytotoxic T-lymphocytes. *Cancer Res*, Jul 15; 57 (14): 2943-2950.

Farzaneh, F., Roberts, S., Mandal, D., Ollier, B., Winters, U., Kitchener, H.C., & Brabin, L. (2006). The IL-10 -1082G polymorphism is associated with clearance of HPV infection. *BJOG*, Aug; 113 (8): 961-964.

Fausch, S.C., Da Silva, D.M., & Kast, W.M. (2003). Differential uptake and cross-presentation of human papillomavirus virus-like particles by dendritic cells and Langerhans cells. *Cancer Res*, Jul 1; 63 (13): 3478-3482.

Favre-Bonvin, A., Reynaud, C., Kretz-Remy, C., & Jalinot, P. (2005). Human papillomavirus type 18 E6 protein binds the cellular PDZ protein TIP-2/GIPC, which is involved in transforming growth factor beta signaling and triggers its degradation by the proteasome. *J Virol*, Apr; 79 (7): 4229-4237.

Fehrmann, F., & Laimins, L.A. (2003). Human papillomaviruses: targeting differentiating epithelial cells for malignant transformation. *Oncogene*, Aug 11; 22 (33): 5201-5207. Review.

Ferber, M.J., Thorland, E.C., Brink, A.A., Rapp, A.K., Phillips, L.A., McGovern, R., Gostout, B.S., Cheung, T.H., Chung, T.K., Fu, W.Y., & Smith, D.I. (2003). Preferential integration of human papillomavirus type 18 near the c-myc locus in cervical carcinoma. *Oncogene*, Oct 16; 22 (46): 7233-7242.

Ferguson, R., Ramanakumar, A.V., Richardson, H., Tellier, P.P., Coutlée, F., Franco, E.L., & Roger, M. (2011). Human leukocyte antigen (HLA)-E and HLA-G polymorphisms in human papillomavirus infection susceptibility and persistence. *Hum Immunol*, Apr; 72 (4): 337-341. doi: 10.1016/j.humimm.2011.01.010. Epub 2011 Jan 20.

Ferguson, R., Ramanakumar, A.V., Koushik, A., Coutlée, F., Franco, E., & Roger, M.; Biomarkers of Cervical Cancer Risk Study Team. (2012). Human leukocyte antigen G polymorphism is associated with an increased risk of invasive cancer of the uterine cervix. *Int J Cancer*, Aug 1; 131 (3): E312-931. doi: 10.1002/ijc.27356. Epub 2012 Jan 3.

Ferreux, E., Lont, A.P., Horenblas, S., Gallee, M.P., Raaphorst, F.M., von Knebel Doeberitz, M., Meijer, C.J., & Snijders, P.J. (2003). Evidence for at least three alternative mechanisms targeting the p16INK4A/cyclin D/Rb pathway in penile carcinoma, one of which is mediated by high-risk human papillomavirus. *J Pathol*, Sep; 201 (1): 109-118.

Fichorova, R.N., & Anderson, D.J. (1999). Differential expression of immunobiological mediators by immortalized human cervical and vaginal epithelial cells. *Biol Reprod*, Feb; 60 (2): 508-514.

Forman, D., de Martel, C., Lacey, C.J., Soerjomataram, I., Lortet-Tieulent, J., Bruni, L., Vignat, J., Ferlay, J., Bray, F., Plummer, M., & Franceschi, S. (2012). Global burden of human papillomavirus and related diseases. *Vaccine*, Nov 20; 30 Suppl 5: F12-23. doi: 10.1016/j.vaccine.2012.07.055. Review.

Frattini, M.G., & Laimins, L.A. (1994). The role of the E1 and E2 proteins in the replication of human papillomavirus type 31b. *Virology*, Nov 1; 204 (2): 799-804.

Funk, J.O., Waga, S., Harry, J.B., Espling, E., Stillman, B., & Galloway, D.A. (1997). Inhibition of CDK activity and PCNA-dependent DNA replication by p21 is blocked by interaction with the HPV-16 E7 oncoprotein. *Genes Dev*, Aug 15; 11 (16): 2090-2100.

Garnett, T.O., Filippova, M., & Duerksen-Hughes, P.J. (2006). Accelerated degradation of FADD and procaspase 8 in cells expressing human papilloma virus 16 E6 impairs TRAIL-mediated apoptosis. *Cell Death Differ*, Nov; 13 (11): 1915-1926. Epub 2006 Mar 10.

Georgopoulos, N.T., Proffitt, J.L., & Blair, G.E. (2000). Transcriptional regulation of the major histocompatibility complex (MHC) class I heavy chain, TAP1 and LMP2 genes by the human papillomavirus (HPV) type 6b, 16 and 18 E7 oncoproteins. *Oncogene*, Oct 5; 19 (42): 4930-4935.

Gewin, L., Myers, H., Kiyono, T., & Galloway, D.A. (2004). Identification of a novel telomerase repressor that interacts with the human papillomavirus type-16 E6/E6-AP complex. *Genes Dev*, Sep 15; 18 (18): 2269-2282.

Ghittoni, R., Accardi, R., Hasan, U., Gheit, T., Sylla, B., & Tommasino, M. (2010). The biological properties of E6 and E7 oncoproteins from human papillomaviruses. *Virus Genes*, Feb; 40 (1): 1-13. doi: 10.1007/s11262-009-0412-8. Epub 2009 Oct 17. Review.

Giroglou, T., Florin, L., Schäfer, F., Streeck, R.E., & Sapp, M. (2001). Human papillomavirus infection requires cell surface heparan sulfate. *J Virol*, Feb; 75 (3): 1565-1570.

Gissmann, L., & zur Hausen, H. (1980). Partial characterization of viral DNA from human genital warts (Condylomata acuminata). *Int J Cancer*, 1980 May 15; 25 (5): 605-609.

Glaunsinger, B.A., Lee, S.S., Thomas, M., Banks, L., & Javier, R. (2000). Interactions of the PDZ-protein MAGI-1 with adenovirus E4-ORF1 and high-risk papillomavirus E6 oncoproteins. *Oncogene*, Nov 2; 19 (46): 5270-5280.

Gravitt, P.E. (2012). Evidence and impact of human papillomavirus latency. *Open Virol J*, 6: 198-203. doi: 10.2174/1874357901206010198. Epub 2012 Dec 28.

Gros, F., Sebti, Y., de Guibert, S., Branger, B., Bernard, M., Fauchet, R., & Amiot, L. (2006). Soluble HLA-G molecules increase during acute leukemia, especially in subtypes affecting monocytic and lymphoid lineages. *Neoplasia*, Mar; 8 (3): 223-230.

Gross, G., & Pfister, H. (2004). Role of human papillomavirus in penile cancer, penile intraepithelial squamous cell neoplasias and in genital warts. *Med Microbiol Immunol*, Feb; 193 (1): 35-44. Epub 2003 Jun 28.

Gaur, U., & Aggarwal, B.B. (2003). Regulation of proliferation, survival and apoptosis by members of the TNF superfamily. *Biochem Pharmacol*, Oct 15; 66 (8): 1403-1408.

Goh, A.M., Coffill, C.R., & Lane, D.P. (2011). The role of mutant p53 in human cancer. *J Pathol*, Jan; 223 (2): 116-126. doi: 10.1002/path.2784. Epub 2010 Oct 25. Review.

Gonzalez, S.L., Stremlau, M., He, X., Basile, J.R., & Münge,r K. (2001). Degradation of the retinoblastoma tumor suppressor by the human papillomavirus type 16 E7 oncoprotein is important for functional inactivation and is separable from proteasomal degradation of E7. *J Virol*, Aug; 75 (16): 7583-7591.

Haedicke, J., & Iftner, T. (2013). Human papillomaviruses and cancer. *Radiother Oncol*, Sep; 108 (3): 397-402. doi: 10.1016/j.radonc.2013.06.004. Epub 2013 Jul 3.

Hagensee, M.E., Koutsky, L.A., Lee, S.K., Grubert, T., Kuypers, J., Kiviat, N.B., & Galloway, D.A. (2000). Detection of cervical antibodies to human papillomavirus type 16 (HPV-16) capsid antigens in relation to detection of HPV-16 DNA and cervical lesions. *J Infect Dis*, Apr; 181 (4): 1234-1239. Epub 2000 Apr 7.

Harley, C.B., Futcher, A.B., & Greide,r C.W. (1990). Telomeres shorten during ageing of human fibroblasts. *Nature*, May 31; 345 (6274): 458-460.

Havard, L., Delvenne, P., Fraré, P., Boniver, J., & Giannini, S.L. (2002). Differential production of cytokines and activation of NF-kappaB in HPV-transformed keratinocytes. *Virology*, Jul 5; 298 (2): 271-285.

Havard, L., Rahmouni, S., Boniver, J., & Delvenne, P. (2005). High levels of p105 (NFKB1) and p100 (NFKB2) proteins in HPV16-transformed keratinocytes: role of E6 and E7 oncoproteins. *Virology*, Jan 20; 331 (2): 357-366.

Hasan, U. A., Bates, E., Takeshita, F., Biliato, A., Accardi, R., Bouvard, V., Mansour, M., Vincent, I., Gissmann, L., Iftner, T., Sideri, M., Stubenrauch, F., & Tommasino, M. (2007). TLR9 expression and function is abolished by the cervical cancer-associated human papillomavirus type 16. *J Immunol*, Mar 1; 178 (5): 3186-3197.

Hasan, U. (2014). Human papillomavirus (HPV) deregulation of Toll-like receptor 9. *Oncoimmunology*, Jan 1; 3 (1): e27257.

Hehlgans, T., & Pfeffer, K. (2005). The intriguing biology of the tumour necrosis factor/tumour necrosis factor receptor superfamily: players, rules and the games. *Immunology*, May; 115 (1): 1-20. Review.

Herrick, J., Conti, C., Teissier, S., Thierry, F., Couturier, J., Sastre-Garau, X., Favre, M., Orth, G., & Bensimon, A. (2005). Genomic organization of amplified MYC genes suggests distinct mechanisms of amplification in tumorigenesis. *Cancer Res*, Feb 15; 65 (4): 1174-1179.

Horvath, C. A., Boulet, G.A., Renoux, V.M., Delvenne, P.O., & Bogers, J.P. (2010). Mechanisms of cell entry by human papillomaviruses: an overview. *Virol J*, Jan 20; 7: 11. doi: 10.1186/1743-422X-7-11. Review.

Huh, K.W., DeMasi, J., Ogawa, H., Nakatani, Y., Howley, P.M., & Münger, K. (2005). Association of the human papillomavirus type 16 E7 oncoprotein with the 600-kDa retinoblastoma protein-associated factor, p600. *Proc Natl Acad Sci U S A*, Aug 9; 102 (32): 11492-11497. Epub 2005 Aug 1.

Huibregtse, J.M., Scheffner, M., & Howley, P.M. (1993). Localization of the E6-AP regions that direct human papillomavirus E6 binding, association with p53, and ubiquitination of associated proteins. *Mol Cell Biol*, Aug; 13 (8): 4918-4927.

Humbey, O., Cairey-Remonnay, S., Guérrini, J.S., Algros, M.P., Mougin, C., Bittard, H., & Aubin, F. (2003). Detection of the human papillomavirus and analysis of the TP53 polymorphism of exon 4 at codon 72 in penile squamous cell carcinomas. *Eur J Cancer*, Mar; 39 (5): 684-690.

Jabbar, S., Strati, K., Shin, M.K., Pitot, H.C., & Lambert, P.F. (2010). Human papillomavirus type 16 E6 and E7 oncoproteins act synergistically to cause head and neck cancer in mice. *Virology*, Nov 10; 407 (1): 60-67. doi: 10.1016/j.virol.2010.08.003. Epub 2010 Aug 24.

James, M. A., Lee, J.H., & Klingelhutz, A.J. (2006). Human papillomavirus type 16 E6 activates NF-kappaB, induces cIAP-2 expression, and protects against apoptosis in a PDZ binding motif-dependent manner. *J Virol*, Jun; 80 (11): 5301-5307.

Jeleń, F., Oleksy, A., Smietana, K., & Otlewski, J. (2003). PDZ domains - common players in the cell signaling. *Acta Biochim Pol*, 50 (4): 985-1017. Review.

Johnson, K. M., Kines, R.C., Roberts, J.N., Lowy, D.R., Schiller, J.T., & Day, P.M. (2009). Role of heparan sulfate in attachment to and infection of the murine female genital tract by human papillomavirus. *J Virol*, Mar; 83 (5): 2067-2074. doi: 10.1128/JVI.02190-08. Epub 2008 Dec 10.

Jones, D. L., Thompson, D.A., & Münger, K. (1997). Destabilization of the RB tumor suppressor protein and stabilization of p53 contribute to HPV type 16 E7-induced apoptosis. *Virology*, Dec 8; 239 (1): 97-107.

Jonjić, S., Babić, M., Polić, B., & Krmpotić, A. (2008). Immune evasion of natural killer cells by viruses. *Curr Opin Immunol*, Feb; 20 (1): 30-38. doi: 10.1016/j.coi.2007.11.002. Review.

Joyce, J. G., Tung, J.S., Przysiecki, C.T., Cook, J.C., Lehman, E.D., Sands, J.A., Jansen, K.U., & Keller, P.M. (1999). The L1 major capsid protein of human papillomavirus type 11 recombinant virus-like particles interacts with heparin and cell-surface glycosaminoglycans on human keratinocytes. *J Biol Chem*, Feb 26; 274 (9): 5810-5822.

Kadish, A. S., Ho, G.Y., Burk, R.D., Wang, Y., Romney, S.L., Ledwidge, R., & Angeletti, R.H. (1997). Lymphoproliferative responses to human papillomavirus (HPV) type 16 proteins E6 and E7: outcome of HPV infection and associated neoplasia. *J Natl Cancer Inst*, Sep 3; 89 (17): 1285-1293.

Kanaya, T., Kyo, S., & Laimins, L.A. (1997). The 5' region of the human papillomavirus type 31 upstream regulatory region acts as an enhancer which augments viral early expression through the action of YY1. *Virology*, Oct 13; 237 (1): 159-169.

Kanodia, S., Fahey, L.M., & Kast, W.M. (2007). Mechanisms used by human papillomaviruses to escape the host immune response. *Curr Cancer Drug Targets*, Feb; 7 (1): 79-89.

Karin, M. (2008). The IkappaB kinase - a bridge between inflammation and cancer. *Cell Res*, Mar; 18 (3): 334-342. doi: 10.1038/cr.2008.30. Review.

Karin, M. (2009). NF-kappaB as a critical link between inflammation and cancer. *Cold Spring Harb Perspect Biol*, Nov; 1 (5): a000141. doi: 10.1101/cshperspect.a000141. Review.

Katzenellenbogen, R.A., Egelkrout, E.M., Vliet-Gregg, P., Gewin, L.C., Gafken, P.R., & Galloway, D.A. (2007). NFX1-123 and poly(A) binding proteins synergistically augment activation of telomerase in human papillomavirus type 16 E6-expressing cells. *J Virol*, Apr; 81 (8): 3786-3796. Epub 2007 Jan 31.

Khan, M. J., Castle, P.E., Lorincz, A.T., Wacholder, S., Sherman, M., Scott, D.R., Rush, B.B., Glass, A.G., & Schiffman, M. (2005). The elevated 10-year risk of cervical precancer and cancer in women with human papillomavirus (HPV) type 16 or 18 and the possible utility of type-specific HPV testing in clinical practice. *J Natl Cancer Inst*, Jul 20; 97 (14): 1072-1079.

Khleif, S. N., DeGregori, J., Yee, C.L., Otterson, G.A., Kaye, F.J., Nevins, J.R., & Howley, P.M. (1996). Inhibition of cyclin D-CDK4/CDK6 activity is associated with an E2F-mediated induction of cyclin kinase inhibitor activity. *Proc Natl Acad Sci U S A*, Apr 30; 93 (9): 4350-4354.

Kim, H. J., Hawke, N., & Baldwin, A.S. (2006). NF-kappaB and IKK as therapeutic targets in cancer. *Cell Death Differ*, May; 13 (5): 738-747.

Kim, H., Kwon, B., & Sin, J.I. (2013). Combined stimulation of IL-2 and 4-1BB receptors augments the antitumor activity of E7 DNA vaccines by increasing Ag-specific CTL responses. *PLoS One*, Dec 31; 8 (12): e83765. doi: 10.1371/journal.pone.0083765. eCollection 2013.

Kim, K., & Lambert, PF. (2002). E1 protein of bovine papillomavirus 1 is not required for the maintenance of viral plasmid DNA replication. *Virology*, Feb 1; 293 (1): 10-14.

Kim, W.Y., Lee, J.W., Choi, J.J., Choi, C.H., Kim, T.J., Kim, B.G., Song, S.Y., & Bae, D.S. (2008). Increased expression of Toll-like receptor 5 during progression of cervical neoplasia. *Int J Gynecol Cancer*, Mar-Apr; 18 (2): 300-305. Epub 2007 Jun 22.

Kim, N. W., Piatyszek, M.A., Prowse, K.R., Harley, C.B., West, M.D., Ho, P.L., Coviello, G.M., Wright, W.E., Weinrich, S.L., & Shay, J.W. (1994). Specific association of human telomerase activity with immortal cells and cancer. *Science*, Dec 23; 266 (5193): 2011-2015.

Kines, R. C., Thompson, C.D., Lowy, D.R., Schiller, J.T., & Day, P.M. (2009). The initial steps leading to papillomavirus infection occur on the basement membrane prior to cell surface binding. *Proc Natl Acad Sci U S A*, Dec 1; 106 (48): 20458-20463. doi: 10.1073/pnas.0908502106. Epub 2009 Nov 17.

Kinoshita, T., Shirasawa, H., Shino, Y., Moriya, H., Desbarats, L., Eilers, M., & Simizu, B. (1997). Transactivation of prothymosin alpha and c-myc promoters by human papillomavirus type 16 E6 protein. *Virology*, May 26; 232 (1): 53-61.

Kiriakidis, S., Andreakos, E., Monaco, C., Foxwell, B., Feldmann, M., & Paleolog, E. (2003). VEGF expression in human macrophages is NF-kappaB-dependent: studies using adenoviruses expressing the endogenous NF-kappaB inhibitor IkappaBalpha and a kinase-defective form of the IkappaB kinase 2. *J Cell Sci*, Feb 15; 116 (Pt 4): 665-674.

Klaes, R., Woerner, S.M., Ridder, R., Wentzensen, N., Duerst, M., Schneider, A., Lotz, B., Melsheimer, P., & von Knebel Doeberitz, M. (1999). Detection of high-risk cervical intraepithelial neoplasia and cervical cancer by amplification of transcripts derived from integrated papillomavirus oncogenes. *Cancer Res*, Dec 15; 59 (24): 6132-6136.

Klaes, R., Friedrich, T., Spitkovsky, D., Ridder, R., Rudy, W., Petry, U., Dallenbach-Hellweg, G., Schmidt, D., & von Knebel Doeberitz, M. (2001). Overexpression of p16(INK4A) as a specific marker for dysplastic and neoplastic epithelial cells of the cervix uteri. *Int J Cancer*, Apr 15; 92 (2): 276-284.

Klingelhutz, A.J., Foster, S.A., & McDougall, J.K. (1996). Telomerase activation by the E6 gene product of human papillomavirus type 16. *Nature*, Mar 7; 380 (6569): 79-82.

Kloover, J.S., Grauls, G.E., Blok, M.J., Vink, C., & Bruggeman, C.A. (2002). A rat cytomegalovirus strain with a disruption of the r144 MHC class I-like gene is attenuated in the acute phase of infection in neonatal rats. *Arch Virol*, Apr; 147 (4): 813-824.

Koh, J., Enders, G.H., Dynlacht, B.D., & Harlow, E. (1995). Tumour-derived p16 alleles encoding proteins defective in cell-cycle inhibition. *Nature*, Jun 8; 375 (6531): 506-510.

Koutsky, L. The epidemiology behind the HPV vaccine discovery. (2009). *Ann Epidemiol*, Apr; 19 (4): 239-244. doi: 10.1016/j.annepidem.2009.01.023. Review.

Laimins, L.A. (1993). The biology of human papillomaviruses: from warts to cancer. *Infect Agents Dis*, Apr; 2 (2): 74-86. Review.

Lam, K.Y., & Chan, K.W. (1999). Molecular pathology and clinicopathologic features of penile tumors: with special reference to analyses of p21 and p53 expression and unusual histologic features. *Arch Pathol Lab Med*, Oct; 123(10): 895-904.

Lazarczyk, M., Cassonnet, P., Pons, C., Jacob, Y., & Favre, M. (2009). The EVER proteins as a natural barrier against papillomaviruses: a new insight into the pathogenesis of human papillomavirus infections. *Microbiol Mol Biol Rev*, Jun; 73 (2): 348-370. doi: 10.1128/MMBR.00033-08. Review.

Le Bon, A., & Tough, D.F. (2002). Links between innate and adaptive immunity via type I interferon. *Curr Opin Immunol*, Aug; 14 (4): 432-436. Review.

Lebre, M.C., van der Aar, A.M., van Baarsen, L., van Capel, T.M., Schuitemaker, J.H., Kapsenberg, M.L., & de Jong, E.C. (2007). Human keratinocytes express functional Toll-like receptor 3, 4, 5, and 9. *J Invest Dermatol*, 2007 Feb; 127 (2): 331-341. Epub 2006 Oct 26.

Lee, C., & Laimins, L.A. (2004). Role of the PDZ domain-binding motif of the oncoprotein E6 in the pathogenesis of human papillomavirus type 31. *J Virol*, Nov; 78 (22): 12366-12377.

Lee, D., Kim, H.Z., Jeong, K.W., Shim, Y.S., Horikawa, I., Barrett, J.C., & Choe, J. (2002). Human papillomavirus E2 down-regulates the human telomerase reverse transcriptase promoter. *J Biol Chem*, Aug 2; 277 (31): 27748-27756. Epub 2002 May 17.

Lee, J.W., Choi, J.J., Seo, E.S., Kim, M.J., Kim, W.Y., Choi, C.H., Kim, T.J., Kim, B.G., Song, S.Y., & Bae, D.S. (2007). Increased toll-like receptor 9 expression in cervical neoplasia. *Mol Carcinog*, Nov; 46 (11): 941-947.

Lefort, K., Mandinova, A., Ostano, P., Kolev, V., Calpini, V., Kolfschoten, I., Devgan, V., Lieb, J., Raffoul, W., Hohl, D., Neel, V., Garlick, J., Chiorino, G., & Dotto, G.P. (2007). Notch1 is a p53 target gene involved in human keratinocyte tumor suppression through negative regulation of ROCK1/2 and MRCKalpha kinases. *Genes Dev*, Mar 1; 21 (5): 562-577.

Le Negrate, G. (2012). Viral interference with innate immunity by preventing NF-κB activity. *Cell Microbiol*, Feb; 14 (2): 168-181. doi: 10.1111/j.1462-5822.2011.01720.x. Epub 2011 Nov 23. Review.

Leptak, C., Ramon y Cajal, S., Kulke, R., Horwitz, B.H., Riese, D.J. 2nd, Dotto, G.P., & DiMaio, D. (1991). Tumorigenic transformation of murine keratinocytes by the E5 genes of bovine papillomavirus type 1 and human papillomavirus type 16. *J Virol.*, Dec; 65 (12): 7078-7083. Erratum in: *J Virol*, 1992 Mar; 66 (3): 1833.

Levine, A.J., & Oren, M. (2009). The first 30 years of p53: growing ever more complex. *Nat Rev Cancer*, Oct; 9 (10): 749-758. doi: 10.1038/nrc2723.

Li, S., Labrecque, S., Gauzzi, M.C., Cuddihy, A.R., Wong, A.H., Pellegrini, S., Matlashewski, G.J., & Koromilas, A.E. (1999). The human papilloma virus (HPV)-18 E6 oncoprotein physically associates with Tyk2 and impairs Jak-STAT activation by interferon-alpha. *Oncogene*, Oct 14; 18 (42): 5727-5737.

Li, X.J., Zhang, X., Lin, A., Ruan, Y.Y., & Yan, W.H. (2012). Human leukocyte antigen-G (HLA-G) expression in cervical cancer lesions is associated with disease progression. *Hum Immunol*, Sep; 73 (9): 946-949. doi: 10.1016/j.humimm.2012.07.041. Epub 2012 Jul 20.

Liu, J., & Thorp, S.C. (2002). Cell surface heparan sulfate and its roles in assisting viral infections. *Med Res Rev*, Jan; 22 (1): 1-25. Review.

Locksley, R.M., Killeen, N., & Lenardo, M.J. (2001). The TNF and TNF receptor superfamilies: integrating mammalian biology. *Cell*, Feb 23; 104 (4): 487-501. Review. No abstract available.

Lopes, A., Bezerra, A..L, Pinto, C.A., Serrano, S.V., de MellO, C.A., & Villa, L.L. (2002). p53 as a new prognostic factor for lymph node metastasis in penile carcinoma: analysis of 82 patients treated with amputation and bilateral lymphadenectomy. *J Urol*, Jul; 168 (1): 81-86.

Loustau, M., Wiendl, H., Ferrone, S., & Carosella, E.D. (2012). HLA-G 2012 conference: the 15-year milestone update. *Tissue Antigens*, Mar; 81 (3): 127-136. doi: 10.1111/tan.12053. Epub 2013 Jan 24.

Macville, M., Schröck, E., Padilla-Nash, H., Keck, C., Ghadimi, B.M., Zimonjic, D., Popescu, N., & Ried, T. (1999). Comprehensive and definitive molecular cytogenetic characterization of HeLa cells by spectral karyotyping. *Cancer Res*, Jan 1; 59 (1): 141-150.

Maglennon, G.A., McIntosh, P., & Doorbar, J. (2011). Persistence of viral DNA in the epithelial basal layer suggests a model for papillomavirus latency following immune regression. *Virology*, Jun 5; 414 (2): 153-163. doi: 10.1016/j.virol.2011.03.019. Epub 2011 Apr 13.

Mantovani, A., Romero, P., Palucka, A.K., & Marincola, F.M. (2008). Tumour immunity: effector response to tumour and role of the microenvironment. *Lancet*, Mar 1; 371 (9614): 771-783. doi: 10.1016/S0140-6736(08)60241-X. Epub 2008 Feb 13.

Martin, D., & Gutkind, J.S. (2008). Human tumor-associated viruses and new insights into the molecular mechanisms of cancer. *Oncogene*, Dec; 27 Suppl 2: S31-42. doi: 10.1038/onc.2009.351. Review.

McBride, A.A. (2013). The papillomavirus E2 proteins. *Virology*, Oct; 445 (1-2): 57-79. doi: 10.1016/j.virol.2013.06.006. Epub 2013 Jul 10. Review.

McKinney, C.C., Hussmann, K.L., & McBride, A.A. (2015). The Role of the DNA Damage Response throughout the Papillomavirus Life Cycle. *Viruses*, May 21; 7 (5): 2450-2469. doi: 10.3390/v7052450.

McIntyre, M.C., Ruesch, M.N., & Laimins, L.A. (1996). Human papillomavirus E7 oncoproteins bind a single form of cyclin E in a complex with cdk2 and p107. *Virology*, Jan 1; 215 (1): 73-82.

McLaughlin-Drubin, M.E., Meyers, J., & Munger, K. (2012). Cancer associated human papillomaviruses. *Curr Opin Virol*, Aug; 2 (4): 459-466. doi: 10.1016/ j.coviro.2012.05.004. Epub 2012 Jun 2. Review.

McMurray, H.R., & McCance, D.J. (2003). Human papillomavirus type 16 E6 activates TERT gene transcription through induction of c-Myc and release of USF-mediated repression. J Virol, Sep; 77 (18): 9852-9861.

Medzhitov, R., & Janeway, C.A. Jr. (1997). Innate immunity: the virtues of a nonclonal system of recognition. *Cell*, Oct 31; 91 (3): 295-298. Review. No abstract available.

Medzhitov, R. (2007). Recognition of microorganisms and activation of the immune response. *Nature*, Oct 18; 449 (7164): 819-826. Review.

Mesri, E.A., Feitelson, M.A., & Munger, K. (2014). Human viral oncogenesis: a cancer hallmarks analysis. *Cell Host Microbe*, Mar 12; 15 (3): 266-282. doi: 10.1016/j.chom.2014.02.011. Review.

Milde-Langosch, K., Riethdorf, S., Kraus-Pöppinghaus, A., Riethdorf, L., & Löning, T. (2001). Expression of cyclin-dependent kinase inhibitors p16MTS1, p21WAF1, and p27KIP1 in HPV-positive and HPV-negative cervical adenocarcinomas. *Virchows Arch*, Jul; 439 (1): 55-61.

Miller, L.S. (2008). Toll-like receptors in skin. *Adv Dermatol*, 24: 71-87. Review.

Miralles-Guri, C., Bruni, L., Cubilla, A.L., Castellsagué, X., Bosch, F.X., & de Sanjosé, S. (2009). Human papillomavirus prevalence and type distribution in penile carcinoma. *J Clin Pathol*, Oct; 62 (10): 870-878. doi: 10.1136/jcp.2008.063149. Epub 2009 Aug 25.

Miller, L.S., & Modlin, R.L. Human keratinocyte Toll-like receptors promote distinct immune responses. *J Invest Dermatol*, 2007 Feb; 127 (2): 262-263. Review.

Mishra, A., Bharti, A.C., Varghese, P., Saluja, D., & Das, B.C. (2006). Differential expression and activation of NF-kappaB family proteins during oral carcinogenesis: Role of high risk human papillomavirus infection. *Int J Cancer*, Dec 15; 119 (12): 2840-2850.

Mizuuchi, M., Hirohashi, Y., Torigoe, T., Kuroda, T., Yasuda, K., Shimizu, Y., Saito, T., & Sato, N. (2012). Novel oligomannose liposome-DNA complex DNA vaccination efficiently evokes anti-HPV E6 and E7 CTL responses. *Exp Mol Pathol*, Feb; 92 (1): 185-190. doi: 10.1016/j.yexmp.2011.10.002. Epub 2011 Oct 15.

Moody, C.A., & Laimins, L.A. (2010). Human papillomavirus oncoproteins: pathways to transformation. *Nat Rev Cancer*, Aug; 10 (8): 550-560. doi: 10.1038/nrc2886. Epub 2010 Jul 1.

Morandi, F., Levreri, I., Bocca, P., Galleni, B., Raffaghello, L., Ferrone, S., Prigione, I., & Pistoia, V. (2007). Human neuroblastoma cells trigger an immunosuppressive program in monocytes by stimulating soluble HLA-G release. *Cancer Res*, Jul 1; 67 (13): 6433-6441.

Morris, P.J., Den,t C.L., Ring, C.J., & Latchman, D.S. (1993). The octamer binding site in the HPV16 regulatory region produces opposite effects on gene expression in cervical and non-cervical cells. *Nucleic Acids Res*, Feb 25; 21 (4): 1019-1023.

Müller, M., Gissmann, L., Cristiano, R.J., Sun, X.Y., Frazer, I.H., Jenson, A.B., Alonso, A., Zentgraf, H., & Zhou, J. (1995). Papillomavirus capsid binding and uptake by cells from different tissues and species. *J Virol*, Feb; 69 (2): 948-954.

Mulvany, N.J., Allen, D.G., & Wilson, S.M. (2008). Diagnostic utility of p16INK4a: a reappraisal of its use in cervical biopsies. *Pathology*, Jun; 40 (4): 335-344. doi: 10.1080/00313020802035907. Review.

Münger, K., Werness, B.A., Dyson, N., Phelps, W.C., Harlow, E., & Howley, P.M. (1989). Complex formation of human papillomavirus E7 proteins with the retinoblastoma tumor suppressor gene product. *EMBO J*, Dec 20; 8 (13): 4099-4105.

Münger, K., Basile, J.R., Duensing, S., Eichten, A., Gonzalez, S.L., Grace, M., & Zacny, V.L. (2001). Biological activities and molecular targets of the human papillomavirus E7 oncoprotein. *Oncogene*, Nov 26; 20 (54): 7888-7898. Review.

Münger, K., Baldwin, A., Edwards, K.M., Hayakawa, H., Nguyen, C.L., Owens, M., Grace, M., & Huh, K. (2004). Mechanisms of human papillomavirus-induced oncogenesis. *J Virol*, Nov; 78 (21): 11451-11460. Review. No abstract available.

Muñoz, N., Bosch, F.X., de Sanjosé, S., Herrero, R., Castellsagué, X., Shah, K.V., Snijders, P.J., & Meijer, C.J.; International Agency for Research on Cancer Multicenter Cervical Cancer Study Group. (2003). Epidemiologic classification of human papillomavirus types associated with cervical cancer. *N Engl J Med*, Feb 6; 348 (6): 518-527.

Muñoz, N., Castellsagué, X., de González, A.B., & Gissmann, L. (2006). Chapter 1: HPV in the etiology of human cancer. *Vaccine*, Aug 31; 24 Suppl 3: S3/1-10. Epub 2006 Jun 23. Review.

Nakagawa, M., Stites, D.P., Patel, S., Farhat, S., Scott, M., Hills, N.K., Palefsky, J.M., & Moscicki, A.B. (2000). Persistence of human papillomavirus type 16 infection is associated with lack of cytotoxic T lymphocyte response to the E6 antigens. *J Infect Dis*, Aug; 182 (2): 595-598. Epub 2000 Jul 28.

Nakao, Y., Yang, X., Yokoyama, M., Ferenczy, A., Tang, S.C., Pater, M.M., & Pater, A. (1997). Induction of p16 during immortalization by HPV 16 and 18 and not during malignant transformation. *Br J Cancer*, 75 (10): 1410-1416.

Nasu, K., & Narahara, H. (2010). Pattern recognition via the toll-like receptor system in the human female genital tract. *Mediators Inflamm*, 2010: 976024. doi: 10.1155/2010/976024. Epub 2010 Apr 11. Review.

Nees, M., Geoghegan, J.M., Hyman, T., Frank, S., Miller, L., & Woodworth, C.D. (2001). Papillomavirus type 16 oncogenes downregulate expression of interferon-responsive genes and upregulate proliferation-associated and NF-kappaB-responsive genes in cervical keratinocytes. *J Virol*, May; 75 (9): 4283-4296.

Nestle, F.O., Di Meglio, P., Qin, J.Z., & Nickoloff, B.J. (2009). Skin immune sentinels in health and disease. *Nat Rev Immunol*, Oct; 9 (10): 679-691. doi: 10.1038/nri2622. Epub 2009 Sep 18. Review.

Nguyen, D.X., Westbrook, T.F., & McCance, D.J. (2002). Human papillomavirus type 16 E7 maintains elevated levels of the cdc25A tyrosine phosphatase during deregulation of cell cycle arrest. *J Virol*, Jan; 76 (2): 619-632.

Nguyen, M.L., Nguyen, M.M., Lee, D., Griep, A.E., & Lambert, P.F. (2003). The PDZ ligand domain of the human papillomavirus type 16 E6 protein is required for E6's induction of epithelial hyperplasia *in vivo*. *J Virol*, Jun; 7 7 (12): 6957-6964.

Nimako, M., Fiander, A.N., Wilkinson, G.W., Borysiewicz, L.K., & Man, S. (1997). Human papillomavirus-specific cytotoxic T lymphocytes in patients with cervical intraepithelial neoplasia grade III. *Cancer Res*, Nov 1; 57 (21): 4855-4861.

O'Brien, P.M., & Campo, M.S. (2002). Evasion of host immunity directed by papillomavirus-encoded proteins. *Virus Res*, Sep; 88 (1-2): 103-117. Review.

O'Brien, P.M., & Campo, M.S. (2003). Papillomaviruses: a correlation between immune evasion and oncogenicity? *Trends Microbiol*, Jul; 11 (7): 300-305. No abstract available.

Oh, S.T., Kyo, S., & Laimins, L.A. (2001). Telomerase activation by human papillomavirus type 16 E6 protein: induction of human telomerase reverse transcriptase expression through Myc and GC-rich Sp1 binding sites. *J Virol*, Jun; 75 (12): 5559-5566.

Ohtsubo, M., Theodoras, A.M., Schumacher, J., Roberts, J.M., & Pagano, M. (1995). Human cyclin E, a nuclear protein essential for the G1-to-S phase transition. *Mol Cell Biol*, May ;15 (5): 2612-2624.

Ozbun, M.A., & Meyers, C. (1997). Characterization of late gene transcripts expressed during vegetative replication of human papillomavirus type 31b. *J Virol*, Jul; 71 (7): 5161-5172.

Paradkar, P.H.1., Joshi, J.V., Mertia, P.N., Agashe, S.V., & Vaidya, R.A. (2014). Role of cytokines in genesis, progression and prognosis of cervical cancer. *Asian Pac J Cancer Prev*, 15 (9): 3851-3864.

Park, J.S., Kim, E.J., Kwon, H.J., Hwang, E.S., Namkoong, S.E., & Um, S.J. (2000). Inactivation of interferon regulatory factor-1 tumor suppressor protein by HPV E7 oncoprotein. Implication for the E7-mediated immune evasion mechanism in cervical carcinogenesis. *J Biol Chem*, Mar 10; 275 (10): 6764-6769.

Park, R.B., & Androphy, E.J. (2002). Genetic analysis of high-risk e6 in episomal maintenance of human papillomavirus genomes in primary human keratinocytes. *J Virol*, Nov; 76 (22): 11359-11364.

Parkin, D.M., & Bray, F. (2006). Chapter 2: The burden of HPV-related cancers. *Vaccine*, Aug 31; 24 Suppl 3: S3/11-25. Review.

Patel, D., Incassati, A., Wang, N., & McCance, D.J. (2004). Human papillomavirus type 16 E6 and E7 cause polyploidy in human keratinocytes and up-regulation of G2-M-phase proteins. *Cancer Res*, Feb 15; 64 (4): 1299-1306.

Patterson, N.A., Smith, J.L., & Ozbun, M.A. (2005). Human papillomavirus type 31b infection of human keratinocytes does not require heparan sulfate. *J Virol*, Jun; 79 (11): 6838-6847.

Pei, X.H., & Xiong, Y. (2005). Biochemical and cellular mechanisms of mammalian CDK inhibitors: a few unresolved issues. *Oncogene*, Apr 18; 24 (17): 2787-2795. Review.

Pelkmans, L., & Helenius, A. (2003). Insider information: what viruses tell us about endocytosis. *Curr Opin Cell Biol*, Aug; 15 (4): 414-422. Review.

Perea, S.E., Massimi, P., & Banks, L. (2000). Human papillomavirus type 16 E7 impairs the activation of the interferon regulatory factor-1. *Int J Mol Med*, Jun; 5 (6): 661-666.

Peter, M., Rosty, C., Couturier, J., Radvanyi, F., Teshima, H., & Sastre-Garau, X. (2006). MYC activation associated with the integration of HPV DNA at the MYC locus in genital tumors. *Oncogene*, Sep 28; 25 (44): 5985-5993. Epub 2006 May 8.

Pett, M., & Coleman, N. (2007). Integration of high-risk human papillomavirus: a key event in cervical carcinogenesis? *J Pathol*, Aug; 212 (4): 356-367. Review.

Phelps, W.C., Yee, C.L., Münger, K., & Howley, P.M. (1988). The human papillomavirus type 16 E7 gene encodes transactivation and transformation functions similar to those of adenovirus E1A. *Cell*, May 20; 53 (4): 539-547.

Pichlmair, A., & Reis e Sousa, C. (2007). Innate recognition of viruses. *Immunity*, Sep; 27 (3): 370-383. Review.

Pikarsky, E., Porat, R.M., Stein, I., Abramovitch, R., Amit, S., Kasem, S., & Gutkovich-Pyest, E. (2004). NF-kappaB functions as a tumour promoter in inflammation-associated cancer. *Nature*, Sep 23; 431 (7007): 461-466. Epub 2004 Aug 25.

Pistoia, V., Morandi, F., Wang, X., & Ferrone, S. (2007). Soluble HLA-G: Are they clinically relevant? *Semin Cancer Biol*, Dec; 17 (6): 469-479. Epub 2007 Jul 31. Review.

Prowse, D.M., Ktori, E.N., Chandrasekaran, D., Prapa, A., & Baithun, S. (2008). Human papillomavirus-associated increase in p16INK4A expression in penile lichen sclerosus and squamous cell carcinoma. *Br J Dermatol*, Feb; 158 (2): 261-265. Epub 2007 Nov 28.

Pyeon, D., Pearce, S.M., Lank, S.M., Ahlquist, P., & Lambert, P.F. (2009). Establishment of human papillomavirus infection requires cell cycle progression. *PLoS Pathog*, Feb; 5 (2): e1000318. doi: 10.1371/journal.ppat.1000318. Epub 2009 Feb 27.

Pyzik, M., Kielczewska, A., & Vidal, S.M. (2008). NK cell receptors and their MHC class I ligands in host response to cytomegalovirus: insights from the mouse genome. *Semin Immunol*, Dec; 20 (6): 331-342. doi: 10.1016/j.smim.2008.09.003. Epub 2008 Oct 22.

Rebmann, V., LeMaoult, J., Rouas-Freiss, N., Carosella, E.D., & Grosse-Wilde, H. (2007). Quantification and identification of soluble HLA-G isoforms. *Tissue Antigens*, Apr; 69 Suppl 1: 143-149.

Renoux, V.M., Bisig, B., Langers, I., Dortu, E., Clémenceau, B., Thiry, M., Deroanne, C., Colige, A., Boniver, J., Delvenne, P., & Jacobs, N. (2011). Human papillomavirus entry into NK cells requires CD16 expression and triggers cytotoxic activity and cytokine secretion. *Eur J Immunol*, Nov; 41 (11): 3240-3252. doi: 10.1002/eji.201141693. Epub 2011 Sep 27.

Richards, R.M., Lowy, D.R., Schiller, J.T., & Day, P.M. (2006). Cleavage of the papillomavirus minor capsid protein, L2, at a furin consensus site is necessary for infection. *Proc Natl Acad Sci U S A*, Jan 31; 103 (5): 1522-1527. Epub 2006 Jan 23.

Rincon-Orozco, B., Halec, G., Rosenberger, S., Muschik, D., Nindl, I., Bachmann, A., Ritter, T.M., Dondog, B., Ly, R., Bosch, F.X., Zawatzky, R., & Rösl, F. (2009). Epigenetic silencing of interferon-kappa in human papillomavirus type 16-positive cells. *Cancer Res*, Nov 15; 69 (22): 8718-8725. doi: 10.1158/0008-5472.CAN-09-0550. Epub 2009 Nov 3.

Roberts, J.N., Buck, C.B., Thompson, C.D., Kines, R., Bernardo, M., Choyke, P.L., Lowy, D.R., & Schiller, J.T. (2007). Genital transmission of HPV in a mouse model is potentiated by nonoxynol-9 and inhibited by carrageenan. *Nat Med*, Jul; 13 (7): 857-861. Epub 2007 Jul 1.

Roden, R.B., Kirnbauer, R., Jenson, A.B., Lowy, D.R., & Schiller, J.T. (1994). Interaction of papillomaviruses with the cell surface. *J Virol*, Nov; 68 (11): 7260-7266.

Romagosa, C., Simonetti, S., López-Vicente, L., Mazo, A., Lleonart, M.E., Castellvi, J., & Ramon y Cajal, S. (2011). p16(Ink4a) overexpression in cancer: a tumor suppressor gene associated with senescence and high-grade tumors. *Oncogene*, May 5; 30 (18): 2087-2097. doi: 10.1038/onc.2010.614. Epub 2011 Feb 7. Review.

Ronco, L.V., Karpova, A.Y., Vidal, M., & Howley, P.M. (1998). Human papillomavirus 16 E6 oncoprotein binds to interferon regulatory factor-3 and inhibits its transcriptional activity. *Genes Dev*, Jul 1; 12 (13): 2061-2072.

Rouas-Freiss, N., Moreau, P., Ferrone, S., & Carosella, E.D. (2005). HLA-G proteins in cancer: do they provide tumor cells with an escape mechanism? *Cancer Res*, Nov 15; 65 (22): 10139-10144.

Ruesch, M.N., & Laimins, L.A. (1997). Initiation of DNA synthesis by human papillomavirus E7 oncoproteins is resistant to p21-mediated inhibition of cyclin E-cdk2 activity. *J Virol*, Jul; 71 (7): 5570-5578.

Ruesch, M.N., & Laimins, L.A. (1998). Human papillomavirus oncoproteins alter differentiation-dependent cell cycle exit on suspension in semisolid medium. *Virology*, Oct 10; 250 (1): 19-29.

Sano, T., Oyama, T., Kashiwabara, K., Fukuda, T., & Nakajima, T. (1998). Expression status of p16 protein is associated with human papillomavirus oncogenic potential in cervical and genital lesions. *Am J Pathol*, Dec; 153 (6): 1741-1748.

Santin, A.D., Hermonat, P.L., Ravaggi, A., Bellone, S., Pecorelli, S., Roman, J.J., Parham, G.P., & Cannon, M.J. (2000). Interleukin-10 increases Th1 cytokine production and cytotoxic potential in human papillomavirus-specific CD8(+) cytotoxic T lymphocytes. *J Virol*, May; 74 (10): 4729-4737.

Sapp, M., & Bienkowska-Haba, M. (2009a). Viral entry mechanisms: human papillomavirus and a long journey from extracellular matrix to the nucleus. *FEBS J*, Dec; 276 (24): 7206-7216. doi: 10.1111/j.1742-4658.2009.07400.x. Epub . Review.

Sapp, M., & Day, P.M. (2009b). Structure, attachment and entry of polyoma- and papillomaviruses. *Virology*, Feb 20; 384 (2): 400-409. doi: 10.1016/j.virol.2008.12.022. Epub 2009 Jan 21. Review.

Scheffner, M., Werness, B.A., Huibregtse, J.M., Levine, A.J., & Howley, P.M. (1990). The E6 oncoprotein encoded by human papillomavirus types 16 and 18 promotes the degradation of p53. *Cell*, Dec 21; 63 (6): 1129-1136.

Scheffner, M., Huibregtse, J.M., Vierstra, R.D., & Howley, P.M. (1993). The HPV-16 E6 and E6-AP complex functions as a ubiquitin-protein ligase in the ubiquitination of p53. *Cell*, Nov 5; 75 (3): 495-505.

Schelhaas, M., Shah, B., Holzer, M., Blattmann, P., Kühling, L., Day, P.M., Schiller, J.T., & Helenius, A. (2012). Entry of human papillomavirus type 16 by actin-dependent, clathrin-

and lipid raft-independent endocytosis. *PLoS Pathog*, 8 (4): e1002657. doi: 10.1371/journal.ppat.1002657. Epub 2012 Apr 19.

Schiffman, M., Castle, P.E., Jeronimo, J., Rodriguez, A.C., & Wacholder, S. (2007). Human papillomavirus and cervical cancer. *Lancet*, Sep 8; 370 (9590): 890-907. Review.

Schulze, A., Mannhardt, B., Zerfass-Thome, K., Zwerschke, W., & Jansen-Dürr, P. (1998). Anchorage-independent transcription of the cyclin A gene induced by the E7 oncoprotein of human papillomavirus type 16. *J Virol*, Mar; 72 (3): 2323-2334.

Sedman, J., & Stenlund, A. (1995). Co-operative interaction between the initiator E1 and the transcriptional activator E2 is required for replicator specific DNA replication of bovine papillomavirus *in vivo* and *in vitro*. *EMBO J*, Dec 15; 14 (24): 6218-6228.

Selinka, H.C., Giroglou, T., Nowak, T., Christensen, N.D., & Sapp, M. (2003). Further evidence that papillomavirus capsids exist in two distinct conformations. *J Virol*, Dec; 77 (24): 12961-12967.

Selinka, H.C., Florin, L., Patel, H.D., Freitag, K., Schmidtke, M., Makarov, V.A., & Sapp, M. (2007). Inhibition of transfer to secondary receptors by heparan sulfate-binding drug or antibody induces noninfectious uptake of human papillomavirus. *J Virol*, Oct; 81 (20): 10970-10980. Epub 2007 Aug 8.

Senba, M., Kumatori, A., Fujita, S., Jutavijittum, P., Yousukh, A., Moriuchi, T., Nakamura, T., & Toriyama, K. (2006). The prevalence of human papillomavirus genotypes in penile cancers from northern Thailand. *J Med Virol*, Oct; 78 (10): 1341-1346.

Senba, M., Buziba, N., Mori, N., Wada, A., Irie, S., & Toriyama, K. (2009a). Detection of human papillomavirus and cellular regulators p16INK4a, p53, and NF-kappaB in penile cancer cases in Kenya. *Acta Virol*, 53 (1): 43-48.

Senba, M., Mori, N., & Wada, A: Oncogenesis of human papillomavirus (HPV). (2009b). In: Tao HE (Ed.), DNA Tumor Viruses. 75-102, New York, Nova Science Publishers, Inc.

Senba, M., Mori, N., & Wada, A. (2009c). Oncogenesis and the link between inflammation and cancer due to human papillomavirus (HPV) infection, and the development of vaccine control strategies. *Cancer Res J*, 2 (4): 307-338. Review

Senba, M., Mori, N., Wada, A., Fujita, S., Yasunami, M., Irie, S., Hayashi, T., Igawa, T., Kanetake, H., Takahara, O., & Toriyama, K. (2010a). Human papillomavirus genotypes in penile cancers from Japanese patients and HPV-induced NF-κB activation. *Oncol Lett*, Mar; 1 (2): 267-272. Epub 2010 Mar 1.

Senba, M., Mori, N., Fujita, S., Jutavijittum, P., Yousukh, A., Toriyama, K., & Wada A. (2010b). Relationship among human papillomavirus infection, p16(INK4a), p53 and NF-κB activation in penile cancer from northern Thailand. *Oncol Lett*, Jul; 1 (4): 599-603. Epub 2010 Jul 1.

Senba, M., Buziba, N., Mori, N., Fujita, S., Morimoto, K., Wada, A., & Toriyama, K. (2011a). Human papillomavirus infection induces NF-κB activation in cervical cancer: A comparison with penile cancer. *Oncol Lett*, Jan; 2 (1): 65-68. Epub 2010 Nov 23.

Senba, M., Mori, N., & Wada, A. (2011b). Oncogenesis of and the Link Between Inflammation and Cancer Due to Human Papillomavirus (HPV) Infection, and the Forthcoming Eradication for Vaccination and the Development of Vaccine Control Strategies. In: Watanabe HS (Ed.), Horizons in Cancer Research Volume 44. 85-115, New York, Nova Science Publishers, Inc.

Senba, M., & Mori, N. (2012). Mechanisms of virus immune evasion lead to development from chronic inflammation to cancer formation associated with human papillomavirus infection. *Oncol Rev*, Oct 5; 6 (2): e17. doi: 10.4081/oncol.2012.e17. eCollection 2012 Oct 2. Review.

Serrano, M., Hannon, G.J., & Beach, D. (1993). A new regulatory motif in cell-cycle control causing specific inhibition of cyclin D/CDK4. *Nature*, Dec 16; 366 (6456): 704-707.

Serrano, M. (1997). The tumor suppressor protein p16INK4a. *Exp Cell Res.*, Nov 25; 237 (1): 7-13. Review.

Shastri, N., Nagarajan, N., Lind, K.C., & Kanaseki, T. (2014). Monitoring peptide processing for MHC class I molecules in the endoplasmic reticulum. *Curr Opin Immunol*, Feb; 26: 123-127. doi: 10.1016/j.coi.2013.11.006. Epub 2013 Dec 11. Review.

Sheu, B.C., Hsu, S.M., Ho, H.N., Lin, R.H., & Huang, S.C. (1999). Tumor immunology--when a cancer cell meets the immune cells. *J Formos Med Assoc*, Nov; 98 (11): 730-735. Review.

Smith, A.E., & Helenius, A. (2004). How viruses enter animal cells. *Science*, Apr 9; 30 4 (5668): 237-242. Review.

Sheu, B.C., Chang, W.C., Lin, H.H., Chow, S.N., & Huang, S.C. (2007). Immune concept of human papillomaviruses and related antigens in local cancer milieu of human cervical neoplasia. *J Obstet Gynaecol Res*, Apr; 33 (2): 103-113. Review.

Silva, I.D., Muniz, Y.C., Sousa, M.C., Silva, K.R., Castelli, E.C., Filho, J.C., Osta, A.P., Lima, M.I., & Simões, R.T. (2013). HLA-G 3'UTR polymorphisms in high grade and invasive cervico-vaginal cancer. *Hum Immunol*, Apr; 74 (4): 452-458. doi: 10.1016/j.humimm.2012.11.025. Epub 2012 Dec 8.

Simões, R.T., Gonçalves, M.A., Castelli, E.C., Júnior, C.M., Bettini, J.S., Discorde, M.L., Duarte, G., Quintana, S.M., Simões, A.L., Moreau, P., Carosella, E.D., Soares, E.G., & Donadi, E.A. (2009). HLA-G polymorphisms in women with squamous intraepithelial lesions harboring human papillomavirus. *Mod Pathol*, Aug; 22 (8): 1075-1082. doi: 10.1038/modpathol.2009.67. Epub 2009 May 1.

Smith, J.L., Campos, S.K., Wandinger-Ness, A., & Ozbun, M.A. (2008). Caveolin-1-dependent infectious entry of human papillomavirus type 31 in human keratinocytes proceeds to the endosomal pathway for pH-dependent uncoating. *J Virol*, Oct; 82 (19): 9505-9512. doi: 10.1128/JVI.01014-08. Epub 2008 Jul 30.

Song, D., Li, H., Li, H., & Dai, J. (2015). Effect of human papillomavirus infection on the immune system and its role in the course of cervical cancer. Cancer Lett, 10: 600-606.

Spillmann, D. (2001). Heparan sulfate: anchor for viral intruders? *Biochimie*, Aug; 83 (8): 811-817.

Spitkovsky, D., Hehner, S.P., Hofmann, T.G., Möller, A., & Schmitz, M.L. (2002). The human papillomavirus oncoprotein E7 attenuates NF-kappa B activation by targeting the Ikappa B kinase complex. *J Biol Chem*, Jul 12; 277 (28): 25576-25582. Epub 2002 May 1.

Spoden, G., Freitag, K., Husmann, M., Boller, K., Sap,p M., Lambert, C., & Florin, L. (2008). Clathrin- and caveolin-independent entry of human papillomavirus type 16--involvement of tetraspanin-enriched microdomains (TEMs). *PLoS One*, Oct 2; 3 (10): e3313. doi: 10.1371/journal.pone.0003313.

Stanley, M.A. (1994). Replication of human papillomaviruses in cell culture. *Antiviral Res*, May; 24 (1): 1-15. Review.

Stanley, M. (2006). Immune responses to human papillomavirus. *Vaccine.*, Mar 30; 24 Suppl 1: S16-22. Review.

Stanley, M. (2010). Pathology and epidemiology of HPV infection in females. *Gynecol Oncol*. May; 117 (2 Suppl): S5-10. doi: 10.1016/j.ygyno.2010.01.024. Review.

Stanley, M.A. (2012). Epithelial cell responses to infection with human papillomavirus. *Clin Microbiol Rev*, Apr; 25 (2): 215-222. doi: 10.1128/CMR.05028-11. Review.

Sterling, J.C., Skepper, J.N., & Stanley, M.A. (1993). Immunoelectron microscopical localization of human papillomavirus type 16 L1 and E4 proteins in cervical keratinocytes cultured *in vivo*. *J Invest Dermatol*, Feb; 100 (2): 154-158.

Steele, J.C., Mann, C.H., Rookes, S., Rollason, T., Murphy, D., Freeth, M.G., Gallimore, P.H., & Roberts, S. (2005). T-cell responses to human papillomavirus type 16 among women with different grades of cervical neoplasia. *Br J Cancer*, Jul 25; 93 (2): 248-259.

Storrs, C.H., & Silverstein, S.J. (2007). PATJ, a tight junction-associated PDZ protein, is a novel degradation target of high-risk human papillomavirus E6 and the alternatively spliced isoform 18 E6. *J Virol*, Apr; 81 (8): 4080-4090. Epub 2007 Feb 7.

Stubenrauch, F., Lim, H.B., & Laimins, L.A. (1998). Differential requirements for conserved E2 binding sites in the life cycle of oncogenic human papillomavirus type 31. *J Virol*, Feb; 72 (2): 1071-1077.

Talora, C., Sgroi, D.C., Crum, C.P., & Dotto, G.P. (2002). Specific down-modulation of Notch1 signaling in cervical cancer cells is required for sustained HPV-E6/E7 expression and late steps of malignant transformation. *Genes Dev*, Sep 1; 16 (17): 2252-2263.

Tan, S.H., Leong, L.E., Walker, P.A., & Bernard, H.U. (1994). The human papillomavirus type 16 E2 transcription factor binds with low cooperativity to two flanking sites and represses the E6 promoter through displacement of Sp1 and TFIID. *J Virol*, Oct; 68 (10): 6411-6420.

Tay, S.K. (2012). Cervical cancer in the human papillomavirus vaccination era. *Curr Opin Obstet Gynecol*, Feb; 24 (1): 3-7. doi: 10.1097/GCO.0b013e32834daed9. Review.

Terai, M., & Burk, R.D. (2002). Felis domesticus papillomavirus, isolated from a skin lesion, is related to canine oral papillomavirus and contains a 1.3 kb non-coding region between the E2 and L2 open reading frames. *J Gen Virol*, 2002 Sep; 83 (Pt 9): 2303-2307.

Theofilopoulos, A.N., Baccala, R., Beutler, B., & Kono, D.H. (2005). Type I interferons (alpha/beta) in immunity and autoimmunity. *Annu Rev Immunol*, 23: 307-336. Review.

Thomas, J.T., Hubert, W.G., Ruesch, M.N., & Laimins, L.A. (1999). Human papillomavirus type 31 oncoproteins E6 and E7 are required for the maintenance of episomes during the viral life cycle in normal human keratinocytes. *Proc Natl Acad Sci USA*, Jul 20; 96 (15): 8449-8454.

Thomas, M., Pim, D., & Banks, L. (1999). The role of the E6-p53 interaction in the molecular pathogenesis of HPV. *Oncogene*, Dec 13; 18 (53): 7690-7700. Review.

Tindle, R.W. (2002). Immune evasion in human papillomavirus-associated cervical cancer. *Nat Rev Cancer*, Jan; 2 (1): 59-65. Review.

Tommasino, M., Adamczewski, J.P., Carlotti, F., Barth, C.F., Manetti, R., Contorni, M., Cavalieri, F., Hunt, T., & Crawford, L. (1993). HPV16 E7 protein associates with the protein kinase p33CDK2 and cyclin A. *Oncogene*, Jan; 8 (1): 195-202.

Tummers, B., & Burg, S.H. (2015). High-risk human papillomavirus targets crossroads in immune signaling. *Viruses*, May 21; 7 (5): 2485-2506. doi: 10.3390/v7052485. Review.

Ustav, M., Ustav, E., Szymanski, P., & Stenlund, A. (1991). Identification of the origin of replication of bovine papillomavirus and characterization of the viral origin recognition factor E1. *EMBO J*, Dec; 10 (13): 4321-4329.

Vambutas, A., Bonagura, V.R., & Steinberg, B.M. (2000). Altered expression of TAP-1 and major histocompatibility complex class I in laryngeal papillomatosis: correlation of TAP-1 with disease. *Clin Diagn Lab Immunol*, Jan; 7 (1): 79-85.

Vambutas, A., DeVoti, J., Pinn, W., Steinberg, B.M., & Bonagura, V.R. (2001). Interaction of human papillomavirus type 11 E7 protein with TAP-1 results in the reduction of ATP-dependent peptide transport. *Clin Immunol*, Oct; 101 (1): 94-99.

van de Weijer ML, Luteijn RD, Wiertz EJ. (2015). Viral immune evasion: Lessons in MHC class I antigen presentation. *Semin Immunol*, Mar; 27 (2): 125-137. doi: 10.1016/j.smim.2015.03.010. Epub 2015 Apr 15.

Veldman, T., Liu, X., Yuan, H., & Schlegel, R. (2003). Human papillomavirus E6 and Myc proteins associate *in vivo* and bind to and cooperatively activate the telomerase reverse transcriptase promoter. *Proc Natl Acad Sci U S A*, Jul 8; 100 (14): 8211-8216. Epub 2003 Jun 23.

Volpers, C., Unckell, F., Schirmacher, P., Streeck, R.E., & Sapp, M. (1995). Binding and internalization of human papillomavirus type 33 virus-like particles by eukaryotic cells. *J Virol*, Jun; 69 (6): 3258-3264.

Wagner, M., Gutermann, A., Podlech, J., Reddehase, M.J., & Koszinowski, U.H. (2002). Major histocompatibility complex class I allele-specific cooperative and competitive interactions between immune evasion proteins of cytomegalovirus. *J Exp Med*, Sep 16; 196 (6): 805-816.

Walboomers, J.M., Jacobs, M.V., Manos, M.M., Bosch, F.X., Kummer, J.A., Shah, K.V., Snijders, P.J., Peto, J., Meijer, C.J., & Muñoz, N. (1999). Human papillomavirus is a necessary cause of invasive cervical cancer worldwide. *J Pathol*, Sep; 189 (1): 12-19.

Wallin, K.L., Wiklund, F., Angström, T., Bergman, F., Stendahl, U., Wadell, G., Hallmans, G., & Dillner, J. (1999). Type-specific persistence of human papillomavirus DNA before the development of invasive cervical cancer. *N Engl J Med.*, Nov 25; 341 (22): 1633-1638.

Wang, C.Y., Cusack, J.C. Jr, Liu, R., & Baldwin, A.S. Jr. (1999). Control of inducible chemoresistance: enhanced anti-tumor therapy through increased apoptosis by inhibition of NF-kappaB. *Nat Med*, Apr; 5 (4): 412-417.

Wang, J.W., & Roden, R.B. (2013). L2, the minor capsid protein of papillomavirus. *Virology.*, Oct; 445 (1-2): 175-86. doi: 10.1016/j.virol.2013.04.017. Epub 2013 May 17. Review.

Watson, R.A., Thomas, M., Banks, L., & Roberts, S. (2003). Activity of the human papillomavirus E6 PDZ-binding motif correlates with an enhanced morphological transformation of immortalized human keratinocytes. *J Cell Sci*, Dec 15; 116 (Pt 24): 4925-4934.

Wang, Y., Liu, X.H., Li, Y.H., & Li, O. (2013). The paradox of IL-10-mediated modulation in cervical cancer. *Biomed Rep*, May; 1 (3): 347-351. Epub 2013 Feb 26. Review.

Weber, J.D., Jeffers, J.R., Rehg, J.E., Randle, D.H., Lozano, G., Roussel, M.F., Sherr, C.J., & Zambetti, G.P. (2000). p53-independent functions of the p19(ARF) tumor suppressor. *Genes Dev*, Sep 15; 14 (18): 2358-2365.

Webster, K., Parish, J., Pandya, M., Stern, P.L., Clarke, A.R., & Gaston, K. (2000). The human papillomavirus (HPV) 16 E2 protein induces apoptosis in the absence of other HPV proteins and via a p53-dependent pathway. *J Biol Chem*, Jan 7; 275 (1): 87-94.

Wentzensen, N., Vinokurova, S., & von Knebel Doeberitz, M. (2004). Systematic review of genomic integration sites of human papillomavirus genomes in epithelial dysplasia and invasive cancer of the female lower genital tract. *Cancer Res*, Jun 1; 64 (11): 3878-3884. Review.

Werness, B.A., Levine, A.J., & Howley, P.M. (1990). Association of human papillomavirus types 16 and 18 E6 proteins with p53. *Science*, Apr 6; 248 (4951): 76-79.

White, E.A., Sowa, M.E., Tan, M.J., Jeudy, S., Hayes, S.D., Santha, S., Münger, K., Harper, J.W., & Howley, P.M. (2012). Systematic identification of interactions between host cell proteins and E7 oncoproteins from diverse human papillomaviruses. *Proc Natl Acad Sci U S A*, Jan 31; 109 (5): E260-267. doi: 10.1073/pnas.1116776109. Epub 2012 Jan 9.

White, M.K., Pagano, J.S., & Khalili, K. (2014). Viruses and human cancers: a long road of discovery of molecular paradigms. *Clin Microbiol Rev*, Jul; 27 (3): 463-481. doi: 10.1128/CMR.00124-13. Review.

Williams, K.J., & Fuki, I.V. (1997). Cell-surface heparan sulfate proteoglycans: dynamic molecules mediating ligand catabolism. *Curr Opin Lipidol*, Oct; 8(5): 253-262. Review. Erratum in: *Curr Opin Lipidol* 1998 Feb; 9 (1) : 80.

Woo, Y.L., van den Hende, M., Sterling, J.C., Coleman, N., Crawford, R.A., Kwappenberg, K.M., Stanley, M.A., & van der Burg, S.H. (2010). A prospective study on the natural course of low-grade squamous intraepithelial lesions and the presence of HPV16 E2-, E6- and E7-specific T-cell responses. *Int J Cancer*, Jan 1; 126 (1): 133-141. doi: 10.1002/ijc.24804.

Woodman, C.B., Collins, S.I., & Young, L.S. (2007). The natural history of cervical HPV infection: unresolved issues. *Nat Rev Cancer*, Jan; 7 (1): 11-22. Review.

Xu, M., Luo, W., Elzi, D.J., Grandori, C., & Galloway, D.A. (2008). NFX1 interacts with mSin3A/histone deacetylase to repress hTERT transcription in keratinocytes. *Mol Cell Biol*, Aug; 28 (15): 4819-4828. doi: 10.1128/MCB.01969-07. Epub 2008 May 27.

Yan, W.H. (2011). HLA-G expression in cancers: potential role in diagnosis, prognosis and therapy. *Endocr Metab Immune Disord Drug Targets*, Mar; 11 (1): 76-89. Review.

Yang, Y.C., Chang, T.Y., Chen, T.C., Lin, W.S., Chang, S.C., & Lee ,Y.J. (2014). Human leucocyte antigen-G polymorphisms are associated with cervical squamous cell carcinoma risk in Taiwanese women. *Eur J Cancer*, Jan; 50 (2): 469-474. doi: 10.1016/j.ejca.2013.10.018. Epub 2013 Nov 18.

Yokoyama, W.M. (2005). Natural killer cell immune responses. *Immunol Res*, 32 (1-3): 317-325. Review.

Yoon, B.S., Kim, Y.T., Kim, J.W., Kim, S.H., Kim, J.H., & Kim, S.W. (2007). Expression of human leukocyte antigen-G and its correlation with interleukin-10 expression in cervical carcinoma. *Int J Gynaecol Obstet*, Jul; 98 (1): 48-53. Epub 2007 May 9.

Yoshida, K., & Miki, Y. (2010). The cell death machinery governed by the p53 tumor suppressor in response to DNA damage. *Cancer Sci*, Apr; 101 (4): 831-835. doi: 10.1111/j.1349-7006.2010.01488.x. Epub 2010 Feb 3. Review.

Yugawa, T., Handa, K., Narisawa-Saito, M., Ohno, S., Fujita, M., & Kiyono T. (2007). Regulation of Notch1 gene expression by p53 in epithelial cells. *Mol Cell Biol*, May; 27 (10): 3732-3742. Epub 2007 Mar 12.

Yugawa, T., & Kiyono, T. (2009). Molecular mechanisms of cervical carcinogenesis by high-risk human papillomaviruses: novel functions of E6 and E7 oncoproteins. *Rev Med Virol*, Mar; 19 (2): 97-113. doi: 10.1002/rmv.605. Review.

Zagouras, P., Stifani, S., Blaumueller, C.M., Carcangiu, M.L., & Artavanis-Tsakonas, S. (1995). Alterations in Notch signaling in neoplastic lesions of the human cervix. *Proc Natl Acad Sci USA*, Jul 3; 92 (14): 6414-6418.

Zerfass-Thome, K., Zwerschke, W., Mannhardt, B., Tindle, R., Botz, J.W., & Jansen-Dürr, P. (1996). Inactivation of the cdk inhibitor p27KIP1 by the human papillomavirus type 16 E7 oncoprotein. *Oncogene*, Dec 5; 13 (11): 2323-2330.

Zhang, H.S., Postigo, A.A., & Dean, D.C. (1999). Active transcriptional repression by the Rb-E2F complex mediates G1 arrest triggered by p16INK4a, TGFbeta, and contact inhibition. *Cell*, Apr 2; 97 (1): 53-61.

Zhao, J., He, S., Minassian, A., Li, J., & Feng, P. (2015). Recent advances on viral manipulation of NF-κB signaling pathway. *Curr Opin Virol*, Sep 15; 15: 103-111. doi: 10.1016/j.coviro.2015.08.013. Review.

Zhao, P., Mao, X., & Talbot, I.C. (2006). Aberrant cytological localization of p16 and CDK4 in colorectal epithelia in the normal adenoma carcinoma sequence. *World J Gastroenterol*, Oct 21; 12 (39): 6391-6396.

Zheng, N., Wang, C.X., Zhang, X., Du, L.T.,, Zha, J., Kan, S.F., Zhu, C.B., Dong, Z.G., Wang, L.L., Wang, S., & Li, W. (2011). Up-regulation of HLA-G expression in cervical premalignant and malignant lesions. *Tissue Antigens*, Mar; 77 (3): 218-224. doi: 10.1111/j.1399-0039.2010.01607.x.

Zhou, Q., Zhu, K., & Cheng, H. (2013). Toll-like receptors in human papillomavirus infection. *Arch Immunol Ther Exp* (Warsz), Jun ; 61 (3): 203-215. doi: 10.1007/s00005-013-0220-7. Epub 2013 Feb 24. Review.

Ziegert, C., Wentzensen, N., Vinokurova, S., Kisseljov, F., Einenkel, J., Hoeckel, M., & von Knebel Doeberitz, M. (2003). A comprehensive analysis of HPV integration loci in anogenital lesions combining transcript and genome-based amplification techniques. *Oncogene*, Jun 19; 22 (25): 3977-3984.

Zielinski, G.D., Snijders, P.J., Rozendaal, L., Daalmeijer, N.F., Risse, E.K., Voorhorst, F.J., Jiwa, N.M., van der Linden, H.C., de Schipper, F.A., Runsink, A.P., & Meijer, C.J. (2003). The presence of high-risk HPV combined with specific p53 and p16INK4a expression patterns points to high-risk HPV as the main causative agent for adenocarcinoma in situ and adenocarcinoma of the cervix. *J Pathol*, Dec; 201 (4): 535-543.

zur Hausen, H., & de Villiers, E.M. (1994). Human papillomaviruses. *Annu Rev Microbiol*, 48: 427-447. Review.

zur Hausen, H. (1996). Papillomavirus infections--a major cause of human cancers. *Biochim Biophys Acta*, Oct 9; 1288 (2): F55-78. Review.

zur Hausen, H. (2000). Papillomaviruses causing cancer: evasion from host-cell control in early events in carcinogenesis. *J Natl Cancer Inst*, May 3; 92 (9): 690-698. Review.

zur Hausen, H. (2002). Papillomaviruses and cancer: from basic studies to clinical application. *Nat Rev Cancer*, May; 2 (5): 342-350. Review.

zur Hausen, H. (2009). Papillomaviruses in the causation of human cancers - a brief historical account. *Virology*, Feb 20; 384 (2): 260-265. doi: 10.1016/j.virol.2008.11.046. Epub 2009 Jan 8. Review.

In: Horizons in Cancer Research. Volume 61
Editor: Hiroto S. Watanabe
ISBN: 978-1-63484-503-8

Chapter 3

MONOCLONAL GAMMOPATHIES: FROM MGUS TO MULTIPLE MYELOMA

Ana Bela Sarmento-Ribeiro[1,2,3,4,*], Catarina Geraldes[1,2,3], Adriana Roque[3] and José Manuel Nascimento Costa[2,5,6]

[1]Oncobiology and Hematology Lab, University Clinic of Haematology and Applied Molecular Biology, Faculty of Medicine, University of Coimbra, Coimbra, Portugal
[2]Center of Investigation in Environment, Genetics and Oncobiology (CIMAGO), University of Coimbra, Coimbra, Portugal
[3]Clinical Hematology Service, Centro Hospitalar Universitário de Coimbra (CHUC), Coimbra, Portugal
[4]Center for Neuroscience and Cell Biology and Institute for Biomedical Imaging and Life Sciences (CNC.IBILI), University of Coimbra, Coimbra, Portugal
[5]University Clinic of Oncology, Faculty of Medicine, University of Coimbra, Coimbra, Portugal
[6]Clinical Oncology Service, Centro Hospitalar Universitário de Coimbra (CHUC), Coimbra, Portugal

ABSTRACT

Monoclonal Gammopathies are a group of hematopoietic system's disorders, which result from the expansion of a B-cell clone that secrets immunoglobulins, also known as plasma cells or lymphoplasmacytic cells. They occur together with serum and/or urinary monoclonal protein production (M-protein, Bence-Jones protein), therefore being called Monoclonal Gammopathies.

Monoclonal Gammopathies' differential diagnosis include various entities, like Multiple Myeloma (MM), Monoclonal Gammopathy of Undetermined Significance (MGUS) and Waldenström's Macroglobulinemia (WM) and also AL Amyloidosis,

* Corresponding author: Ana Bela Sarmento-Ribeiro, MD, PhD, Adress: Faculty of Medicine, University of Coimbra, Azinhaga de Sta Comba-Celas, 3000-548 Coimbra, Portugal, E-mail: absarmento@fmed.uc.pt Tm: 00351917835675.

Solitary Plasmacytoma, POEMS Syndrome and Heavy Chain Disease, but only MM and MGUS will be described in this chapter.

MM is a mature B cell neoplasm that represents 1% of all neoplasms and 10% of hematologic neoplasms. It is characterized by the abnormal proliferation of monoclonal plasma cells in bone marrow that secret monoclonal immunoglobulin that is detected in the serum and/or urine. There are other pathologies with these characteristics but MM distinguishes itself for having specific diagnosis criteria and typical lesion of the target organs like osteolytic lesions, renal insufficiency, anemia and hypercalcemia (CRAB symptoms). MM is most often diagnosed during an evaluation for unrelated problems, although it can present with bone pain or a pathologic fracture.

Current models assume that MM pathogenesis involve a multistep transformation process. Several cellular and molecular mechanisms are involved in the characteristic aberrant proliferation and apoptosis in MM. The first pathogenic event is Monoclonal Gammopathy of Undetermined Significance (MGUS), a premalignant lesion that frequently evolves to MM through diverse molecular mechanisms. The earliest changes, that thought to occur in germinal center B cells, include complex genetic and/or epigenetic events, such as primary translocations involving the Immunoglobulin heavy chain (IgH) gene and multiple trissomies. Chromosome translocations lead, directly or indirectly, to cyclin-D dysregulation, which contributes to higher cells susceptibility to proliferative stimuli, leading to a selective expansion. Activating mutations of *N-* or *K-RAS* appear to mark the progression from MGUS to MM, among others.

Besides, somatic mutations, epigenetic regulation and bone marrow´s microenvironment are also important in the initiation and disease progression. However, many of the biologic processes in MM remain to be defined. Complex interactions between the MM cells and the microenvironment clearly play important roles in the pathogenesis of the disease including the induction of angiogenesis, the suppression of cell-mediated immunity, and the development of paracrine signaling loops involving cytokines such as interleukin-6 and vascular endothelial growth factor (VEGF) and other multiple signaling pathways mediated by NF-kB (nuclear factor-k B-cell) and IGF1 (insulin growth factor 1). All these mechanisms are crucial to tumor cell proliferation, growth, angiogenesis, invasion, metastasis, bone destruction and protection from spontaneous and drug-induces apoptosis.

Although MM progression is observed mainly within the BM during the early stages of the disease, these mechanisms promote extramedullary spreading during the terminal stage of the disease and malignant cells can be detected in peripheral blood of many patients. Furthermore, the resultant interactions of myeloma cells, bone marrow stromal cells and microvessels contribute to persistence of the tumor and its resistance to drugs.

Recently the existence of a clonal cellular subpopulation in MM relatively resistant to therapy was described. This clonal cellular subpopulation has the capacity of self-renewal that is identical to the stem cells. The identification and characterization of these MM stem cells can lead to important information about the molecular pathogenesis and the progression from MGUS to MM. On the other hand, it is thought that MM stem cells can be responsible of therapeutic failure as they share highly conserved phylogenetic pathways with stem cells, pathways that favor cell survival.

The knowledge of MM biology has led to the development of new drugs directed to the molecular profile that had improved patient´s survival.

1. INTRODUCTION

Monoclonal gammopathies (MG) constitute a group of disorders, derived from the expansion of a malignant B-cell clone (plasma cells or lymphoplasmacytic cells) that secrets immunoglobulins, with the consequent presence of the monoclonal protein in serum and/or in urine [1].

MG includes different entities such as monoclonal gammopathy of undetermined significance (MGUS), smouldering multiple myeloma (SMM) and multiple myeloma (MM) (the three of them integrating different points of the same spectrum) and some other diseases with different characteristics such as Waldenström's Macroglobulinemia, AL Amyloidosis, Solitary Plasmacytoma, POEMS Syndrome and Heavy Chain Disease [1].

International Myeloma Working Group (IMWG) has established actualized diagnostic criteria and classification for monoclonal gammopathies [2]:

The diagnosis of ***Non-IgM MGUS*** requires all the following criteria: serum monoclonal protein (non-IgM type) lower than 30 g/L; clonal bone marrow plasma cells lower than 10% and the absence of amyloidosis and CRAB features (hypercalcemia, renal failure, anemia, and bone lesions) that can be attributed to the underlying plasma proliferative cell disorder [2]. The diagnosis of ***IgM MGUS*** requires also a serum IgM monoclonal protein inferior to 30 g/L and bone marrow lymphoplasmacytic infiltration inferior to 10% and also the absence of evidence of anemia, constitutional symptoms, hyperviscosity, lymphadenopathy, hepatosplenomegaly, or other end-organ damage that can be attributed to the underlying lymphoproliferative disorder [2]. ***Light chain MGUS*** diagnostic criteria are the abnormal free light-chains (FLC) ratio (<0.26 or >1.65), increased level of the appropriate involved light chain (increased κ FLC in patients with a ratio superior to 1.65 and increased λ FLC in patients with a ratio inferior to 0.26); no immunoglobulin heavy chain expression on immunofixation; absence of CRAB symptoms or amyloidosis that can be attributed to the plasma cell proliferative disorder, clonal bone marrow plasma cells lower than 10% and urinary monoclonal protein inferior to 500 mg/24 h [2].

Revised criteria for ***smouldering multiple myeloma*** (SMM) are serum monoclonal protein (IgG or IgA) superior or equal to 30 g/L or urinary monoclonal protein superior or equal to 500 mg per 24 h and/or 10 to 60% of clonal bone marrow plasma cells and absence of myeloma defining events or amyloidosis. As with MGUS, the diagnosis needs the absence of CRAB features attributable to the clonal plasma cell proliferative disorder, but the thresholds for monoclonal protein level and bone marrow plasma cell percentage are different [2, 3].

Criteria for ***multiple myeloma*** has been also revised recently [2] and includes: clonal bone marrow plasma cells superior or equal to 10% or biopsy-proven bony or extramedullary plasmacytoma and any one or more of the myeloma defining events [evidence of end organ damage that can be attributed to the underlying plasma cell proliferative disorder, specifically hypercalcemia (serum calcium >1 mg/dL higher than the upper limit of normal or >11 mg/dL); renal insufficiency (creatinine clearance <40 mL per min or serum creatinine >2 mg/dL); anemia (hemoglobin >20 g/L below the lower limit of normal or a <100 g/L); bone lesions (presence of osteolytic bone lesions or the presence of osteoporosis with compression fractures attributable to the underlying clonal plasma cell disorder.)] or any one or more of the biomarkers of malignancy (clonal bone marrow plasma cell percentage superior or equal to 60%; involved: uninvolved serum FLC ratio ≥100; more than one focal lesions on MRI studies) [2].

Solitary plasmocytoma is defined as a biopsy-proven solitary lesion of bone or soft tissue with evidence of clonal plasma cells; normal bone marrow with no evidence of clonal plasma cells; normal skeletal survey and magnetic resonance or computerized tomography of spine and pelvis (except for the primary solitary lesion); absence of CRAB criteria that can be attributed to a lymphoplasma cell proliferative disorder [2].

POEMS syndrome is a paraneoplastic syndrome due to an underlying plasma cell neoplasm (monoclonal gammopathy), besides the presence of polyneuropathy, organomegaly, endocrinopathy and skin changes. The diagnosis is made with three of the major criteria (polyradiculoneuropathy, clonal plasma cell disorder, sclerotic bone lesions, elevated vascular endothelial growth factor, and the presence of Castleman disease), two of which must include polyradiculoneuropathy and clonal plasma cell disorder, and at least one of the minor criteria (organomegaly, endocrinopathy, characteristic skin changes, papilledema, extravascular volume overload, and thrombocytosis) [2, 4].

Systemic amyloidosis criteria are the presence of an amyloid-related systemic syndrome (renal, liver, heart, gastrointestinal tract, or peripheral nerve involvement), positive amyloid staining by Congo red in any tissue (fat aspirate, bone marrow, or organ biopsy), evidence that amyloid is light-chain-related established by direct examination (mass spectrometry-based proteomic analysis, or immune-electron-microscopy) of the amyloid substance, and evidence of a monoclonal plasma cell proliferative disorder (serum or urine monoclonal protein, abnormal free light-chain ratio, or clonal plasma cells in the bone marrow) [2].

In individuals older than 50 years, the incidence of MG is 3.2%. This value increases with age, being more frequent in males and blacks. In addition to be associated with these diseases, the production of M component may also occur in benign diseases such as autoimmune diseases (rheumatoid arthritis, scleroderma, Hashimoto's thyroiditis), skin (*pyoderma gangrenosum*) and liver (hepatitis, cirrhosis), and infectious (bacterial endocarditis, *Mycobacterium tuberculosis* infection) [1].

In this chapter we will only described MM and MGUS. MM represents 1% of all neoplasms and 10% of hematologic neoplasms. MGUS is a common condition affecting about 3% of individuals over the age of 70 years and having an incidence that increases with age [5, 6].

2. Physiopathology and Evolution

Current models assume that MM pathogenesis involve a multistep transformation process. Several cellular and molecular mechanisms are involved in the characteristic aberrant proliferation and apoptosis in MM [7-10]. The first pathogenic event is Monoclonal Gammopathy of Undetermined Significance (MGUS), a premalignant lesion that frequently evolves to MM through diverse molecular mechanisms [11, 12]. The earliest changes, that thought to occur in germinal center B cells, include complex genetic and/or epigenetic events, such as primary translocations involving the Immunoglobulin heavy chain (IgH) gene and multiple trissomies. Chromosome translocations lead, directly or indirectly, to cyclin-D dysregulation, which contributes to higher cells susceptibility to proliferative stimuli, leading to a selective expansion. Activating mutations of *N*- or *K-RAS* appear to mark the progression from MGUS to MM, among others [7, 13]. Besides that, somatic mutations, epigenetic regulation and bone marrow's microenvironment are also important in the initiation and disease progression [7].

Although MM progression is observed mainly within the BM during the early stages of the disease, these mechanisms promote extramedullary spreading during the terminal stage of the disease and malignant cells can be detected in peripheral blood of many patients. Furthermore, the resultant interactions of myeloma cells, bone marrow stromal cells and microvessels contribute to persistence of the tumor and its resistance to drugs [7, 8, 10, 14, 15].

Recently the existence of a clonal cellular subpopulation in MM relatively resistant to therapy was described. This clonal cellular subpopulation has the capacity of self-renewal that is identical to the stem cells. The identification and characterization of these MM stem cells can lead to important information about the molecular pathogenesis and the progression from MGUS to MM. On the other hand, it is thought that MM stem cells can be responsible of therapeutic failure as they share highly conserved phylogenetic pathways with stem cells, pathways that favor cell survival [13, 16].

Although it is known that MGUS precedes almost universally the development of MM, with a lifelong rate of malignant transformation of 1% per year, the molecular basis of this transformation remains unclear. It have been hypothesized that neoplastic bone marrow microenvironment has a determinant role on this evolution [5, 6, 11, 13, 17]. Meanwhile, several laboratory and clinical predictive factors of neoplastic evolution of MGUS to MM have been identified [18].

Some of main characteristics are the concentration of the monoclonal protein and its evolution (an increase in the serum monoclonal protein level by at least 10% on two successive evaluations within a 6-month period has been associated with a 65% probability of progression into SMM) [2, 19], the isotype of immunoglobulin (higher if non-IgG), serum free light-chain (FLC) ratio (the presence of an abnormal FLC ratio, and the extent to which the FLC ratio is abnormal) [20], presence of immunoparesis, bone marrow plasmacytosis (infiltration of bone marrow by malignant plasma cells exceeding 5%), presence of cytogenetic abnormalities and/or DNA aneuploidy (especially translocation t(4;14), 1q gain, and deletion 17p) [2, 21, 22] and the proportion of phenotypically clonal plasma cells [in MGUS, a substantial proportion of polyclonal plasma cells persist, whereas in MM almost all plasma cells (>95%) are clonal] and suppression of polyclonal normal bone marrow plasma cells) [7, 23-26].

Progression rate of non-IgM MGUS to MM is about 1% per year, mainly to multiple myeloma, solitary plasmacytoma or AL amyloidosis [2]. In the event of progression, IgM immunoglobulin MGUS (IgM MGUS) usually evolves to Waldenström macroglobulinemia or AL amyloidosis, but in rare instances IgM MGUS can progress to multiple myeloma (IgM myeloma), with a progression rate of 1.5% [2, 27]. The progression rate of light-chain MGUS is about 0.3% per year (lower when compared to full immunoglobulin-producing MGUS), mainly to light chain MM, or AL amyloidosis [2, 20]. By the other side, about 80% of multiple myeloma originates from non-IgM immunoglobulin MGUS (non-IgM MGUS), and 20% from light-chain immunoglobulin MGUS [2].

Although MM being dependent of bone marrow and restrained to it mainly during the early stages of the disease, sometimes it can spread to extramedullary locations, such as spleen, liver, and extracellular spaces and could finally be detected in peripheral blood of many patients [10]. Extramedullary MM is a more aggressive tumor that sometimes is associated with primary or secondary plasma cells leukemia [10].

2.1. Intraclonal Heterogeneity in Multiple Myeloma

Molecular studies have contributed not only to characterize genes and cellular pathways altered in MM, but also for demonstrating that the intraclonal heterogeneity is a common feature of this pathology [28-31]. This heterogeneity adds complexity to the progression of MM, since the genetic changes are not acquired in a linear fashion, but random, following different routes with branches, like the "Darwin Evolution Theory of Species." This model of development of MM through different and complex paths with multiple "branches" translates a simplified representation form of numerous cellular and molecular pathways that may be involved in the progression of MM and development of resistance to therapy [28-31] (Figure 1). It is important to understand that MM different clones co-exist as part of a dynamic equilibrium and compete for limited resources. The analogy with the Darwinian theory explains the selection of subclones of plasma cells that have competitive advantage in survival conferred by genetic and/or epigenetic changes that random have being acquired [28-31]. The concept of intraclonal heterogeneity is fundamental to understanding MM evolution, since the genes and pathways deregulated in predominantly clonal population are probably not common in the other subclones present. These could justify the resistance to therapy and relapse often seen in patients with MM, as a result of progression of the minority clones [28-32].

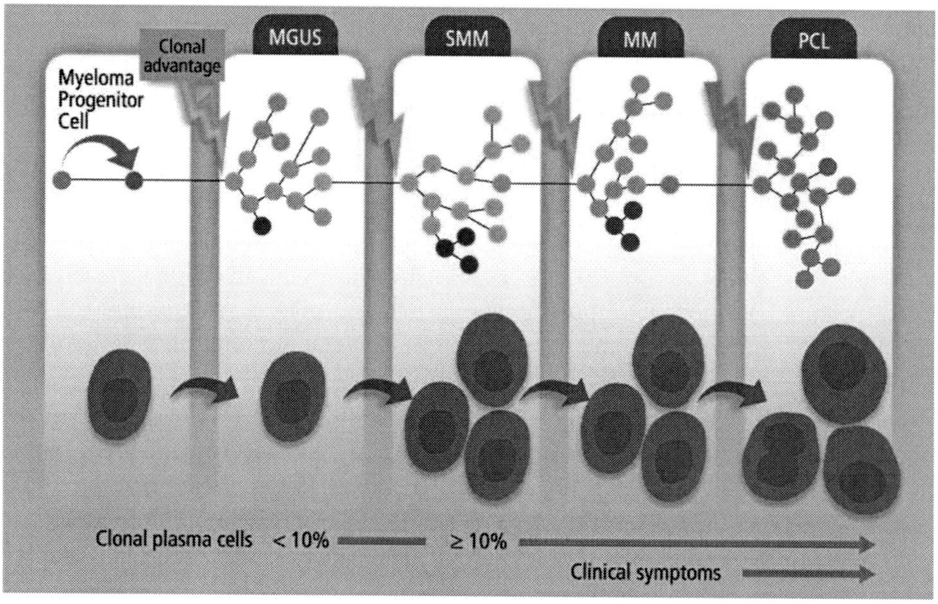

Figure 1. Clonal evolution in Multiple Myeloma – MGUS develops from a MM progenitor cell and can evolve to SMM, MM and plasma cell leukemia, a transformation marked by heterogeneity between clones. *(In Geraldes C., 2015, adapted from Morgan et al., 2012)* [29].

2.2. Genetics and Epigenetics from MGUS to MM

The genetic changes that occur in the evolution of MGUS for leukemia plasma can be classified as primary events, which contribute to immortalization of plasma cells, or secondary, responsible for disease progression. This classification facilitates the division of MM into two groups reflecting two different oncogenetic ways of evolution: a primary phase characterized by chromosomal gains (hyperdiploid) and another by structural changes (non-hyperdiploid) involving in most cases, translocation of genes encoding immunoglobulin heavy chain (IgH) in locus 14q32 translocated with other genes localized in other chromosomes (in particular, 4, 6, 11, 16 and 20). These translocations occur due to an aberrant recombination in lymph nodes germinal centers and lead to a subsequent oncogenes deregulation (Figure 2) [9, 10, 33-35].

Heterogeneity between clones is a frequent characteristic in MM as referred. This finding has several consequences in diagnosis and treatment, not only because genetic alterations are acquired in an aleatory way, but also because altered genes in the dominant clone are not common to the others, which can contribute to resistance to therapeutics [28, 29, 31].

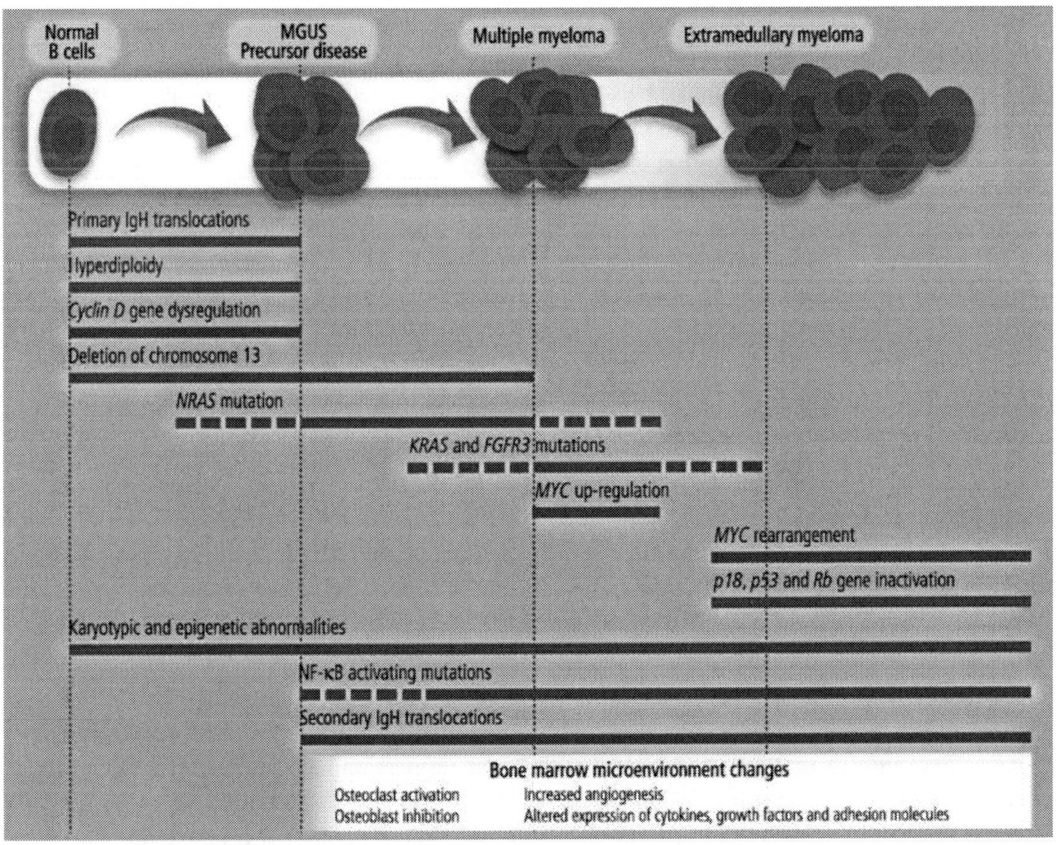

Figure 2. Genetic and epigenetics alterations in MM development - The transition of germinal center B cells to a premalignant clone (MGUS) includes primary translocations such as immunoglobulin heavy chain gene (IgH), hyperdiploidy and chromosome 13 deletions, that lead to cyclin D gene deregulation. Secondary translocations that include *MYC* (8q24), *MAFB* (20q12) and *IRF4* (6p25) are common in MM and rare in MGUS. *RAS* and *FGFR3* genes mutations, *MYC* deregulation and *p18*, *p53* and *pRb* inactivation are exclusive of MM. (*In Geraldes C., 2015, adapted from Kuehl & Bergsagel, 2002 and Palumbo & Anderson, 2011*) [36, 37].

Clonal heterogeneity and genomic instability worsen during the transformation of MGUS in SMM and consequently MM, which had been proved by array comparative genomic hybridization, whole-exome sequencing, and whole-genome sequencing [13, 18, 21, 28, 29, 38-40]. This instability and clonal evolution can be potentiated by several therapies such as alkylating agents and lenalidomide [13, 41].

Genetic alterations in MM spectrum can be classified as primary, when participate in plasma cells immortalization or secondary, when are responsible for disease progression [10]. Primary genetic events culminate in cell cycle deregulation in G1/S transition by cyclin D gene hyper-expression, and are followed by karyotype instability that promotes secondary mutations [34].

The first pathogenic event, which include the transition of germinal center B cells to a premalignant clone (MGUS), appears to occur in the germinal center during the processes of isotype class switching and somatic hypermutation, which are mutation prone [13]. It includes genetic and epigenetic events and involves primary translocations between IgH gene, hyperdiploidity and deletions of chromosome 13 that lead, directly or indirectly, to cyclin D gene deregulation, as mentioned [10, 41]. Current models, based on the immunoglobulin heavy chain (*IgH*) variable region sequencing in MM cells, suggest that MM pathogenesis involve a multistep transformation process, and that dysregulated expression of cyclin D might be an universal event in MM transformation and other neoplasms [42].

Patients with premalignant plasma cell dyscrasia like MGUS and SMM also carry these initial mutations, namely IgH translocations, 13q14 and 17p13 deletions, and additional copies of 1q21, which suggests that they are necessary, although not sufficient, in MM pathogenesis [43, 44]. Although translocations involving 14q32 are associate to early stages in MM progression, namely MGUS and SMM (in which are present in 35-50% of the cases), some variants can be associated to progression and secondary translocations [10, 44, 45].

Late oncogenic events are thought to occur in the bone marrow, after the original cancer clone is completely differentiated into a long-lived plasma cell [2, 11, 13, 29]. Secondary translocations that include *MYC* (8q24), *MAFB* (20q12) and *IRF4* (6p25) genes are common in MM but rare in MGUS and another ones like *RAS* or *FGFR3* genes mutations, *MYC* (v-myc avian myelocytomatosis viral) deregulation and *p18*, *p53* and *pRb* inactivation are exclusive of MM [10, 41]. Activating mutations of *N-RAS (*neuroblastoma RAS viral) or *K-RAS* (Kirsten rat sarcoma RAS viral) seems to be a hallmark of progression from MGUS to MM [13, 29, 39].

There are two different subgroups of chromosomal alterations in MM pathogenesis in which concerning to oncogenic evolution. The first (hyperploid) is characterized by gain of chromosomes and constitutes 40% to 60% of cases, exhibit mainly trisomy of odd chromosomes (3, 5, 7, 9, 11, 15, 19, and 21) [36, 44]. The commonest primary translocations in MM are t(4;14) and t(11;14) while t(14;16), t(6;14) and t(14;20) are less common [46]. The latter (non-hyperploid) presents translocations and other structural rearrangements, mainly translocations between *IgH* (14q32) and other genes located in chromosomes 4, 6, 11, 16 and 20, such has *MAF* (v-maf avian muscle aponeurotic fibrosarcoma oncogene homolog), *MAFB*, MM SET domain (*MMSET*), fibroblast growth factor receptor 3 (FGFR3), and cyclins D1 and D3[9, 10, 33, 36, 44]. It leads to an aberrant recombination of class switching in germinal center and consequently to oncogene deregulation by controller of *IgH*, contributing to higher cells susceptibility to proliferative stimuli [13, 29, 39].

Genetic anomalies associated with worse outcome are the translocations involving the immunoglobulin heavy chain locus on chromosome 14 – t(4;14), t(14;16) and t(4;20), del(17p), complete or partial deletions of chromosome 13, and amplification of 1q [28]. Some other alterations are associated with a better prognosis due to a longer duration of response to therapy and improved survival, such as the presence of hyperdiploidy (3, 5, 7, 9, 11, 15, 19 and 21 chromosome trissomy), t(11;14), or t(6;14) [28, 31].

2.2.1. Genetic Alterations in MM

The primary translocations most frequently observed in MM are t (4; 14) and t (11; 14); the less common include t (14; 16), t (6; 14) and (14; 20). These translocations are associated with overexpression of oncogenes, including D group cyclins (*D1*, *D2*, *D3*), members of *MAF* family (*MAF A*, *MAF B* and *C-MAF*), myeloma SET domain protein (*MMSET*) and fibroblast growth factor receptor 3 (*FGFR3*), which demonstrated influence in prognosis [46-48].

The secondary translocations occur, in general, later in the development of MM and instead the primary translocations, are independent of recombination related to the immunoglobulin class switching. The most frequent secondary translocation involves rearrangements at 8q24 *locus* [49]. Typically the deregulated gene is the secondary translocations *c MYC* with a key role in cell growth and proliferation [50]. Its overexpression is associated with an unfavorable prognosis, advanced stages of the disease and high β2-microglobulin levels [51].

t(4;14)

t(4;14) occurs in 15% of new diagnosed MM and is associated with bad prognosis[52, 53]. It leads to the overexpression of fibroblast growth factor receptor 3 *(FGFR3)* and multiple myeloma SET domain containing protein, *MMSET (WHSC1/NSD2)* [52, 54].

FGFR3, localized in chromosome 4, encodes a tyrosine kinase transmembrane receptor that participates in cell proliferation, differentiation and migration [55]. MMSET protein is overexpressed in MM patients with t(4;14) and is a major epigenetic regulator in MM with t(4;14) by its role in chromatin condensation. Loss of *MMSET* expression modifies adhesion, suppresses growth, and results in apoptosis in MM cells. Genes affected by high levels of *MMSET* are implicated in *p53* pathway, cell cycle regulation, and integrin signaling and their regulation required functional histone methyl-transferase activity of *MMSET* [56].

Its adverse effect in prognosis can be overcome by bortezomib and lenalidomide and *FGFR3* inhibitors are being studied [52].

t(11;14)

t(11;14) is present in 15 to 17% of MM patients and is one of most common translocation[57]. IgH-mediated translocations can activate *CCND1* (11q13) and *CCND3* (6p21)[58]. Normal B and plasma cells do not express *CCND1*, but about 60% of MGUS or MM tumors without a primary *IgH* translocation express *CCND1*, and the other 40% show *CCND2* increased expression compared with normal plasma cells [10, 45].

CCND1 participates in cell cycle regulation and in association with *CDK4* (cyclin dependent kinase 4) and *CDK6* (cyclin dependent kinase 6) phosphorylates retinoblastoma protein (*Rb*), that regulates G1/S transition, stimulating cell cycle progression [59].

Because the expression of cyclin D1 is more common than the t(11;14), it was suggested that genetic amplification mechanisms and trissomy 11 can have a role on it. The impact of t(11;14) in prognosis is not completely clarified with discordant results [31, 57].

t(14;16)

t(14;16) occurs in approximately 5% to 10% of MM and overlaps *IgH* gene switch region and *c-MAF* gene (16p23), leading to hyperexpression of *c-MAF*[44, 60]. It was also described in MGUS, and could be present in early phases of disease [44].

Dysregulation of expression of the transcription factor MAF causes increased expression of many genes, including *CCND2*, a gene involved in cell cycle G1/S transition (which promotes progression in cell cycle) and adhesion molecules as B7-integrin (an adhesion molecule that binds E-cadherin expressed in bone marrow stromal cells). It allows tumor cell to interact with microenvironment, by increasing VEGF (vascular endothelial growth factor) secretion that potentiated bone lesions [60, 61]. However, a retrospective study has revealed that t(14;16) has no impact in prognosis [62].

t(14;18)

t(14;18) involves the *BCL-2* locus and appears in 2% to 3% of MM patients. *BCL-XL* and *MCL-1* are similarly upregulated in MM via the interleukin IL-6–signal transducer and activator of transcription 3 (STAT3) axis [13]. Overexpression of the antiapoptotic BCL-2 proteins correlates with resistance to apoptosis and it seems to be predictive of treatment failure with interferon [13, 63]. Recent studies suggest that the process of isotype switching and somatic hypermutation can persist after progression of MGUS to MM and terminal differentiation in plasma cells [13].

Chromossome 1

Additional copies of 1q are found in 35 to 40% of newly diagnosed MM patients and frequently are associated with deletions of 1p, contributing to an adverse prognosis [40, 45].

Gain of 1q copies are associated with upregulation of genes involved in intracellular protein transport such as *ARF1* and *COPA (*important to vesicle-mediated transport from the endoplasmic reticulum to the Golgi complex) and *RABIF* and *RAB3GAP2* (related to the Rab GTPases, that regulate membrane-vesicle transport) [58, 64].

The alterations of 1q21 region is more frequent in relapsed MM and plasma cell leukemia[63, 65] and involve several oncogenes such as *CKS1B*, *ANP32E*, *BCL-9* and *PDZK1*[29, 66]. Gains of its additional copies are associated with adverse prognosis [63], namely when involves *ANP32E*, a 2A phosphatase inhibitor, that has a role in chromatin remodeling and transcription regulation [66]. When there is a gain of 1q, there are a downregulation of genes important to protein translation such as *RPLP2*, *RPL21*, and *FAU* and an up-regulation of genes that participate in endoplasmic reticulum stress-induced responses such as *CLN3* (chaperone), *UBAP2L and UBE2Q1* (ubiquitin cycle), *PSMD4* (involved in degradation of proteasome), and *CASP4* (that initiates apoptosis in this situation) [67, 68].

Partial or total deletions of 1p are present in 30% of MM patients and are also associated to an adverse prognosis [66], mainly if there are compromising of 1p12 (that encodes tumor suppressor gene *FAM46C*) and 1p32.3 (that encodes *FIF1*, a participant in FAS pathway, and *CDKN2C*, a cyclin-dependent kinase 4(CDK4) involved in cell cycle regulation) [28, 31, 66].

del(13)

Chromosome 13 deletion (mainly deletion of 13q) is detected in 50% of MM, specially non-hyperdyploid [31] and is more common in MM than in SMM or MGUS [44, 51]. Different studies had revealed that in this situation, tumor suppressor gene *RB1* is under express, compromising cell cycle regulation [66] and can be associated with an adverse prognosis when detected by cytogenetics [51].

del(17p)

Alelic deletions of 17p and point mutations of tumor suppressor gene *p53* are the most common genetic alterations seen in cancer [69], but p53 mutations are found only in 3% of MM and hemizigotic deletions in 10% [44]. p53 encodes a protein that is involved in cell cycle control, programmed cell death, senescence, differentiation, transcription, replication, DNA repair and genomic stability maintenance [69].

These alterations constitutes an adverse prognosis factor, which is associated with an aggressive phenotype, disease outside of bone marrow and evolution to plasma cell leukemia [51, 70-72]. Although genetic instability is a characteristic of MM and contributes to accumulation of genetic alterations during disease progression, DNA repairing genes such as *p53* (only mutated in about 10% of MM cases) and *PARP1* (poly ADP ribose polymerase-1) that encodes an enzyme involved in single strand breaks, are not frequently mutated. However, increase expression of *PARP1* is associated with a worst prognosis, allowing the classification of the disease as high risk [73].

Del(8p)

The del(8p) is present in 19 to 24% of MM cases and corresponds to an adverse prognosis [66]. In this case, *TRAIL* (tumour necrosis factor-related apoptosis-inducing ligand) receptor gene expression is decreased leading to a decreased sensibility of tumor cells to apoptosis and surveillance of NK cells and T cytotoxic cells [74].

Other Chromosomic Alterations

Other chromosomic deletions in tumor suppressor genes are important in MM transformation, with the majority of them being involved in NK-kB pathway.

Del(14q) that compromises *TRAF3 gene*, is present in 38% of MM cases; del(16q) is described in 35-50% of MM patients and leads to loss of function of *CYLD* and *WWOX* genes; del(11q) corresponds to 7% of MM and interests *BIRC2* and *BIRC3* genes [66].

Overactivation of transcription factors paired box 5 (*PAX5*), involved in the early process of B lymphocyte development, and interferon-regulating factor 4 (*IRF-4*), a modulator of innate and adaptive immunity, have also been reported as having an important role in MM pathogenesis [13, 75].

The pathogenic role and significance of other genes such as *FAM46C* (family with sequence similarity 46, member C), *SP140* (SP140 nuclear body protein), *SP100* (SP100 nuclear antigen), *ROBO1* (receptor roundabout 1), *EGR1* (transcription factor early growth response 1), remains unknown [13, 38].

2.2.2. Epigenetic Alterations

Epigenetics is related with the modulation of gene expression by other means than from alteration of DNA sequence and has an important role in several pathologies, including tumorigenesis [13, 76-78]. The more frequently studied epigenetic alterations are DNA methylation, post-translation histone modifications and regulation based in microRNA (Figure 3) [79].

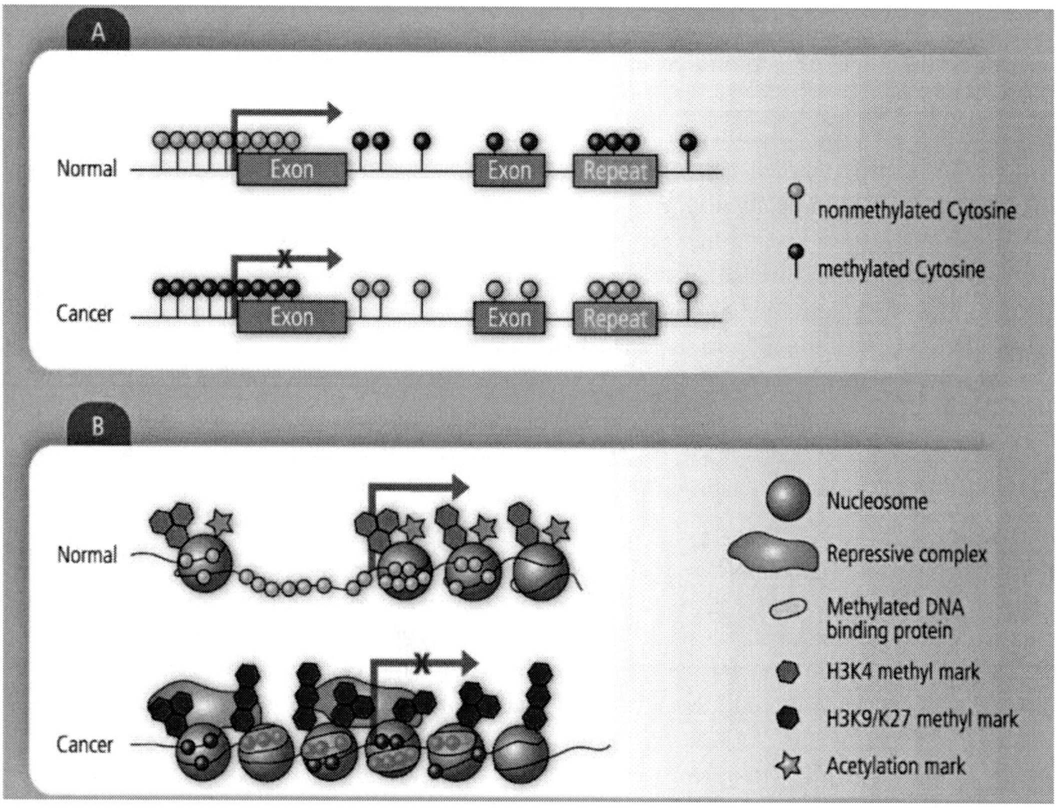

Figure 3. DNA methylation (A) and modifications of histones (B) as major epigenetic modulators. *(Adapted from Geraldes C., 2015).*

Epigenetics seems to have an important role in clonal evolution of neoplasms and in the natural history of cancer being important in MM initiation and progression [76, 80]. It is also involved in the response to drugs or radiation, and could constitute a potential therapeutic approach to cancer prevention and treatment [78]. Furthermore, epigenetic modification is one of the ways by which cancer cells can adapt to environment changes [81]. Reversibility of epigenetic alterations (by DNA hypomethylating agents and histone deacetylases inhibitors) is a fragile point of cancer cells defense mechanisms, because hypermethylated tumoral suppressor genes can be reactivated, inhibiting cell growth [81].

DNA methylation has an important role in gene activity control and nuclear architecture. It is characterized by the transference of a methyl group (-CH3) from S-adenosylmethionine to the carbon-5 of cytosines localized in CpG islands (associated to 5' regulator region of genes, normally non-methylated) and is catalyzed by DNA-methyltransferases (DNMTs) - DNMT1 (maintains methylation during cell division), DNMT3A and DNMT3B (methylation *de novo* in non-methylated areas) [82]. Maintenance of methylation status can have an important role in chromosome integrity preservation, avoiding instability.

DNA methylation do not occur isolated as a marker of epigenetic modulation, being frequently associated with N-terminal histone modifications. Histones storage epigenetic information occurs through post-translational modifications such as lysine acetylation, arginine and lysine methylation and serine phosphorylation [81].

Table 1. Methylated genes in Multiple Myeloma

Biological process	**Gene**	Frequency of methylation in MM primary samples	References
Cell cycle regulation	*Cyclin-dependent kinase 4 inhibitor B (CDKN2B, p15)*	5-30%	[84-87]
	Cyclin-dependent kinase 4 inhibitor 2A (CDKN2A, p16)	7-53%	[84-89]
Apoptosis regulation	*Death-associated protein kinase 1 (DAPK)*	5-77%	[84-87]
	BCL2/adenovirus E1B 19 kDa protein-interacting protein 3 (BNIP)	5-13%	[85, 90]
	B-cell CLL/lymphoma 7C (BCL 7c)	21%	[90]
	Growth Arrest and DNA Damage inducible y (GADD45)	19%	[90]
DNA reparation	*Methylated-DNA-protein-cysteine methyltransferase (MGMT)*	2-4%	[84-87]
Tumor suppression	*Tumor protein 73 (TP73)*	12-45%	[84-87]
Signal transduction	*Suppressor of cytokine signaling 1,3 (SOCS-1, -3)*	45-50%	[84-87, 91, 92]
	Spleen tyrosine kinase (SYK)	38%	[91]
	Dexamethasone-induced Ras-related protein 1 (RASD1)	8%	[93]
	Deleted in liver cancer-1 (DLC-1)	2-15%	[94]
	Ras association domain-containing protein 1A (RASSF1A)	2-15%	[86, 87]
	Stratifin (SFN)	100%	[95]
Wnt pathway	*Wnt inhibitory factor 1 (WIF1)*	22%	[89]
	Secreted frizzled-related protein 1, 2, 4, 5 (sFRP1, 2, 4, 5)	4-50%	[89, 96]
	Dickkopf-related protein 1, 3 (DKK1, 3)	16-32%	[89, 97]
	Adenomatous polyposis coli (APC)	18%	[89]
Osteogenesis	*Secreted protein acidic and rich in cysteine (SPARC)*	8%	[90]
Growth factor signaling	*Transforming growth factor beta-receptor 2 (TGFBR2)*	45%	[95]
Cell adhesion	*Cadherin 1 (CDH1, E-cadherin)*	30-80%	[84-87, 95]
	Gap junction alpha-1 protein (GJA1)	23%	[90]
	A-kinase anchor protein 12 (AKAP12)	13%	[90]
Transcription repression	*Hypermethylated in cancer 1 (HIC1)*	70%	[95]
Translation regulation	*Cytoplasmic polyadenylation element-binding protein 1 (CPEB1)*	50%	[90]
Transcription factor	*Interferon regulatory factor 8 (IRF8)*	10%	[98]

MicroRNAs (miRNAs) are noncoding RNAs that regulate global gene expression and could be epigenetically regulated. miRNAs can function synergistically to repress target genes, and their dysregulation can contribute to the initiation and progression of a variety of cancers [79].

In cancer, global reduction of methylation results from hypomethylation of repetitive sequences and introns. This global DNA hypomethylation contributes to cancer because contributes to chromosomal instability, transposable elements reactivation and imprinting loss. Paradoxally, other regions are hypermethylated, such as promoter regions of CpG islands of tumor suppressor genes, which leads to gene inactivation [81].

DNA methylation profiles can be useful for distinguishing MGUS from other plasma cells disorders. Some tumor suppressor genes are hypomethylated early in the course of MM, with evidence that methylation increases during the process of MM evolution, culminating in plasma cell leukemia [83]. Besides that, hypermethylation of CpG islands in promoter regions of genes involved in cell cycle regulation, cell death and dissemination give to neoplastic plasma cell growth and survival advantages which leads to progression to MM (Table 1) [84].

The etiology of disruption of DNA methylation in MM is not clear, but several studies suggest that it could be related with DNMTs, and *DNMT1* is overexpressed in MM, by pathways initiated by *STAT3* and activated by IL-6 [99].

Epigenetic silencing of *p15* (INK4B) and *p16* (INK4A) genes, that belong to INK4 family of cyclin dependent kinases inhibitors (involved in cell cycle regulation, inhibiting progression from G1 to S phase, are commonly methylated in MM [100]. These genes leads to activation of cell cycle by overexpression of cyclin dependent kinases (CDK) 4 and 6 and, consequently, stimulate plasma cells proliferation and MM progression. Inactivation of *p16* by hypermethylation is present in 7 to 53% of MM patients and is associated not only to progression from MGUS to MM but also with MM prognosis [84-87, 101].

DAPK (Death-Associated Protein Kinase) in a serine/threonine kinase regulated by calcium/calmodulin that stimulates apoptosis. It is methylated in 5 to 77% of MM patients (similar frequency in MGUS) and this is also associate with worst response to therapy and overall survival [84, 85, 89]

In eukaryotes, chromatin is composed by several nucleosomes – consisting of a segment of DNA wound in sequence around eight histone protein cores [102]. Histones properties changes interfere with nucleosome architecture and regulate gene transcription, replication and recombination. Histone N and C terminal tails suffer several modifications such as acetylation, phosphorylation, methylation and ubiquitination of different amino acids, by histone acetyltransferases (HAT), histone deacetylates (HDAC) and histone methyltransferases, which will allow gene activation or silencing [103]. Histone acetylation reduces affinity between histone and DNA, exposing chromatin to transcription factors and to other proteins that bind DNA. Consequently, acetylation is associated with increased transcription and deacetylation inhibits transcription. The process is specific for different locus and reversible [103]. In this way, alterations in the balance between HAT e HDAC lead to cancer development [104].

Until today, there are few information about the relation between histone modifications and MM pathogenesis. Alteration in *MMSET* gene via t(4;14) results in aberrant histone methylation, with an increasing transcription of several oncogenes and altered expression of *p53* and other genes involved in apoptosis, cell cycle regulation, DNA repair and adhesion

[13, 76, 77, 105]. *MMSET* silencing affects negatively survival and MM plasma cells adhesion [56].

Pharmacological modulation with histone methylation inhibitors 3-Deazaneplanocin or HDAC inhibitors like LBH-589 leads to silenced genes re-expression, and *in vitro* and *in vivo* reduction of MM cells survival [106].

Histone methylation and acetylation are altered in MM, with histone deacetylases being hyperactive in MM, resulting in globally increased gene transcription, and aberrant methylation of specific loci in several genes such as *SPARC*, *BNIP3*, *DLC-1*, *DAPK*, *CDH-1*, *TGFβR2* and *p16*. These are associated with adverse prognosis [84, 86, 90, 94, 95] and others such as *RASD1* are related with resistance to therapy, namely to dexamethasone [93].

Furthermore, bromodomains exert an epigenetic function via their direct interaction with acetylated lysine residues. The bromo and extra-terminal (*BET*) family of bromodomains was recently proved to induce *MYC* expression in MM and proved to be a potential drug target in anti-MM therapy [13, 107].

MicroRNAs are small sequences of non-codifying RNA (16-24 pairs of bases), that regulate gene expression by inducing messenger RNA or inhibiting its translation and their regulator functions are frequently altered in cancer, as previously referred. MicroRNAs are related with epigenetic mechanisms because DNA methylation and histone modifications also regulate miRNA expression and microRNAs can also regulate epigenetic control intervenients [108, 109]. The study of microRNA by microarray analysis has identified alterations in the expression of several miRNAs in MGUS and MM, culminating in increased proliferation and resistance to apoptosis. The overexpression of miR-21, miR-32, miR-17-92, miR-106b, miR-181a, miR-181b, miR-221, miR-222, and miR-382 (miR-32 and miR-17-92 are only upregulated in MM, suggesting a role in the latter phases of evolution) and under-expression of miR-15a and miR-16 [13, 110].

2.3. Proliferation and Survival Pathways – The Role of Microenvironment

The pathophysiology and malignant growth of multiple myeloma (MM) are mainly govern by genetic and epigenetic defects within the tumor and through the interaction between myeloma cells and the bone marrow microenvironment (BMM). This interaction leads to the activation of multiple signaling pathways that promote the proliferation, survival and expansion of the malignant clone and stimulate neoangiogenesis and osteoclastogenesis (Figure 4). The knowledge of the prominent pathways involved in MM pathogenesis contributes to the identification of potential prognostic biomarkers and targets to find directed therapies [7, 9, 15, 111, 112].

The majority of the myeloma stimulating growth factors activate the RAS/MAPK signal transduction pathway, whereas the STAT3 pathway is primarily stimulated by IL-6 and IL-6-related cytokines. Other pathways activated by various bone marrow-derived cytokines and chemokines may contribute to the proliferation and survival of MM cells as the phosphatidyl/inositol3-kinase/AKT/mTOR (PI3K/AKT/mTOR) and nuclear factor-kappa B (NF-kB) [7, 113-115].

through the IL-6/JAK (Janus kinase)/STAT3, and tumor necrosis factor TNF- α/canonical nuclear factor NF-kB pathways [13, 132].

Loss of function of cell cycle inhibitors genes when associated to increasing of proto-oncogene expression, seems to have an important role in cell cycle dysregulation, such as *CDKN2C (p18)* expression, which is reduced [by del(1p]*CDKN2A (p16)* inactivation (by changes in DNA methylation) and RB1 inactivation [by del(13) or inactivating mutation] that can leads to G1/S transition dysregulation [66, 101, 133].

The balance between pro-apoptotic and anti-apoptotic members of the B-cell CLL/lymphoma 2 (*BCL-2*) family of proteins is key to determine the cell fate. Cancer cells frequently show upregulation of antiapoptotic members such as *BCL-2*, *BCL-XL* (BCL2-like 1), and *MCL-1* (myeloid cell leukemia 1), or downregulation of the proapoptotic modulators (*BAX*, *BID*, *BAD*, *BAK*, *BCL-XS)*. BMI-1 (that inhibits the expression of the pro-apoptotic *BIM* gene) is overexpressed in MM plasma cells, and BMI-1 silencing reduces cell survival [134].

Constitutive signaling pathway activated by transcription factor X-box binding protein 1 (*XBP-1*), a key molecule in guiding commitment and differentiation to plasma cells, and a downstream effector of the endoplasmic reticulum to nucleus signaling 1 (*ERN1*) branch of the unfolded protein response, was shown to be pathogenic and correlated with poor prognosis [13, 135]. Lack of *XBP-1* lead to turn away from a prior commitment of plasma cells fate, decreased immunoglobulin production, escape from proteasome inhibitor–induced death, and eventually therapeutic failure and disease relapse [13, 71]. XBP1s acts as an independent prognostic marker and can be used with β2 microglobulin and t(4;14), in order to identify patients with a poor outcome, and also as a predictor of thalidomide response [135].

2.4. Bone Marrow Microenvironment

Tumor cells do not grow isolated and they establish close relationship with their neighbors, its microenvironment, being this microenvironment very important for tumor survival and progression configuring one of the hallmarks of cancer [13, 136, 137].

Unlike solid malignancies, in which the places of primary lesion and metastasis are different, in MM, the bone marrow is the place of origin and spreading of neoplastic component and microenvironment. So, bone marrow is an interesting study niche in MM pathogenesis, because this is the center of control of cancer cell proliferation, resistance to apoptosis, trafficking and homing.

Bone marrow microenvironment has an heterogeneous composition, with osteoblasts and osteoclasts, endothelial cells, fibroblasts, stromal cells, adipocytes, macrophages, dendritic cells and lymphocytes, having all of them a role in MM pathogenesis (Figure 5) [13].

However, the role of bone marrow microenvironment in the progression of MGUS to SMM and consequently to active MM remains unknown [13, 138]. It is known that exists a signaling loop between MM cells and the cells that make up bone marrow microenvironment, however they are different (in cell and molecular composition) between MM patients and healthy individuals [7, 13, 18]. Besides the molecular alterations, anomalies in the interactions between MM plasm cells and microenvironment and altered angiogenesis are characteristic of MM progression [10, 41].

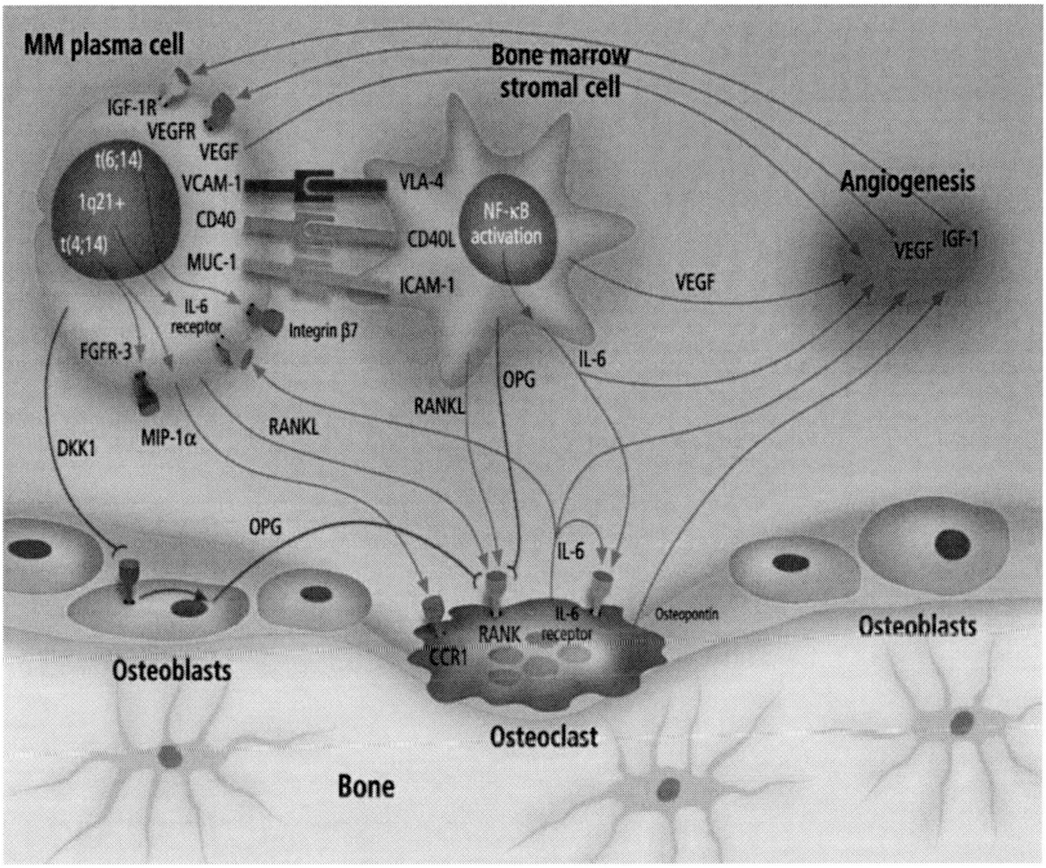

Figure 5. Bone marrow microenvironment in multiple myeloma – Interaction between MM plasma cells and bone marrow stoma cells is mediated by several adhesion molecules such as VCAM-1 (vascular-cell adhesion molecule 1) and VLA-4 (very-late antigen 4). This interaction increases growth factor production and proangiogenic cytokines such as IL-6 (Interleukin-6) and VEGF (vascular endothelial growth factor), that stimulate plasma cells and angiogenesis. Osteoclastogenesis is caused by an altered balance between RANK (receptor activator of nuclear factor kB) and OPG (osteoprotegerin), with diminished production of OPG. Osteoclast, activated by stroma cells, can maintain angiogenesis by themselves, secreting osteopontin. By other side, osteoblastogenesis is diminished due to DKK1 (dikkhopf homolog 1) secretion by malignant plasma cells. MUC-1 - Mucin 1. IGF-1 - Insulin-like growth factor 1. ICAM-1 – intercellular adhesion molecule. (In Geraldes C, 2015; adapted from Palumbo & Anderson, 2011) [36].

Similar to other cancers with bone-metastatic potential, MM cells localize near osteoblasts and vascular endothelium cells, hijacking the bone marrow niche, the main support of hematopoiesis in healthy patients [139].

MM patients bone marrow microenvironment is hypoxic, which leads to an increased expression of hypoxia inducible factor 1α *(HIF-1α)* and *VEGFA* and consequently to neoangiogenesis, building an intersection between osteoblastic and perivascular niches that affects hematopoietic stem cells function involving mesenchymal stromal and endothelial cells (Figure 6) [140, 141]. *HIF-1α* seems to have an important role in MM pathogenesis, and studies *in vitro* has shown that it is necessary to MM cells proliferation and survival [142]. The spread of MM into the peripheral blood involves the decrease of E-cadherin expression, and, consequently, the adhesion of MM cells to the bone marrow, that contributes to entrance or homing of MM cells into other sites of the bone marrow by increasing the expression of CXCR4 [143]. Besides that, hypoxia also contributes to epithelial-to-mesenchymal transition in MM[143, 144] and consequently to disease progression, and appears to induce a stem-like phenotype[144]. Chronic hypoxia also has shown to increase exosome synthesis by MM cells, with up-regulation of miR-135b [145]. All these properties of HIF-1α can configure it as different and promisor therapeutic target in MM.

Some studies using drugs that modulate hypoxia (such as TH-302) showed effects in MM, inducing apoptosis of the MM cells within the bone marrow microenvironment and decreasing paraprotein secretion, which provides a potential new treatment option for MM [146].

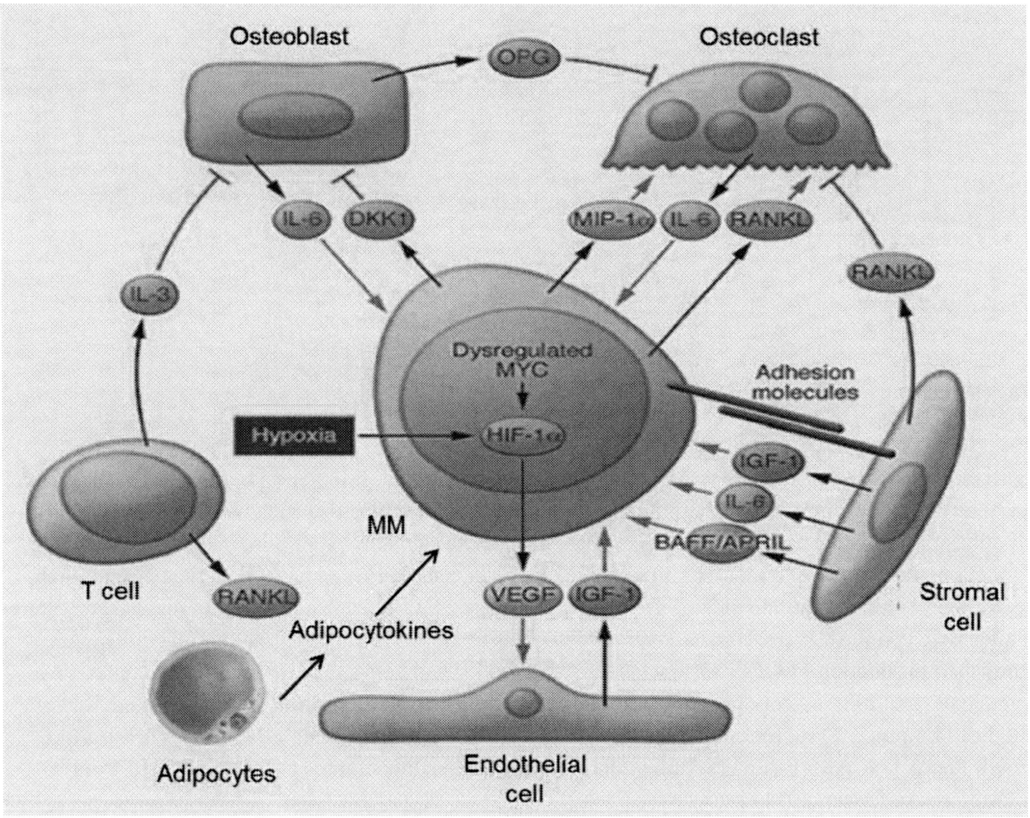

Figure 6. The role of hypoxia and interactions of BM microenvironment with MM cells. External stimuli, such as hypoxia and internal signals resulting from dysregulated MYC, stimulate HIF-1α and VEGF secretion, which in turn stimulate endothelial cells to secrete IGF-1. IL-6 and other critical survival and growth factors are produced by more than one kind of BM cell. The bone remodeling is partially explained by an increase in osteoclast activity (mediated by RANKL/RANK interactions, decreased osteoprotegerin (OPG), and increased MIP-1α) and a decrease in osteoblast activity (mediated by DKK1 and IL-3). The resultant increase in osteoclast activity stimulates the survival and growth of MM cells which can be also activated by some adipocytokines relased by the adipocytes (Adapted from *Kuehl*, *2012*) [10].

Bone Marrow Stem Cells

Bone marrow stem cells are a major constituent of the bone marrow compartment, and have an important role in supporting and nourishing hematopoietic cells [147].

MM and normal bone marrow stem cells are different in terms of function, and support MM proliferation, resistance to apoptosis, drug resistance, migration, and invasion by direct cell-to-cell contact and paracrine mechanisms by the cytokines and chemokines secretion [138].

The interaction of bone marrow stem cells with MM cells by the connection of vascular cell adhesion molecule 1 /integrin b1 (VCAM1/ITGB1), intercellular adhesion molecule 1 /integrin b2 (ICAM1/ITGB2), and mucin 1 cell surface–associated (MUC1) pathways triggers several signaling cascades, with consequently activation of MAPK1 pathway in MM cells, and both NF-kB and MAPK1 pathways in bone marrow stem cells. This leads to myelomagenesis supporting by the secretion of proliferative, antiapoptotic, and chemotactic cytokines such as IL-6, IL-3, IL-1 β, IL-11, M-CSF (macrophage colony-stimulating factor), TNF-a, TNF-β, VEGF and SDF-1 (stroma-derived factor 1 a), creating a favorable environment to MM plasma cells [13, 138, 148].

NF-kB and its related transcription factors have an important role in MM pathogenesis and its excessive activation is due to stimuli in bone marrow microenvironment, such as TNFa, IL-1 β, BAFF and APRIL [114, 149]. The connection between MM plasma cells and bone marrow stem cells leads to NF-kB activation and increases IL-6 secretion, which is reduced by the specific NF-kB inhibition by IkB kinase [149]. This relationship leads to drug resistance namely to alkylating and intercalating agents by a p21-dependent and NF-kB–independent mechanism due to the engagement of the NOTCH1 receptor on MM cells by bone marrow stem cells [13, 138, 150].

CXCL12 (SDF-1a) produced by bone marrow stem cells is the ligand of CXCR4 expressed by MM cells [149]. CXCL12 have a role in homing and trafficking of MM cells, by inducing bone marrow cells IL-6 and VEGF secretion and activation of signaling pathways such as ERK, PI3-K/AKT and NF-kB, promoting MM cells proliferation, neoangiogenesis, and resistance to therapy, namely dexamethasone [151, 152].

Mesenchymal Stem Cells

Mesenchymal stem cells maintain the capacity to self-renewal and differentiation into a several cell types, namely fibroblasts, adipocytes, chondrocytes, and osteoblast and osteocytes and *in vitro* are precursors of bone marrow stem cells [7, 153].

Studies comparing MM-mesenchymal stem cells and mesenchymal stem cells derivate from normal individuals reveal differences in which concerns to genomic background and cytokine production, although it is not yet clear if these differences are acquired or intrinsic and if they are correlated to the phenotype [154]. Mesenchymal stem cells from myeloma patients have increasing production of cytokines such as VEGFA, IL-6, IL-1 beta, and TNF, that induces MM cells proliferation and osteoblastic function and differentiation [155].

Cancer cells and microenvironment cells exchange macromolecules, including nucleic acid, via exosomes and microvesicles [156]. Multiple myeloma cells may uptake miRs from exosome produced by bone marrow stem cells and mesenchymal cells and their exosome content differs between healthy and MM patients, namely with decreased levels of the oncosuppressor miR-15a [157, 158]. Exosomes seem to have an important role in the promotion of tumorigenesis by MM-mesenchymal stem cells by the transferring of oncogenic factors such as IL-6, chemokine (C-C motif) ligand 2 (CCL2) and fibronectin, and by having lower levels of antioncogenic factors [13, 157, 158] and possibly genetic material [159].

Exosomes released by MM-mesenchymal stem cells have also a different pattern of miRs, namely a lower level of the oncosuppressor miR-15a and higher levels of miR-135b (resulting in decreased SMAD family member 5 (SMAD5) expression and impaired capacity of osteoblasts differentiation) [157, 158, 160, 161]. Pre-clinical studies have revealed that the exposure of MM cells to exosomes secreted by MM mesenchymal stem cells induced MM cells proliferation and increased bone marrow homing, while exosomes from healthy individuals have an antitumorigenic effect on MM cells [157].

In vitro studies_suggest that myeloma cells exert a major role in the function of mesenchymal stem cells, but healthy and MM mesenchymal stem cells respond differently to this interaction, with both responding similarly in which concerns to upregulation of genes involved in MM chemotaxis, neoangiogenesis, osteoclasts induction, and osteoblasts inhibition. However, only in MM mesenchymal cells the modulation of genes associated with ribosome function, the ubiquitin-proteasome pathway, and the non-canonical WNT pathway are present [140].

The Osteoblastic/Osteoclastic Niche

Osteoblasts are responsible for formation of new bone, counterbalancing the function of osteoclasts, that resorbing bone, that in physiological circumstances are in equilibrium, in order to maintain bone mass [162, 163]. Osteoclasts are multinucleated cells that participate in bone reabsorption, under osteoblast regulation [163].

Bone marrow mesenchymal stem cells differentiate in osteoblasts after stimulation by paracrine (TGF-β and bone morphogenetic proteins) and endocrine (parathyroid hormone, glucocorticoid hormones, and estrogens) stimuli, being the transcription factor Runt-related transcription factor 2 (RUNX2), one of the most important regulator of osteoblastic differentiation and the canonical WNT pathway relevant in osteoblastogenesis [13, 140].

In physiological situation, osteoblasts localize in the endosteum in the transition between trabecular bone and red marrow, where they support the hematopoietic stem cells [164]. The osteoblastic niche has an important role in the regulation of hematopoietic stem cell and self-renewal and in hematopoiesis. Different mechanisms are involved in the communication between stem cells and osteoblasts, namely soluble cytokines, adhesion molecules, and signal pathways such as the Wnt, Notch, and parathyroid hormone pathways [140, 155, 165].

Bone destruction manifesting with osteopenia, lytic lesions, and eventually pathological fractures is the hallmark of MM, due to the high capacity of malignant plasma cells to induce a severe imbalance of bone remodeling. MM cells favor osteoclastogenesis and inhibiting osteoblastogenesis [155, 165]. MM cells suppress osteoblast formation and function, leading to impairment of bone formation and the development of osteolytic lesions by different pathways including downregulation of RUNX2 in myeloma stem cells and differentiated osteoblasts progenitors; increased production of WNT pathway inhibitors, such as dick-kopf WNT signaling pathway inhibitor 1 (DKK1); secretion of anti-osteoblastic factors such as TGF-beta and hepatocyte growth factor; and constitutive activation of the NOTCH pathway [140, 155, 165]. By the other side, increased osteoclastogenesis in MM is mainly determined by the soluble composition of the bone marrow milieu, can also existing a differentiation of some hematopoietic cells into osteoclasts [155, 165].

RANK/RANKL signaling pathway has an important role in normal and malignant bone remodeling. RANK is a transmembrane receptor from TNF receptor family, present in osteoclasts progenitors' surface. RANKL, is a membrane-bound protein in bone marrow stem cells and osteoblasts, also secreted by activated lymphocytes. Their expression is induced by cytokines that stimulate bone reabsorption such as parathormone, 1,25-(OH)2D3 and prostaglandins. When RANKL binds RANK, induces osteoclast differentiation from their progenitors. Besides that, RANK stimulates osteoclasts survival by induce NF-kB and kinase JUN-terminal pathways [166].

Osteoprotegerin (OPG) is a RANKL soluble decoy receptor, produced by osteoblasts, also from TNF receptor family, that blocks RANKL-RANK binding and diminishes osteoclastogenesis [167]. RANKL/OPG ratio is reduced in healthy individuals and increased in MM patients due to increasing of RANKL and decreasing of OPG [167, 168]. RANKL and OPG levels correlate with MM activity, severity of bone disease and adverse prognosis and can be used as therapeutic targets [169]. MM plasma cells themselves produce RANKL which can exacerbate bone disease together with the increase of circulating pro-osteoclastic cytokines such as MIP-1 alpha, IL-6, IL-7, and IL-3, favoring osteoclastic activity and leading to osteoblasts apoptosis [170, 171].

Osteoblasts has also a role in MM proliferation supported by increasing the secretion of IL-6 and inhibition of apoptotic stimulus through the releasing of osteoprotegerin that protects against TNF-related apoptosis-inducing ligand/Apo2 ligand (TRAIL) [170, 172]. Osteoblasts has also a role in MM pathogenesis promotion through the secretion of IL-6 and osteopontin, which stimulate MM cells proliferation and angiogenesis [171].

The Vascular/Endothelial Niche

Neoangiogenesis and increased vessel are hallmarks of MGUS and SMM transformation in MM. They also are independent negative prognosis factors, after hematopoietic stem cell transplant [173].

By one side, constitutive activation of HIF-1alpha, aberrant expression of HIF-2 and elevated levels of VEGF-A, hepatocyte growth factor, and syndecan-1 promote angiogenesis in MM. By the other side increased tumor burden and loss of an inhibitor of angiogenesis during evolution from MGUS to MM are the major determinants of increased microvessel density in MM patients [13, 174].

MM associated endothelial cells displays a gene expression profile different from those associated to MGUS with upregulation of chemotactic, neo-angiogenetic, and pro-proliferative factors such as CXCL12 [175]. VEGF stimulates FLT-1 phosphorylation and activation of MEK/ERK e PI3-K/PKC pathways in MM plasma cells, leading to increasing of proliferation and migration [176].

Lymphocytes

Another hallmark of cancer[136] that MM cells exhibit is the capacity of escaping from immunologic surveillance by inducing immune tolerance and T-cell anergy, which is corroborated by the benefic role of the graft-*versus*-myeloma effect in allogeneic hematopoietic stem cell transplant in MM [177].

Microenvironment lymphocyte composition is different between MM and normal bone marrow [177], which can be related not only with pathogenesis but also with MM progression and prognosis. Th17 cells (stimulated by IL-6 and TGF- beta) [178], a subset of CD4+ T helper lymphocytes, are abundant on MM patients bone marrow and suppress cancer immune surveillance by secreting cytokines like IL-17 and IL-10. They also stimulate osteoclast's activity contributing to MM bone lesions and possibly by stimulating angiogenesis and attracting myeloid-derived suppressor cells [178, 179]. Also regulator T cells seems to have a similar immunosuppressive function on cytotoxic T cells and antigen-presenting cells by IL-10 and TGF-beta secretion, and proved to be a worse prognosis factor in MM patients [15]. Resident cytotoxic CD8+ T cells in MM bone marrow have different characteristics, namely in which concerns to T-cell receptor (TCR) co-receptor molecules, with increase of PD-1, that has an inhibitory function and contributes to immunologic tolerance [180], which could be therapeutic targets.

Both Th17 cells [178] and CD8+ T cells[165] stimulate osteoclasts activity contributing to MM bone lesions by increasing RANKL and decreasing interferon-gamma secretion.

In MM patients, natural killer (NK) cells have an increasing activity by downregulating NK group 2D (NKG2D) activating receptor and upregulating the inhibitory co-receptor PD-1 [15].

During the transformation to MM from MGUS, cells shed major histocompatibility complex class I polypeptide-related sequence A (MICA) that although can function as a ligand for NKG2D which stimulate NK cell–mediated lysis. When it is soluble contributes to immune surveillance escape in MM [181], increased by lower amounts of type I NK-T cells [182]. Besides that, during MM progression and relapse, it have been described a NK-T deficiency cells [182], whose replacement can have therapeutic impact [183].

Other Cells

Myeloid-derived suppressor cells result from an arrest of myeloid precursors differentiation in MM, due to chronic inflammation [184] and constitute an heterogeneous population of immature myeloid precursors with an immunosuppressive function, inhibiting lymphocytes proliferation. These contribute to MM pathogenesis by differentiating into osteoclasts [185] due to a RANKL-rich milieu and into tumor-associated macrophages [186]. Tumor-associated macrophages, that can also result from differentiation of circulating monocytes attracted to cancer cells via chemoattractants, have an important role into MM pathogenesis and progression mainly due to the secretion of pro-MM cytokines such as IL-6, TNFα and IL-1β, IL-10 (that suppresses T cells function), VEGF-A and nitric oxide (important to angiogenesis and endothelial cells differentiation) [187]. The binding of IL-6 to its receptor on the MM cells triggers a signaling to MAPK/JAK2/STAT3 and PI3K/AKT pathways, leading to MM cells proliferation and survival, as referred [13].

Insulin growth factor-1 (IGF-1) has an important pro-survival function by increasing telomerase activity and upregulating antiapoptotic molecules (such as the surviving cellular FADD-like IL-1 beta–converting enzyme (FLICE)-inhibitory protein (c-FLIP), X-linked inhibitor of apoptosis protein (XIAP), cellular inhibitor of apoptosis 2 (cIAP-2), and BCL-2–related protein A1 (BFL1) via the PI3K/AKT, MAPK, and NF- kB pathways[188]. When IGF-1 is secreted in bone marrow microenvironment induce NF-kB activation in MM cells and absence of binding of IGF-1 to its receptor, initiate apoptosis [115].

IL-6 is an important proliferative factor to plasma cells but with a relation between its levels and disease evolution, with higher levels in MM patients, mainly in those with osteolytic lesions [189, 190]. IL-6 is produced by bone marrow stem cells and osteoclasts due to stimulation from neoplastic plasma cells and CD45+ plasma cells has a positive response to IL-6 [191]. IL-6 binds gp80 (CD80, IL6R) expressed by MM plasma cells and induces phosphorylation and homodimerization of gp130 [192] and consequently activation of RAS/RAF/MAPK, MEK/ERK, JAK/STAT and PI3-K/AKT signaling pathways, that induce MM plasma cells growth and survival and potentiate resistance to therapy [193, 194].

Extracellular matrix plays an active role in supporting MM cells growth and survival. Fibroblasts differentiate from mesenchymal stem cells and are the base of the support and structure of tissues. In cancer, they infiltrate microenvironment and have an active role in the promotion of tumor spreading. Consequently, not only MM cells induce fibroblasts proliferation but also these fibroblasts promote angiogenesis and MM progression,. This occur because they produce a different group of extra-cellular proteins during the evolution from MGUS to MM, such as integrin alpha5 beta5, periostin, matrix metalloproteinase 2 (MMP2), platelet-derived growth factor receptor b, laminin a4, plasminogen activator inhibitor-1, lysyl-hydroxylase 2, prolyl 4-hydroxylase 1, nidogen-2, c-type mannose receptor 2, and basigin [195, 196]. Also hyaluronan and fibronectin have shown to mediate drug resistance in MM [197]. Syndecan-1 (CD138), a type I transmembrane heparan sulfate proteoglycan, is expressed by MM cells, and the proteolytic cleavage of extracellular matrix has impact in MM pathophysiology, with high-levels of this molecule correlating with a worse prognosis [198].

Adipocytes also have a role in MM proliferation, survival, and migration mainly due to leptin or resistin [18, 199].

Conclusion

Understanding of the genomic landscape of MM and the role of bone marrow microenvironment have important immediate repercussions for patient care because an improved in knowledge of the molecular mechanisms of MM pathogenesis will develop more efficacious biomarkers and target therapies [13]. The heterogeneity observed in MM patients outcomes result from a differential evolution of complex genetic and epigenetic abnormalities that involve the malignant myeloma cell as well as the bone marrow microenvironment that lead to disease progression. Gene-expression profiling (GEP) can be used to study the molecular basis for resistance to chemotherapy through global assessment of molecular alterations [64].

One of the major difficulties in multiple myeloma is that, unlike other malignancies, the disease definition is clinic-pathological; it needs overt clinical manifestations of serious end organ damage, such as osteolytic bone lesions and renal failure, before the diagnosis can be made. This problem has ensured that patients cannot get early therapy to prevent organ damage, and also prevented any attempts of cancer treatment at a stage when it is in its most susceptible microenvironment-dependent state [2]. To interfere before the development of end-organ damage in multiple myeloma, biomarkers are needed that accurately identify the subset of patients with SMM who have biological malignancy and are at imminent risk of progression [2, 12, 20, 24, 25].

MM stem cells receive both tumor cell (autocrine) and paracrine signals from a variety of cells in the tumor microenvironment. Collectively, these signals govern the self-renewal and survival of the MM stem cells, the maintenance of its cancer stem cell state and, the acquisition of drug resistance [200]. Genetic heterogeneity inside the tumor, and additional heterogeneity between tumors, contributes to the emergence of drug resistance [10].

The knowledge of all this mechanisms could contribute to the development of new prognostic markers and therapeutic strategies to circumvent chemoresistance in MM.

References

[1] Cook, L; Macdonald, DH. Management of paraproteinaemia. *Postgrad Med J*, 2007, 83(978), 217-223.

[2] Rajkumar, SV; Dimopoulos, MA; Palumbo, A; Blade, J; Merlini, G; Mateos, MV; Kumar, S; Hillengass, J; Kastritis, E; Richardson, P; et al., International Myeloma Working Group updated criteria for the diagnosis of multiple myeloma. *Lancet Oncol*, 2014, 15(12), e538-548.

[3] Rajkumar, SV; Landgren, O; Mateos, MV. Smoldering multiple myeloma. *Blood*, 2015, 125(20), 3069-3075.

[4] Dispenzieri, A. POEMS syndrome: Update on diagnosis, risk-stratification, and management. *Am J Hematol*, 2015, 90(10), 951-962.

[5] Kyle, RA; Therneau, TM; Rajkumar, SV; Larson, DR; Plevak, MF; Offord, JR; Dispenzieri, A; Katzmann, JA; Melton, LJ. 3rd: Prevalence of monoclonal gammopathy of undetermined significance. *N Engl J Med*, 2006, 354(13), 1362-1369.

[6] Kyle, RA; Durie, BG; Rajkumar, SV; Landgren, O; Blade, J; Merlini, G; Kroger, N; Einsele, H; Vesole, DH; Dimopoulos, M; et al., Monoclonal gammopathy of undetermined significance (MGUS) and smoldering (asymptomatic) multiple myeloma: IMWG consensus perspectives risk factors for progression and guidelines for monitoring and management. *Leukemia*, 2010, 24(6), 1121-1127.

[7] Bianchi, G; Anderson, KC. Understanding biology to tackle the disease: Multiple myeloma from bench to bedside, and back. *CA Cancer J Clin*, 2014, 64(6), 422-444.

[8] Furukawa, Y; Kikuchi, J. Molecular pathogenesis of multiple myeloma. *Int J Clin Oncol*, 2015, 20(3), 413-422.

[9] Klein, B; Seckinger, A; Moehler, T; Hose, D. Molecular pathogenesis of multiple myeloma: chromosomal aberrations, changes in gene expression, cytokine networks, and the bone marrow microenvironment. *Recent Results Cancer Res*, 2011, 183, 39-86.

[10] Kuehl, WM; Bergsagel, PL. Molecular pathogenesis of multiple myeloma and its premalignant precursor. *J Clin Invest*, 2012, 122(10), 3456-3463.

[11] Landgren, O; Kyle, RA; Pfeiffer, RM; Katzmann, JA; Caporaso, NE; Hayes, RB; Dispenzieri, A; Kumar, S; Clark, RJ; Baris, D; et al., Monoclonal gammopathy of undetermined significance (MGUS) consistently precedes multiple myeloma: a prospective study. *Blood*, 2009, 113(22), 5412-5417.

[12] Landgren, O; Waxman, AJ. Multiple myeloma precursor disease. *Jama*, 2010, 304(21), 2397-2404.

[13] Bianchi, G; Munshi, NC. Pathogenesis beyond the cancer clone(s) in multiple myeloma. *Blood*, 2015, 125(20), 3049-3058.

[14] Attar-Schneider, O; Zismanov, V; Dabbah, M; Tartakover-Matalon, S; Drucker, L; Lishner, M. Multiple myeloma and bone marrow mesenchymal stem cells' crosstalk: Effect on translation initiation. *Mol Carcinog*, 2015.

[15] Kawano, Y; Moschetta, M; Manier, S; Glavey, S; Gorgun, GT; Roccaro, AM; Anderson, KC; Ghobrial, IM. Targeting the bone marrow microenvironment in multiple myeloma. *Immunol Rev*, 2015, 263(1), 160-172.

[16] Matsui, W; Wang, Q; Barber, JP; Brennan, S; Smith, BD; Borrello, I; McNiece, I; Lin, L; Ambinder, RF; Peacock, C; et al., Clonogenic multiple myeloma progenitors: stem cell properties, and drug resistance. *Cancer Res*, 2008, 68(1), 190-197.

[17] Weiss, BM; Kuehl, WM. Advances in understanding monoclonal gammopathy of undetermined significance as a precursor of multiple myeloma. *Expert Rev Hematol*, 2010, 3(2), 165-174.

[18] Bianchi, G; Ghobrial, IM. Biological and Clinical Implications of Clonal Heterogeneity and Clonal Evolution in Multiple Myeloma. *Curr Cancer Ther Rev*, 2014, 10(2), 70-79.

[19] Perez-Persona, E; Mateo, G; Garcia-Sanz, R; Mateos, MV; de Las Heras, N; de Coca, AG; Hernandez, JM; Galende, J; Martin-Nunez, G; Barez, A; et al., Risk of progression in smouldering myeloma and monoclonal gammopathies of unknown significance: comparative analysis of the evolution of monoclonal component and multiparameter flow cytometry of bone marrow plasma cells. *Br J Haematol*, 2010, 148(1), 110-114.

[20] Dispenzieri, A; Kyle, RA; Katzmann, JA; Therneau, TM; Larson, D; Benson, J; Clark, RJ; Melton, LJ; 3rd, Gertz, MA; Kumar, SK; et al., Immunoglobulin free light chain ratio is an independent risk factor for progression of smoldering (asymptomatic) multiple myeloma. *Blood*, 2008, 111(2), 785-789.

[21] Rajkumar, SV; Gupta, V; Fonseca, R; Dispenzieri, A; Gonsalves, WI; Larson, D; Ketterling, RP; Lust, JA; Kyle, RA; Kumar, SK. Impact of primary molecular cytogenetic abnormalities and risk of progression in smoldering multiple myeloma. *Leukemia*, 2013, 27(8), 1738-1744.

[22] Neben, K; Jauch, A; Hielscher, T; Hillengass, J; Lehners, N; Seckinger, A; Granzow, M; Raab, MS; Ho, AD; Goldschmidt, H; et al., Progression in smoldering myeloma is independently determined by the chromosomal abnormalities del(17p), t(4;14), gain 1q, hyperdiploidy, and tumor load. *J Clin Oncol*, 2013, 31(34), 4325-4332.

[23] Cesana, C; Klersy, C; Barbarano, L; Nosari, AM; Crugnola, M; Pungolino, E; Gargantini, L; Granata, S; Valentini, M; Morra, E. Prognostic factors for malignant transformation in monoclonal gammopathy of undetermined significance and smoldering multiple myeloma. *J Clin Oncol*, 2002, 20(6), 1625-1634.

[24] Landgren, O; Kyle, RA; Rajkumar, SV. From myeloma precursor disease to multiple myeloma: new diagnostic concepts and opportunities for early intervention. *Clin Cancer Res*, 2011, 17(6), 1243-1252.

[25] Mailankody, S; Mena, E; Yuan, CM; Balakumaran, A; Kuehl, WM; Landgren, O. Molecular and biologic markers of progression in monoclonal gammopathy of undetermined significance to multiple myeloma. *Leuk Lymphoma*, 2010, 51(12), 2159-2170.

[26] Perez-Persona, E; Vidriales, MB; Mateo, G; Garcia-Sanz, R; Mateos, MV; de Coca, AG; Galende, J; Martin-Nunez, G; Alonso, JM; de Las Heras, N; et al., New criteria to identify risk of progression in monoclonal gammopathy of uncertain significance and smoldering multiple myeloma based on multiparameter flow cytometry analysis of bone marrow plasma cells. *Blood*, 2007, 110(7), 2586-2592.

[27] Schuster, SR; Rajkumar, SV; Dispenzieri, A; Morice, W; Aspitia, AM; Ansell, S; Kyle, R; Mikhael, J. IgM multiple myeloma: disease definition, prognosis, and differentiation from Waldenstrom's macroglobulinemia. *Am J Hematol*, 2010, 85(11), 853-855.

[28] Chapman, MA; Lawrence, MS; Keats, JJ; Cibulskis, K; Sougnez, C; Schinzel, AC; Harview, CL; Brunet, JP; Ahmann, GJ; Adli, M; et al., Initial genome sequencing and analysis of multiple myeloma. *Nature*, 2011, 471(7339), 467-472.

[29] Morgan, GJ; Walker, BA; Davies, FE. The genetic architecture of multiple myeloma. *Nat Rev Cancer*, 2012, 12(5), 335-348.

[30] Egan, JB; Shi, CX; Tembe, W; Christoforides, A; Kurdoglu, A; Sinari, S; Middha, S; Asmann, Y; Schmidt, J; Braggio, E; et al., Whole-genome sequencing of multiple myeloma from diagnosis to plasma cell leukemia reveals genomic initiating events, evolution, and clonal tides. *Blood*, 2012, 120(5), 1060-1066.

[31] Prideaux, SM; Conway O'Brien, E; Chevassut, TJ. The genetic architecture of multiple myeloma. *Adv Hematol*, 2014, 2014, 864058.

[32] Anderson, KC; Carrasco, RD. Pathogenesis of myeloma. *Annu Rev Pathol*, 2011, 6, 249-274.

[33] Chesi, M; Bergsagel, PL. Molecular pathogenesis of multiple myeloma: basic and clinical updates. *Int J Hematol*, 2013, 97(3), 313-323.

[34] Sawyer, JR. The prognostic significance of cytogenetics and molecular profiling in multiple myeloma. *Cancer Genet*, 2011, 204(1), 3-12.

[35] Herve, AL; Florence, M; Philippe, M; Michel, A; Thierry, F; Kenneth, A; Jean-Luc, H; Nikhil, M; Stephane, M. Molecular heterogeneity of multiple myeloma: pathogenesis, prognosis, and therapeutic implications. *J Clin Oncol*, 2011, 29(14), 1893-1897.

[36] Palumbo, A; Anderson, K. Multiple myeloma. *N Engl J Med*, 2011, 364(11), 1046-1060.

[37] Kuehl, WM; Bergsagel, PL. Multiple myeloma: evolving genetic events and host interactions. *Nat Rev Cancer*, 2002, 2(3), 175-187.

[38] Bolli, N; Avet-Loiseau, H; Wedge, DC; Van Loo, P; Alexandrov, LB; Martincorena, I; Dawson, KJ; Iorio, F; Nik-Zainal, S; Bignell, GR; et al., Heterogeneity of genomic evolution and mutational profiles in multiple myeloma. *Nat Commun*, 2014, 5, 2997.

[39] Faiman, B. Myeloma genetics and genomics: practice implications and future directions. *Clin Lymphoma Myeloma Leuk*, 2014, 14(6), 436-440.

[40] Walker, BA; Wardell, CP; Melchor, L; Brioli, A; Johnson, DC; Kaiser, MF; Mirabella, F; Lopez-Corral, L; Humphray, S; Murray, L; et al., Intraclonal heterogeneity is a critical early event in the development of myeloma and precedes the development of clinical symptoms. *Leukemia*, 2014, 28(2), 384-390.

[41] Palumbo, A; Bringhen, S; Kumar, SK; Lupparelli, G; Usmani, S; Waage, A; Larocca, A; van der Holt, B; Musto, P; Offidani, M; et al., Second primary malignancies with lenalidomide therapy for newly diagnosed myeloma: a meta-analysis of individual patient data. *Lancet Oncol*, 2014, 15(3), 333-342.

[42] Nahi, H; Sutlu, T; Jansson, M; Alici, E; Gahrton, G. Clinical impact of chromosomal aberrations in multiple myeloma. *J Intern Med*, 2011, 269(2), 137-147.

[43] Lopez-Corral, L; Gutierrez, NC; Vidriales, MB; Mateos, MV; Rasillo, A; Garcia-Sanz, R; Paiva, B; San Miguel, JF. The progression from MGUS to smoldering myeloma and eventually to multiple myeloma involves a clonal expansion of genetically abnormal plasma cells. *Clin Cancer Res*, 2011, 17(7), 1692-1700.

[44] Fonseca, R; Barlogie, B; Bataille, R; Bastard, C; Bergsagel, PL; Chesi, M; Davies, FE; Drach, J; Greipp, PR; Kirsch, IR; et al., Genetics and cytogenetics of multiple myeloma: a workshop report. *Cancer Res*, 2004, 64(4), 1546-1558.

[45] Fonseca, R; Bergsagel, PL; Drach, J; Shaughnessy, J; Gutierrez, N; Stewart, AK; Morgan, G; Van Ness, B; Chesi, M; Minvielle, S; et al., International Myeloma Working Group molecular classification of multiple myeloma: spotlight review. *Leukemia*, 2009, 23(12), 2210-2221.

[46] Decaux, O; Lode, L; Magrangeas, F; Charbonnel, C; Gouraud, W; Jezequel, P; Attal, M; Harousseau, JL; Moreau, P; Bataille, R; et al., Prediction of survival in multiple myeloma based on gene expression profiles reveals cell cycle and chromosomal instability signatures in high-risk patients and hyperdiploid signatures in low-risk patients: a study of the Intergroupe Francophone du Myelome. *J Clin Oncol*, 2008, 26(29), 4798-4805.

[47] Zhan, F; Huang, Y; Colla, S; Stewart, JP; Hanamura, I; Gupta, S; Epstein, J; Yaccoby, S; Sawyer, J; Burington, B; et al., The molecular classification of multiple myeloma. *Blood*, 2006, 108(6), 2020-2028.

[48] Stewart, AK; Bergsagel, PL; Greipp, PR; Dispenzieri, A; Gertz, MA; Hayman, SR; Kumar, S; Lacy, MQ; Lust, JA; Russell, SJ; et al., A practical guide to defining high-risk myeloma for clinical trials; patient counseling and choice of therapy. *Leukemia*, 2007, 21(3), 529-534.

[49] Gabrea, A; Martelli, ML; Qi, Y; Roschke, A; Barlogie, B; Shaughnessy, JD; Jr. Sawyer, JR; Kuehl, WM. Secondary genomic rearrangements involving immunoglobulin or MYC loci show similar prevalences in hyperdiploid and nonhyperdiploid myeloma tumors. *Genes Chromosomes Cancer*, 2008, 47(7), 573-590.

[50] Dang, CV. MYC on the path to cancer. *Cell*, 2012, 149(1), 22-35.

[51] Avet-Loiseau, H; Li, C; Magrangeas, F; Gouraud, W; Charbonnel, C; Harousseau, JL; Attal, M; Marit, G; Mathiot, C; Facon, T; et al., Prognostic significance of copy-number alterations in multiple myeloma. *J Clin Oncol*, 2009, 27(27), 4585-4590.

[52] Kalff, A; Spencer, A. The t(4;14) translocation and FGFR3 overexpression in multiple myeloma: prognostic implications and current clinical strategies. *Blood Cancer J*, 2012, 2, e89.

[53] Chang, H; Sloan, S; Li, D; Zhuang, L; Yi, QL; Chen, CI; Reece, D; Chun, K; Keith Stewart, A. The t(4;14) is associated with poor prognosis in myeloma patients undergoing autologous stem cell transplant. *Br J Haematol*, 2004, 125(1), 64-68.

[54] Chesi, M; Nardini, E; Lim, RS; Smith, KD; Kuehl, WM; Bergsagel, PL. The t(4;14) translocation in myeloma dysregulates both FGFR3 and a novel gene, MMSET, resulting in IgH/MMSET hybrid transcripts. *Blood*, 1998, 92(9), 3025-3034.

[55] Turner, N; Grose, R. Fibroblast growth factor signalling: from development to cancer. *Nat Rev Cancer*, 2010, 10(2), 116-129.

[56] Martinez-Garcia, E; Popovic, R; Min, DJ; Sweet, SM; Thomas, PM; Zamdborg, L; Heffner, A; Will, C; Lamy, L; Staudt, LM. et al., The MMSET histone methyl transferase switches global histone methylation and alters gene expression in t(4;14) multiple myeloma cells. *Blood*, 2011, 117(1), 211-220.

[57] Chang, H; Qi, XY; Stewart, AK. t(11;14) does not predict long-term survival in myeloma. In: *Leukemia. Volume*, *19*, edn. England; 2005: 1078-1079.

[58] Zhou, Y; Barlogie, B; Shaughnessy, JD; Jr. The molecular characterization and clinical management of multiple myeloma in the post-genome era. *Leukemia*, 2009, 23(11), 1941-1956.

[59] Bartek, J; Lukas, J. DNA repair: Cyclin D1 multitasks. In: *Nature.*, Volume 474, edn. England, 2011, 171-172.

[60] Hurt, EM; Wiestner, A; Rosenwald, A; Shaffer, AL; Campo, E; Grogan, T; Bergsagel, PL; Kuehl, WM; Staudt, LM. Overexpression of c-maf is a frequent oncogenic event in multiple myeloma that promotes proliferation and pathological interactions with bone marrow stroma. *Cancer Cell*, 2004, 5(2), 191-199.

[61] Yeung, J; Chang H. Genomic aberrations and immunohistochemical markers as prognostic indicators in multiple myeloma. *J Clin Pathol*, 2008, 61(7), 832-836.

[62] Avet-Loiseau, H; Malard, F; Campion, L; Magrangeas, F; Sebban, C; Lioure, B; Decaux, O; Lamy, T; Legros, L; Fuzibet, JG. et al., Translocation t(14;16) and multiple myeloma: is it really an independent prognostic factor? *Blood*, 2011, 117(6), 2009-2011.

[63] Shaughnessy, JD; Jr. Zhan, F; Burington, BE; Huang, Y; Colla, S; Hanamura, I; Stewart, JP; Kordsmeier, B; Randolph, C; Williams, DR. et al., A validated gene expression model of high-risk multiple myeloma is defined by deregulated expression of genes mapping to chromosome 1. *Blood*, 2007, 109(6), 2276-2284.

[64] Johnson, SK; Heuck, CJ; Albino, AP; Qu, P; Zhang, Q; Barlogie, B; Shaughnessy, JD; Jr. The use of molecular-based risk stratification and pharmacogenomics for outcome prediction and personalized therapeutic management of multiple myeloma. *Int J Hematol*, 2011, 94(4), 321-333.

[65] Hanamura, I; Stewart, JP; Huang, Y; Zhan, F; Santra, M; Sawyer, JR; Hollmig, K; Zangarri, M; Pineda-Roman, M; van Rhee, F; et al., Frequent gain of chromosome band 1q21 in plasma-cell dyscrasias detected by fluorescence in situ hybridization: incidence increases from MGUS to relapsed myeloma and is related to prognosis and disease progression following tandem stem-cell transplantation. *Blood*, 2006, 108(5), 1724-1732.

[66] Walker, BA; Leone, PE; Chiecchio, L; Dickens, NJ; Jenner, MW; Boyd, KD; Johnson, DC; Gonzalez, D; Dagrada, GP; Protheroe, RK; et al., A compendium of myeloma-associated chromosomal copy number abnormalities and their prognostic value. *Blood*, 2010, 116(15), e56-65.

[67] Fabris, S; Ronchetti, D; Agnelli, L; Baldini, L; Morabito, F; Bicciato, S; Basso, D; Todoerti, K; Lombardi, L; Lambertenghi-Deliliers, G; et al., Transcriptional features of multiple myeloma patients with chromosome 1q gain. In: *Leukemia.* Volume, 21, edn. England, 2007, 1113-1116.

[68] Carew, JS; Nawrocki, ST; Krupnik, YV; Dunner, K; Jr. McConkey, DJ; Keating, MJ; Huang, P. Targeting endoplasmic reticulum protein transport: a novel strategy to kill malignant B cells and overcome fludarabine resistance in CLL. *Blood*, 2006, 107(1), 222-231.

[69] Hainaut, P; Hollstein, M. p53 and human cancer: the first ten thousand mutations. *Adv Cancer Res*, 2000, 77, 81-137.

[70] Fonseca, R; Blood, E; Rue, M; Harrington, D; Oken, MM; Kyle, RA; Dewald, GW; Van Ness, B; Van Wier, SA; Henderson, KJ; et al., Clinical and biologic implications of recurrent genomic aberrations in myeloma. *Blood*, 2003, 101(11), 4569-4575.

[71] Leung-Hagesteijn, C; Erdmann, N; Cheung, G; Keats, JJ; Stewart, AK; Reece, DE; Chung, KC; Tiedemann, RE. Xbp1s-negative tumor B cells and pre-plasmablasts mediate therapeutic proteasome inhibitor resistance in multiple myeloma. *Cancer Cell*, 2013, 24(3), 289-304.

[72] Tiedemann, RE; Mao, X; Shi, CX; Zhu, YX; Palmer, SE; Sebag, M; Marler, R; Chesi, M; Fonseca, R; Bergsagel, PL; et al., Identification of kinetin riboside as a repressor of CCND1 and CCND2 with preclinical antimyeloma activity. *J Clin Invest*, 2008, 118(5), 1750-1764.

[73] Neri, P; Ren, L; Gratton, K; Stebner, E; Johnson, J; Klimowicz, A; Duggan, P; Tassone, P; Mansoor, A; Stewart, DA; et al., Bortezomib-induced "BRCAness" sensitizes multiple myeloma cells to PARP inhibitors. *Blood*, 2011, 118(24), 6368-6379.

[74] Takeda, K; Smyth, MJ; Cretney, E; Hayakawa, Y; Kayagaki, N; Yagita, H; Okumura, K. Critical role for tumor necrosis factor-related apoptosis-inducing ligand in immune surveillance against tumor development. *J Exp Med*, 2002, 195(2), 161-169.

[75] Cobaleda, C; Schebesta, A; Delogu, A; Busslinger, M. Pax5: the guardian of B cell identity and function. *Nat Immunol*, 2007, 8(5), 463-470.

[76] Baylin, SB; Jones, PA. A decade of exploring the cancer epigenome - biological and translational implications. *Nat Rev Cancer*, 2011, 11(10), 726-734.

[77] Dimopoulos, K; Gimsing, P; Gronbaek, K. The role of epigenetics in the biology of multiple myeloma. *Blood Cancer J*, 2014, 4, e207.

[78] Jeltsch, A. Epigenetics Europe conference. Munich, Germany, 8-9 September 2011. *Epigenomics*, 2011, 3(6), 693-695.

[79] Melo, SA; Esteller, M. A precursor microRNA in a cancer cell nucleus: get me out of here! *Cell Cycle*, 2011, 10(6), 922-925.

[80] Baylin, SB. Stem cells, cancer, and epigenetics. In: *StemBook.* edn. Cambridge (MA): Harvard Stem Cell Institute Copyright: (c) 2009 Stephen B. Baylin, 2008.

[81] Esteller, M. Epigenetics in cancer. *N Engl J Med*, 2008, 358(11), 1148-1159.

[82] Okano, M; Bell, DW; Haber, DA; Li, E. DNA methyltransferases Dnmt3a and Dnmt3b are essential for de novo methylation and mammalian development. *Cell*, 1999; 99(3), 247-257.

[83] Salhia, B; Baker, A; Ahmann, G; Auclair, D; Fonseca, R; Carpten, J. DNA methylation analysis determines the high frequency of genic hypomethylation and low frequency of hypermethylation events in plasma cell tumors. *Cancer Res*, 2010, 70(17), 6934-6944.

[84] Galm, O; Wilop, S; Reichelt, J; Jost, E; Gehbauer, G; Herman, JG; Osieka, R. DNA methylation changes in multiple myeloma. *Leukemia*, 2004, 18(10), 1687-1692.

[85] Braggio, E; Maiolino, A; Gouveia, ME; Magalhaes, R; Souto Filho, JT; Garnica, M; Nucci, M; Renault, IZ. Methylation status of nine tumor suppressor genes in multiple myeloma. *Int J Hematol*, 2010, 91(1), 87-96.

[86] Seidl, S; Ackermann, J; Kaufmann, H; Keck, A; Nosslinger, T; Zielinski, CC; Drach, J; Zochbauer-Muller, S. DNA-methylation analysis identifies the E-cadherin gene as a potential marker of disease progression in patients with monoclonal gammopathies. *Cancer*, 2004, 100(12), 2598-2606.

[87] Stanganelli, C; Arbelbide, J; Fantl, DB; Corrado, C; Slavutsky, I. DNA methylation analysis of tumor suppressor genes in monoclonal gammopathy of undetermined significance. *Ann Hematol*, 2010, 89(2), 191-199.

[88] Khong, T; Sharkey, J; Spencer, A. The effect of azacitidine on interleukin-6 signaling and nuclear factor-kappaB activation and its *in vitro* and *in vivo* activity against multiple myeloma. *Haematologica*, 2008, 93(6), 860-869.

[89] Chim, CS; Liang, R; Fung, TK; Choi, CL; Kwong, YL. Epigenetic dysregulation of the death-associated protein kinase/p14/HDM2/p53/Apaf-1 apoptosis pathway in multiple myeloma. *J Clin Pathol*, 2007, 60(6), 664-669.

[90] Heller, G; Schmidt, WM; Ziegler, B; Holzer, S; Mullauer, L; Bilban, M; Zielinski, CC; Drach, J; Zochbauer-Muller, S. Genome-wide transcriptional response to 5-aza-2'-deoxycytidine and trichostatin a in multiple myeloma cells. *Cancer Res*, 2008, 68(1), 44-54.

[91] Reddy, J; Shivapurkar, N; Takahashi, T; Parikh, G; Stastny, V; Echebiri, C; Crumrine, K; Zochbauer-Muller, S; Drach, J; Zheng, Y; et al., Differential methylation of genes that regulate cytokine signaling in lymphoid and hematopoietic tumors. *Oncogene*, 2005, 24(4), 732-736.

[92] Wilop, S; van Gemmeren, TB; Lentjes, MH; van Engeland, M; Herman, JG; Brummendorf, TH; Jost, E; Galm, O. Methylation-associated dysregulation of the suppressor of cytokine signaling-3 gene in multiple myeloma. *Epigenetics*, 2011, 6(8), 1047-1052.

[93] Nojima, M; Maruyama, R; Yasui, H; Suzuki, H; Maruyama, Y; Tarasawa, I; Sasaki, Y; Asaoku, H; Sakai, H; Hayashi, T; et al., Genomic screening for genes silenced by DNA methylation revealed an association between RASD1 inactivation and dexamethasone resistance in multiple myeloma. *Clin Cancer Res*, 2009, 15(13), 4356-4364.

[94] Song, YF; Xu, R; Zhang, XH; Chen, BB; Chen, Q; Chen, YM; Xie, Y. High-frequency promoter hypermethylation of the deleted in liver cancer-1 gene in multiple myeloma. *J Clin Pathol*, 2006, 59(9), 947-951.

[95] de Carvalho, F; Colleoni, GW; Almeida, MS; Carvalho, AL; Vettore, AL. TGFbetaR2 aberrant methylation is a potential prognostic marker and therapeutic target in multiple myeloma. *Int J Cancer*, 2009, 125(8), 1985-1991.

[96] Jost, E; Gezer, D; Wilop, S; Suzuki, H; Herman, JG; Osieka, R; Galm, O. Epigenetic dysregulation of secreted Frizzled-related proteins in multiple myeloma. *Cancer Lett*, 2009, 281(1), 24-31.

[97] Kocemba, KA; Groen, RW; van Andel, H; Kersten, MJ; Mahtouk, K; Spaargaren, M; Pals, ST. Transcriptional silencing of the Wnt-antagonist DKK1 by promoter methylation is associated with enhanced Wnt signaling in advanced multiple myeloma. *PLoS One*, 2012, 7(2), e30359.

[98] Tshuikina, M; Jernberg-Wiklund, H; Nilsson, K; Oberg, F. Epigenetic silencing of the interferon regulatory factor ICSBP/IRF8 in human multiple myeloma. *Exp Hematol*, 2008, 36(12), 1673-1681.

[99] Hodge, DR; Peng, B; Cherry, JC; Hurt, EM; Fox, SD; Kelley, JA; Munroe, DJ; Farrar, WL. Interleukin 6 supports the maintenance of p53 tumor suppressor gene promoter methylation. *Cancer Res*, 2005, 65(11), 4673-4682.

[100] Hannon, GJ; Beach, D. p15INK4B is a potential effector of TGF-beta-induced cell cycle arrest. *Nature*, 1994, 371(6494), 257-261.

[101] Gonzalez-Paz, N; Chng, WJ; McClure, RF; Blood, E; Oken, MM; Van Ness, B; James, CD; Kurtin, PJ; Henderson, K; Ahmann, GJ; et al., Tumor suppressor p16 methylation

in multiple myeloma: biological and clinical implications. *Blood*, 2007, 109(3), 1228-1232.

[102] Shukla, V; Vaissiere, T; Herceg, Z. Histone acetylation and chromatin signature in stem cell identity and cancer. *Mutat Res*, 2008, 637(1-2), 1-15.

[103] Jenuwein, T; Allis, CD. Translating the histone code. *Science*, 2001, 293(5532), 1074-1080.

[104] Sun, XJ; Man, N; Tan, Y; Nimer, SD; Wang, L. The Role of Histone Acetyltransferases in Normal and Malignant Hematopoiesis. *Front Oncol*, 2015, 5, 108.

[105] Kaiser, MF; Johnson, DC; Wu, P; Walker, BA; Brioli, A; Mirabella, F; Wardell, CP; Melchor, L; Davies, FE; Morgan, GJ. Global methylation analysis identifies prognostically important epigenetically inactivated tumor suppressor genes in multiple myeloma. *Blood*, 2013, 122(2), 219-226.

[106] Kalushkova, A; Fryknas, M; Lemaire, M; Fristedt, C; Agarwal, P; Eriksson, M; Deleu, S; Atadja, P; Osterborg, A; Nilsson, K; et al., Polycomb target genes are silenced in multiple myeloma. *PLoS One*, 2010, 5(7), e11483.

[107] Delmore, JE; Issa, GC; Lemieux, ME; Rahl, PB; Shi, J; Jacobs, HM; Kastritis, E; Gilpatrick, T; Paranal, RM; Qi, J; et al., BET bromodomain inhibition as a therapeutic strategy to target c-Myc. *Cell*, 2011, 146(6), 904-917.

[108] Sato, F; Tsuchiya, S; Meltzer, SJ; Shimizu, K. MicroRNAs and epigenetics. *Febs j*, 2011, 278(10), 1598-1609.

[109] Fabbri, M; Calin, GA. Epigenetics and miRNAs in human cancer. *Adv Genet*, 2010, 70, 87-99.

[110] Pichiorri, F; Suh, SS; Ladetto, M; Kuehl, M; Palumbo, T; Drandi, D; Taccioli, C; Zanesi, N; Alder, H; Hagan, JP; et al., MicroRNAs regulate critical genes associated with multiple myeloma pathogenesis. *Proc Natl Acad Sci U S A*, 2008, 105(35), 12885-12890.

[111] Shay, G; Hazlehurst, L; Lynch, CC. Dissecting the multiple myeloma-bone microenvironment reveals new therapeutic opportunities. *J Mol Med (Berl)*, 2015.

[112] Wang, N; Bartlow, P; Ouyang, Q; Xie, XQ. Recent advances in antimultiple myeloma drug development. *Pharm Pat Anal*, 2014, 3(3), 261-277.

[113] Tsuyama, N; Ishikawa, H; Abroun, S; Liu, S; Li, FJ; Otsuyama, K; Zheng, X; Obata, M; Taniguchi, O; Kawano, MM. The regulatory mechanism of IL-6-dependent proliferation of human myeloma cells. *Hematology*, 2003, 8(6), 409-411.

[114] Annunziata, CM; Davis, RE; Demchenko, Y; Bellamy, W; Gabrea, A; Zhan, F; Lenz, G; Hanamura, I; Wright, G; Xiao, W; et al., Frequent engagement of the classical and alternative NF-kappaB pathways by diverse genetic abnormalities in multiple myeloma. *Cancer Cell*, 2007, 12(2), 115-130.

[115] Mitsiades, CS; Mitsiades, N; Poulaki, V; Schlossman, R; Akiyama, M; Chauhan, D; Hideshima, T; Treon, SP; Munshi, NC; Richardson, PG. et al., Activation of NF-kappaB and upregulation of intracellular anti-apoptotic proteins via the IGF-1/Akt signaling in human multiple myeloma cells: therapeutic implications. *Oncogene*, 2002, 21(37), 5673-5683.

[116] de la Puente, P; Muz, B; Azab, F; Luderer, M; Azab, AK. Molecularly targeted therapies in multiple myeloma. *Leuk Res Treatment*, 2014, 2014, 976567.

[117] Chng, WJ; Gonzalez-Paz, N; Price-Troska, T; Jacobus, S; Rajkumar, SV; Oken, MM; Kyle, RA; Henderson, KJ; Van Wier, S; Greipp, P; et al., Clinical and biological

significance of RAS mutations in multiple myeloma. In: Leukemia. Volume, 22, edn. England, 2008, 2280-2284.

[118] Rasmussen, T; Haaber, J; Dahl, IM; Knudsen, LM; Kerndrup, GB; Lodahl, M; Johnsen, HE; Kuehl, M. Identification of translocation products but not K-RAS mutations in memory B cells from patients with multiple myeloma. *Haematologica*, 2010, 95(10), 1730-1737.

[119] Bharti, AC; Shishodia, S; Reuben, JM; Weber, D; Alexanian, R; Raj-Vadhan, S; Estrov, Z; Talpaz, M; Aggarwal, BB. Nuclear factor-kappaB and STAT3 are constitutively active in CD138^{+} cells derived from multiple myeloma patients, and suppression of these transcription factors leads to apoptosis. *Blood*, 2004, 103(8), 3175-3184.

[120] Kawano, M; Hirano, T; Matsuda, T; Taga, T; Horii, Y; Iwato, K; Asaoku, H; Tang, B; Tanabe, O; Tanaka, H; et al., Autocrine generation and requirement of BSF-2/IL-6 for human multiple myelomas. *Nature*, 1988, 332(6159), 83-85.

[121] Carroll, RG; Martin, SJ. Autophagy in multiple myeloma: what makes you stronger can also kill you. *Cancer Cell*, 2013, 23(4), 425-426.

[122] Peterson, TR; Laplante, M; Thoreen, CC; Sancak, Y; Kang, SA; Kuehl, WM; Gray, NS; Sabatini, DM. DEPTOR is an mTOR inhibitor frequently overexpressed in multiple myeloma cells and required for their survival. *Cell*, 2009, 137(5), 873-886.

[123] Chaturvedi, MM; Sung, B; Yadav, VR; Kannappan, R; Aggarwal, BB. NF-kappaB addiction and its role in cancer: 'one size does not fit all.' *Oncogene*, 2011, 30(14), 1615-1630.

[124] Basseres, DS; Baldwin, AS. Nuclear factor-kappaB and inhibitor of kappaB kinase pathways in oncogenic initiation and progression. *Oncogene*, 2006, 25(51), 6817-6830.

[125] Keats, JJ; Fonseca, R; Chesi, M; Schop, R; Baker, A; Chng, WJ; Van Wier, S; Tiedemann, R; Shi, CX; Sebag, M; et al., Promiscuous mutations activate the noncanonical NF-kappaB pathway in multiple myeloma. *Cancer Cell*, 2007, 12(2), 131-144.

[126] Tai, YT; Li, XF; Breitkreutz, I; Song, W; Neri, P; Catley, L; Podar, K; Hideshima, T; Chauhan, D; Raje, N; et al., Role of B-cell-activating factor in adhesion and growth of human multiple myeloma cells in the bone marrow microenvironment. *Cancer Res*, 2006, 66(13), 6675-6682.

[127] Tai, YT; Anderson, KC. Targeting B-cell maturation antigen in multiple myeloma. *Immunotherapy*, 2015.

[128] Wegener, E; Krappmann, D. Dynamic protein complexes regulate NF-kappaB signaling. *Handb Exp Pharmacol*, 2008(186), 237-259.

[129] Ben-Neriah, Y; Karin, M. Inflammation meets cancer, with NF-kappaB as the matchmaker. *Nat Immunol*, 2011, 12(8), 715-723.

[130] Cvek, B; Dvorak, Z. The value of proteasome inhibition in cancer. Can the old drug, disulfiram, have a bright new future as a novel proteasome inhibitor? *Drug Discov Today*, 2008, 13(15-16), 716-722.

[131] Nakanishi, C; Toi, M. Nuclear factor-kappaB inhibitors as sensitizers to anticancer drugs. *Nat Rev Cancer*, 2005, 5(4), 297-309.

[132] Hideshima, T; Mitsiades, C; Ikeda, H; Chauhan, D; Raje, N; Gorgun, G; Hideshima, H; Munshi, NC; Richardson, PG; Carrasco, DR; et al., A proto-oncogene BCL6 is up-regulated in the bone marrow microenvironment in multiple myeloma cells. *Blood*, 2010, 115(18), 3772-3775.

[133] Leone, PE; Walker, BA; Jenner, MW; Chiecchio, L; Dagrada, G; Protheroe, RK; Johnson, DC; Dickens, NJ; Brito, JL; Else, M; et al., Deletions of CDKN2C in multiple myeloma: biological and clinical implications. *Clin Cancer Res*, 2008, 14(19), 6033-6041.

[134] Jagani, Z; Wiederschain, D; Loo, A; He, D; Mosher, R; Fordjour, P; Monahan, J; Morrissey, M; Yao, YM; Lengauer, C; et al., The Polycomb group protein Bmi-1 is essential for the growth of multiple myeloma cells. *Cancer Res*, 2010, 70(13), 5528-5538.

[135] Bagratuni, T; Wu, P; Gonzalez de Castro, D; Davenport, EL; Dickens, NJ; Walker, BA; Boyd, K; Johnson, DC; Gregory, W; Morgan, GJ; et al., XBP1s levels are implicated in the biology and outcome of myeloma mediating different clinical outcomes to thalidomide-based treatments. *Blood*, 2010, 116(2), 250-253.

[136] Hanahan, D; Weinberg, RA. Hallmarks of cancer: the next generation. *Cell*, 2011, 144(5), 646-674.

[137] Quail, DF; Joyce, JA. Microenvironmental regulation of tumor progression and metastasis. *Nat Med*, 2013, 19(11), 1423-1437.

[138] Hideshima, T; Mitsiades, C; Tonon, G; Richardson, PG; Anderson, KC. Understanding multiple myeloma pathogenesis in the bone marrow to identify new therapeutic targets. *Nat Rev Cancer*, 2007, 7(8), 585-598.

[139] Xie, Y; Yin, T; Wiegraebe, W; He, XC; Miller, D; Stark, D; Perko, K; Alexander, R; Schwartz, J; Grindley, JC; et al., Detection of functional haematopoietic stem cell niche using real-time imaging. *Nature*, 2009, 457(7225), 97-101.

[140] Garcia-Gomez, A; De Las Rivas, J; Ocio, EM; Diaz-Rodriguez, E; Montero, JC; Martin, M; Blanco, JF; Sanchez-Guijo, FM; Pandiella, A; San Miguel, JF; et al., Transcriptomic profile induced in bone marrow mesenchymal stromal cells after interaction with multiple myeloma cells: implications in myeloma progression and myeloma bone disease. *Oncotarget*, 2014, 5(18), 8284-8305.

[141] Colla, S; Storti, P; Donofrio, G; Todoerti, K; Bolzoni, M; Lazzaretti, M; Abeltino, M; Ippolito, L; Neri, A; Ribatti, D; et al., Low bone marrow oxygen tension and hypoxia-inducible factor-1alpha overexpression characterize patients with multiple myeloma: role on the transcriptional and proangiogenic profiles of CD138(+) cells. In: Leukemia. Volume, 24, edn. England, 2010, 1967-1970.

[142] Borsi, E; Perrone, G; Terragna, C; Martello, M; Zamagni, E; Tacchetti, P; Pantani, L; Brioli, A; Dico, AF; Zannetti, BA. et al., HIF-1alpha inhibition blocks the cross talk between multiple myeloma plasma cells and tumor microenvironment. *Exp Cell Res*, 2014, 328(2), 444-455.

[143] Azab, AK; Hu, J; Quang, P; Azab, F; Pitsillides, C; Awwad, R; Thompson, B; Maiso, P; Sun, JD; Hart, CP; et al., Hypoxia promotes dissemination of multiple myeloma through acquisition of epithelial to mesenchymal transition-like features. *Blood*, 2012, 119(24), 5782-5794.

[144] Muz, B; de la Puente, P; Azab, F; Luderer, M; Azab, AK. Hypoxia promotes stem cell-like phenotype in multiple myeloma cells. In: Blood Cancer J. Volume, 4, edn. United States; 2014, e262.

[145] Umezu, T; Tadokoro, H; Azuma, K; Yoshizawa, S; Ohyashiki, K; Ohyashiki, JH. Exosomal miR-135b shed from hypoxic multiple myeloma cells enhances angiogenesis by targeting factor-inhibiting HIF-1. *Blood*, 2014, 124(25), 3748-3757.

[146] Hu, J; Handisides, DR; Van Valckenborgh, E; De Raeve, H; Menu, E; Vande Broek, I; Liu, Q; Sun, JD; Van Camp, B; Hart, CP; et al., Targeting the multiple myeloma hypoxic niche with TH-302, a hypoxia-activated prodrug. *Blood*, 2010, 116(9), 1524-1527.

[147] Bianco, P; Gehron Robey, P. Marrow stromal stem cells. *J Clin Invest*, 2000, 105(12), 1663-1668.

[148] Edwards, CM; Zhuang, J; Mundy, GR. The pathogenesis of the bone disease of multiple myeloma. *Bone*, 2008, 42(6), 1007-1013.

[149] Hideshima, T; Chauhan, D; Hayashi, T; Podar, K; Akiyama, M; Gupta, D; Richardson, P; Munshi, N; Anderson, KC. The biological sequelae of stromal cell-derived factor-1alpha in multiple myeloma. *Mol Cancer Ther*, 2002, 1(7), 539-544.

[150] Nefedova, Y; Cheng, P; Alsina, M; Dalton, WS; Gabrilovich, DI. Involvement of Notch-1 signaling in bone marrow stroma-mediated de novo drug resistance of myeloma and other malignant lymphoid cell lines. *Blood*, 2004, 103(9), 3503-3510.

[151] Alsayed, Y; Ngo, H; Runnels, J; Leleu, X; Singha, UK; Pitsillides, CM; Spencer, JA; Kimlinger, T; Ghobrial, JM; Jia, X; et al., Mechanisms of regulation of CXCR4/SDF-1 (CXCL12)-dependent migration and homing in multiple myeloma. *Blood*, 2007, 109(7), 2708-2717.

[152] Sanz-Rodriguez, F; Hidalgo, A; Teixido, J. Chemokine stromal cell-derived factor-1alpha modulates VLA-4 integrin-mediated multiple myeloma cell adhesion to CS-1/ fibronectin and VCAM-1. *Blood*, 2001, 97(2), 346-351.

[153] Olechnowicz, SW; Edwards, CM. Contributions of the host microenvironment to cancer-induced bone disease. *Cancer Res*, 2014, 74(6), 1625-1631.

[154] Garayoa, M; Garcia, JL; Santamaria, C; Garcia-Gomez, A; Blanco, JF; Pandiella, A; Hernandez, JM; Sanchez-Guijo, FM; del Canizo, MC; Gutierrez, NC; et al., Mesenchymal stem cells from multiple myeloma patients display distinct genomic profile as compared with those from normal donors. *Leukemia*, 2009, 23(8), 1515-1527.

[155] Toscani, D; Bolzoni, M; Accardi, F; Aversa, F; Giuliani, N. The osteoblastic niche in the context of multiple myeloma. *Ann N Y Acad Sci*, 2015, 1335, 45-62.

[156] Camussi, G; Deregibus, MC; Tetta, C. Tumor-derived microvesicles and the cancer microenvironment. *Curr Mol Med*, 2013, 13(1), 58-67.

[157] Roccaro, AM; Sacco, A; Maiso, P; Azab, AK; Tai, YT; Reagan, M; Azab, F; Flores, LM; Campigotto, F; Weller, E; et al., BM mesenchymal stromal cell-derived exosomes facilitate multiple myeloma progression. *J Clin Invest*, 2013, 123(4), 1542-1555.

[158] Wang, W; Corrigan-Cummins, M; Barber, EA; Saleh, LM; Zingone, A; Ghafoor, A; Costello, R; Zhang, Y; Kurlander, RJ; Korde, N; et al., Aberrant Level of miRNAs in Bone Marrow Microenvironment and Peripheral Blood of Myeloma Patients and Disease Progression. *J Mol Diagn*, 2015.

[159] Wang, J; Hendrix, A; Hernot, S; Lemaire, M; De Bruyne, E; Van Valckenborgh, E; Lahoutte, T; De Wever, O; Vanderkerken, K; Menu, E. Bone marrow stromal cell-derived exosomes as communicators in drug resistance in multiple myeloma cells. *Blood*, 2014, 124(4), 555-566.

[160] Calvo, KR; Landgren, O; Roccaro, AM; Ghobrial, IM. Role of microRNAs from monoclonal gammopathy of undetermined significance to multiple myeloma. *Semin Hematol*, 2011, 48(1), 39-45.

[161] Xu, S; Cecilia Santini, G; De Veirman, K; Vande Broek, I; Leleu, X; De Becker, A; Van Camp, B; Vanderkerken, K; Van Riet, I. Upregulation of miR-135b is involved in the impaired osteogenic differentiation of mesenchymal stem cells derived from multiple myeloma patients. *PLoS One*, 2013, 8(11), e79752.

[162] Harada, S; Rodan, GA. Control of osteoblast function and regulation of bone mass. *Nature*, 2003, 423(6937), 349-355.

[163] Yamashita, T; Takahashi, N; Udagawa, N. New roles of osteoblasts involved in osteoclast differentiation. *World J Orthop*, 2012, 3(11), 175-181.

[164] Zhang, J; Niu, C; Ye, L; Huang, H; He, X; Tong, WG; Ross, J; Haug, J; Johnson, T; Feng, JQ et al., Identification of the haematopoietic stem cell niche and control of the niche size. *Nature*, 2003, 425(6960), 836-841.

[165] Giuliani, N; Rizzoli, V. Myeloma cells and bone marrow osteoblast interactions: role in the development of osteolytic lesions in multiple myeloma. *Leuk Lymphoma*, 2007, 48(12), 2323-2329.

[166] Hsu, H; Lacey, DL; Dunstan, CR; Solovyev, I; Colombero, A; Timms, E; Tan, HL; Elliott, G; Kelley, MJ; Sarosi, I. et al., Tumor necrosis factor receptor family member RANK mediates osteoclast differentiation and activation induced by osteoprotegerin ligand. *Proc Natl Acad Sci U S A*, 1999, 96(7), 3540-3545.

[167] Roux, S, Meignin, V; Quillard, J; Meduri, G; Guiochon-Mantel, A; Fermand, JP; Milgrom, E; Mariette, X. RANK (receptor activator of nuclear factor-kappaB) and RANKL expression in multiple myeloma. *Br J Haematol*, 2002, 117(1), 86-92.

[168] Pearse, RN; Sordillo, EM; Yaccoby, S; Wong, BR; Liau, DF; Colman, N; Michaeli, J; Epstein, J; Choi, Y. Multiple myeloma disrupts the TRANCE/osteoprotegerin cytokine axis to trigger bone destruction and promote tumor progression. *Proc Natl Acad Sci U S A*, 2001, 98(20), 11581-11586.

[169] Terpos, E; Szydlo, R; Apperley, JF; Hatjiharissi, E; Politou, M; Meletis, J; Viniou, N; Yataganas, X; Goldman, JM; Rahemtulla, A. Soluble receptor activator of nuclear factor kappaB ligand-osteoprotegerin ratio predicts survival in multiple myeloma: proposal for a novel prognostic index. *Blood*, 2003, 102(3), 1064-1069.

[170] Abe, M; Hiura, K; Wilde, J; Shioyasono, A; Moriyama, K; Hashimoto, T; Kido, S; Oshima, T; Shibata, H; Ozaki, S; et al., Osteoclasts enhance myeloma cell growth and survival via cell-cell contact: a vicious cycle between bone destruction and myeloma expansion. *Blood*, 2004, 104(8), 2484-2491.

[171] Roodman, GD. Pathogenesis of myeloma bone disease. *Leukemia*, 2009, 23(3), 435-441.

[172] Karadag, A; Oyajobi, BO; Apperley, JF; Russell, RG; Croucher, PI. Human myeloma cells promote the production of interleukin 6 by primary human osteoblasts. *Br J Haematol*, 2000, 108(2), 383-390.

[173] Kumar, S; Witzig, TE; Timm, M; Haug, J; Wellik, L; Kimlinger, TK; Greipp, PR; Rajkumar, SV. Bone marrow angiogenic ability and expression of angiogenic cytokines in myeloma: evidence favoring loss of marrow angiogenesis inhibitory activity with disease progression. *Blood*, 2004, 104(4), 1159-1165.

[174] Andersen, NF; Standal, T; Nielsen, JL; Heickendorff, L; Borset, M; Sorensen, FB; Abildgaard, N. Syndecan-1 and angiogenic cytokines in multiple myeloma, correlation with bone marrow angiogenesis and survival. *Br J Haematol*, 2005, 128(2), 210-217.

[175] Ria, R; Todoerti, K; Berardi, S; Coluccia, AM; De Luisi, A; Mattioli, M; Ronchetti, D; Morabito, F; Guarini, A; Petrucci, MT; et al., Gene expression profiling of bone marrow endothelial cells in patients with multiple myeloma. *Clin Cancer Res*, 2009, 15(17), 5369-5378.

[176] Podar, K; Tai, YT; Davies, FE; Lentzsch, S; Sattler, M; Hideshima, T; Lin, BK; Gupta, D; Shima, Y; Chauhan, D; et al., Vascular endothelial growth factor triggers signaling cascades mediating multiple myeloma cell growth and migration. *Blood*, 2001, 98(2), 428-435.

[177] Braga, WM; Atanackovic, D; Colleoni, GW. The role of regulatory T cells and TH17 cells in multiple myeloma. *Clin Dev Immunol*, 2012, 2012, 293479.

[178] Noonan, K; Marchionni, L; Anderson, J; Pardoll, D; Roodman, GD; Borrello, I. A novel role of IL-17-producing lymphocytes in mediating lytic bone disease in multiple myeloma. *Blood*, 2010, 116(18), 3554-3563.

[179] Bailey, SR; Nelson, MH; Himes, RA; Li, Z; Mehrotra, S; Paulos, CM. Th17 cells in cancer: the ultimate identity crisis. *Front Immunol*, 2014, 5, 276.

[180] Song, W; van der Vliet, HJ; Tai, YT; Prabhala, R; Wang, R; Podar, K; Catley, L; Shammas, MA; Anderson, KC; Balk, SP; et al., Generation of antitumor invariant natural killer T cell lines in multiple myeloma and promotion of their functions via lenalidomide: a strategy for immunotherapy. *Clin Cancer Res*, 2008, 14(21), 6955-6962.

[181] Giuliani, N; Colla, S; Sala, R; Moroni, M; Lazzaretti, M; La Monica, S; Bonomini, S; Hojden, M; Sammarelli, G; Barille, S; et al., Human myeloma cells stimulate the receptor activator of nuclear factor-kappa B ligand (RANKL) in T lymphocytes: a potential role in multiple myeloma bone disease. *Blood*, 2002, 100(13), 4615-4621.

[182] Vivier, E; Ugolini, S; Blaise, D; Chabannon, C; Brossay, L. Targeting natural killer cells and natural killer T cells in cancer. *Nat Rev Immunol*, 2012, 12(4), 239-252.

[183] Richter, J; Neparidze, N; Zhang, L; Nair, S; Monesmith, T; Sundaram, R; Miesowicz, F; Dhodapkar, KM; Dhodapkar, MV. Clinical regressions and broad immune activation following combination therapy targeting human NKT cells in myeloma. *Blood*, 2013, 121(3), 423-430.

[184] Gabrilovich, DI; Nagaraj, S. Myeloid-derived suppressor cells as regulators of the immune system. *Nat Rev Immunol*, 2009, 9(3), 162-174.

[185] Zhuang, J; Zhang, J; Lwin, ST; Edwards, JR; Edwards, CM; Mundy, GR; Yang, X. Osteoclasts in multiple myeloma are derived from Gr-1+CD11b+myeloid-derived suppressor cells. *PLoS One*, 2012, 7(11), e48871.

[186] Mantovani, A; Germano, G; Marchesi, F; Locatelli, M; Biswas, SK. Cancer-promoting tumor-associated macrophages, new vistas and open questions. *Eur J Immunol*, 2011, 41(9), 2522-2525.

[187] Scavelli, C; Nico, B; Cirulli, T; Ria, R; Di Pietro, G; Mangieri, D; Bacigalupo, A; Mangialardi, G; Coluccia, AM; Caravita, T; et al., Vasculogenic mimicry by bone marrow macrophages in patients with multiple myeloma. *Oncogene*, 2008, 27(5), 663-674.

[188] Qiang, YW; Kopantzev, E; Rudikoff, S. Insulinlike growth factor-I signaling in multiple myeloma: downstream elements, functional correlates, and pathway cross-talk. *Blood*, 2002, 99(11), 4138-4146.

[189] Solary, E; Guiguet, M; Zeller, V; Casasnovas, RO; Caillot, D; Chavanet, P; Guy, H; Mack, G. Radioimmunoassay for the measurement of serum IL-6 and its correlation with tumour cell mass parameters in multiple myeloma. *Am J Hematol*, 1992, 39(3), 163-171.

[190] Sati, HI; Apperley, JF; Greaves, M; Lawry, J; Gooding, R; Russell, RG; Croucher, PI. Interleukin-6 is expressed by plasma cells from patients with multiple myeloma and monoclonal gammopathy of undetermined significance. *Br J Haematol*, 1998, 101(2), 287-295.

[191] Ishikawa, H; Tsuyama, N; Kawano, MM. Interleukin-6-induced proliferation of human myeloma cells associated with CD45 molecules. *Int J Hematol*, 2003, 78(2), 95-105.

[192] Matsuda, T; Takahashi-Tezuka, M; Fukada, T; Okuyama, Y; Fujitani, Y; Tsukada, S; Mano, H; Hirai, H; Witte, ON; Hirano, T. Association and activation of Btk and Tec tyrosine kinases by gp130, a signal transducer of the interleukin-6 family of cytokines. *Blood*, 1995, 85(3), 627-633.

[193] Hideshima, T; Nakamura, N; Chauhan, D; Anderson, KC. Biologic sequelae of interleukin-6 induced PI3-K/Akt signaling in multiple myeloma. *Oncogene*, 2001, 20(42), 5991-6000.

[194] Tu, Y; Gardner, A; Lichtenstein, A. The phosphatidylinositol 3-kinase/AKT kinase pathway in multiple myeloma plasma cells: roles in cytokine-dependent survival and proliferative responses. *Cancer Res*, 2000, 60(23), 6763-6770.

[195] Slany, A; Haudek-Prinz, V; Meshcheryakova, A; Bileck, A; Lamm, W; Zielinski, C; Gerner, C; Drach, J. Extracellular matrix remodeling by bone marrow fibroblast-like cells correlates with disease progression in multiple myeloma. *J Proteome Res*, 2014, 13(2), 844-854.

[196] Frassanito, MA; Rao, L; Moschetta, M; Ria, R; Di Marzo, L; De Luisi, A; Racanelli, V; Catacchio, I; Berardi, S; Basile, A; et al., Bone marrow fibroblasts parallel multiple myeloma progression in patients and mice: *in vitro* and *in vivo* studies. *Leukemia*, 2014, 28(4), 904-916.

[197] Vincent, T; Mechti, N. Extracellular matrix in bone marrow can mediate drug resistance in myeloma. *Leuk Lymphoma*, 2005, 46(6), 803-811.

[198] Yang, Y; Yaccoby, S; Liu, W; Langford, JK; Pumphrey, CY; Theus, A; Epstein, J; Sanderson, RD. Soluble syndecan-1 promotes growth of myeloma tumors *in vivo*. *Blood*, 2002, 100(2), 610-617.

[199] Caers, J; Deleu, S; Belaid, Z; De Raeve, H; Van Valckenborgh, E; De Bruyne, E; Defresne, MP; Van Riet, I; Van Camp, B; Vanderkerken, K. Neighboring adipocytes participate in the bone marrow microenvironment of multiple myeloma cells. In: Leukemia. Volume, 21, edn. England, 2007, 1580-1584.

[200] Franqui-Machin, R; Wendlandt, EB; Janz, S; Zhan, F; Tricot, G. Cancer stem cells are the cause of drug resistance in multiple myeloma: fact or fiction? *Oncotarget*, 2015.

In: Horizons in Cancer Research. Volume 61
Editor: Hiroto S. Watanabe
ISBN: 978-1-63484-503-8

Chapter 4

CHOLINE METABOLISM AND INTRACELLULAR SIGNALING IN CANCER

Sandi A. Kwee*[1,2,*]*, MD, PhD
[1]The Queen's Medical Center, Hamamatsu/Queen's PET Imaging Center and Cyclotron Laboratory, Honolulu, HI, US
[2]The University of Hawaii John A. Burns School of Medicine, Honolulu, HI, US

ABSTRACT

Evidence supporting increased choline kinase expression and activity in a variety of human cancers has ignited interest in the development of techniques for assaying the citidine-diphosphocholine (Kennedy) pathway for phosphatidylcholine synthesis as a means of cancer detection and therapeutic monitoring. *In-vivo* molecular imaging modalities such as positron emission tomography (PET) and magnetic resonance spectroscopic imaging are now available for measuring the metabolic constituents of this pathway, emerging into the clinical oncology setting as a potential way to gauge tumor proliferative activity based on the essential role of this pathway for cell membrane synthesis. However, many studies have not been able to consistently show a correlation between cell proliferation and tissue measures of choline phospholipid synthesis, raising the possibility that increases in tumor choline metabolism are reflective of other aspects of tumor biology. This chapter reviews the role of choline metabolites as second messengers in cellular pathways leading to enhanced cell survival, migration, and proliferation to explore the possibility that *in-vivo* imaging of choline metabolism can be used to obtain readouts of cell signal transduction in cancer.

Keywords: choline, fluorocholine, signal transduction, cancer

---

* Corresponding author: Sandi Kwee, MD, PhD. 1301 Punchbowl St. Honolulu, HI 96814. Phone: (808) 691-5466, fax: (808) 537-7813, e-mail: kwee@hawaii.edu.

Interestingly, anti-proliferative agents can induce a decrease in intracellular phosphocholine, along with an increase in GPC level, as has been observed in breast cancer cells after treatment with chemotherapeutic agents such as paclitaxel, vincristine, colchicine, and nocodazole [14]. Docetaxel, an anti-microtubule agent used to treat breast and prostate cancer, has also been shown to decrease phosphocholine and increase GPC levels in breast cancer xenografts [15]. These concomitant changes in phosphocholine and GPC levels may be the result of a decline in tumor proliferative activity (leading to decreased phosphocholine levels) coinciding with an increase in cell membrane turnover (leading to increased GPC levels) as a consequence of mitotic disruptions caused by these agents. If measurable *in vivo*, these changes in the levels of choline metabolites could conceivably serve as biomarkers of clinical therapeutic response to cancer chemotherapy.

In-Vivo Measurement of Choline Metabolism

The recognition that choline metabolism is frequently upregulated in cancer and other diseases has fueled the development of molecular imaging techniques for assessing tissue choline metabolism *in vivo*. One technique that is currently in use clinically for assessing *in-vivo* choline metabolism is based on the implementation of proton (^{1}H) or 31-phosphorus (^{31}P) MRS on standard clinical MR imaging devices. In living tissue, this technique can simultaneously interrogate the status of multiple metabolic processes by discriminating the presence of a variety of free molecules, including choline, creatine, lactate, myoinositol, and glutamine. However, while multiple distinct choline metabolites are identifiable *in vitro* using high-resolution ^{1}H-MRS, the lower signal to noise ratio and limited separation of the chemical shift spectra afforded by *in vivo* MRS at the magnetic field strengths currently available for use in the clinical setting causes peaks in the spectra produced by intracellular choline, phosphocholine, GPC, and free phosphatidylcholine to appear overlapped (Figure 3). As a result, only a single spectral peak commonly referred to as "total choline" can be reliably distinguished on the *in-vivo* MRS spectra, representing a summation of signals from several molecules bearing the choline moiety [16]. While ^{31}P-MRS, which is based on interrogating phosphorous nuclei rather than hydrogen, can also differentiate between several distinct choline metabolites *in vitro*, this technique is limited *in vivo* to distinguishing only between phosphomonoesters and phosphodiesters (with an even lower sensitivity compared with ^{1}H MRS) [11]. These limitations in differentiating between various choline metabolites, if not surmounted, may hamper the potential clinical utility of *in vivo* MRS, since the alterations in phosphocholine and GPC metabolism resulting from cancer treatments may not necessarily be reflected by the change in "total choline" [17, 18]. Nonetheless, because of its unique ability to simultaneously assess a wide array of chemical moieties, it remains a valuable technique for inspecting the biochemistry of tumors *in vivo*.

Molecular PET Imaging of Choline Metabolism

Another technique that is available for assessing tissue choline metabolism *in vivo* is based on positron emission tomography (PET), a scintigraphic technology for detecting and measuring the transport and metabolism of biochemical tracers labeled with short-lived positron-emitter isotopes. Both carbon-11 labeled and fluorine-18 labeled substrates of CK have been developed for *in vivo* PET imaging of tissue phosphocholine synthesis [19, 20].

The most well-studied of the [^{18}F]-labeled derivatives of choline, fluoromethylcholine (FCH), is a specific substrate for CK that is metabolically trapped in the cytoplasm by phosphorylation to produce [^{18}F]-phosphofluorocholine (phospho-FCH) at rates approaching the endogenous activity of this enzyme [21]. Because phospho-FCH is resistant to further metabolism, it accumulates within the cytoplasm, unlike carbon-11 choline which is further metabolized to betaine or other CDP-choline metabolites. This may result in PET images of tumors with very high tumor-to-background ratios even in organs with high constitutive choline metabolism such as the liver (Figure 4). The metabolic trapping of FCH may also allow static PET to serve as biomarkers of *in vivo* CK activity or phosphocholine synthesis.

Because "total choline" measured by MRS *in vivo* does reflect contributions from multiple distinct choline metabolites, it may not come as a surprise if this spectroscopic measure correlates poorly with PET measures of tissue choline metabolism in some disease instances.

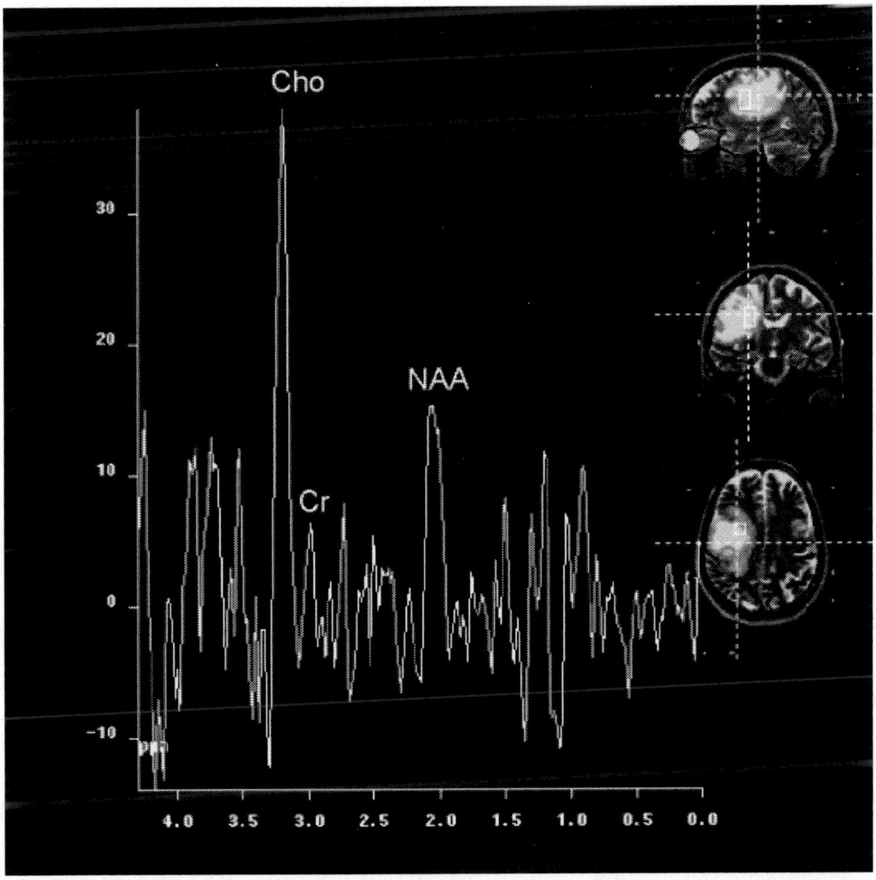

Figure 3. *In-vivo* 1H-magnetic resonance spectroscopy. Single-voxel spectroscopy of malignant glioma showing increased total choline at 3.18 ppm and decreased N-acetyl-aspartate at 1.98 ppm. Individual choline metabolites such as phosphocholine or glycerophosphocholine are not distinguishable on *in-vivo* proton spectroscopy.

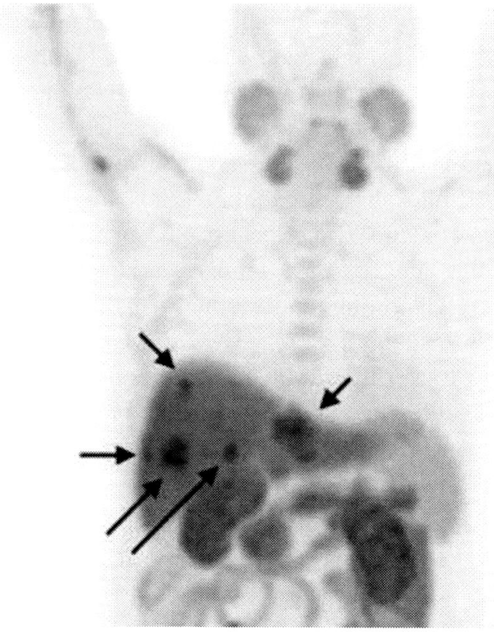

Figure 4. PET image showing increased choline metabolism in liver cancer. Maximum intensity pixel PET image rendering depicts the biological distribution of fluorine-18 fluorocholine, a radiolabeled analog of choline, at approximately 30 minutes after its intravenous injection. Multiple rounded foci of increased activity (arrows) are evident in the liver. Biopsy confirmed the presence of multifocal hepatocellular carcinoma.

For example, the results of FCH PET and ^{1}H-MRS imaging of a benign "tumefactive" demyelinating brain lesion may appear "discordant" in that that such lesions may not show significant FCH uptake despite significantly increased levels of total choline metabolites measured by *in vivo* ^{1}H-MRS imaging [22]. These apparently discordant MRS and PET findings may be the consequence of increased cell membrane turnover (leading to increased free choline and GPC) in the absence of significantly increased membrane proliferation (which would be reflected by an increase in phosphocholine levels and therefore increased FCH uptake). This may in fact be what is occurring metabolically in demyelinating disease.

In contrast, malignant high-grade gliomas can demonstrate a direct correspondence between tumor FCH uptake on PET and increased total choline metabolite levels on MRS. In such tissues, increased tumoral FCH uptake would be expected as reflecting an increased production of phosphocholine to meet the anabolic demands of increased tumor cell membrane synthesis [22]. Based on these examples, MRS imaging and PET might serve as complementary imaging modalities in the clinical diagnostic setting.

Tumor detection based on the intracellular trapping of FCH by the mechanism of phosphorylation is analogous to the metabolic fate of [^{18}F]-fluorodeoxy-D-glucose (FDG). FDG is the most widely used clinical PET imaging agent. Although FDG PET has useful clinical applications in neurology and cardiovascular disease, it was its role in oncology for detecting, diagnosing, and staging cancer that fueled the growth of PET in clinical practice over the past 20 years. FDG is a radiolabeled glucose analog that undergoes intracellular phosphorylation by hexokinase to produce 6-phospho-FDG, enabling PET to produce images reflecting the first enzymatic step of glycolysis. While increased glycolysis in malignancy (i.e., the Warburg effect) is associated with aggressive biological behavior in some cancers, there is little evidence to suggest that glycolytic compounds are no more than metabolic substrates in this regard [23].

In contrast, phospholipids are recognized as often serving dual functional and structural roles, and have been implicated as effector molecules in the activation of potent mitogenic pathways such as those involving protein kinase C, mitogen activated protein kinase (MAPK) and phosphatidylinositol 3-kinase (PI3K) [24-26]. Therefore, in cancer, it is worth considering whether the increased metabolism of choline in tumors is indicative of pathway activation in addition to, or rather than, phospholipid membrane proliferation.

While biochemical similarities between FCH and FDG exist, these two compounds clearly serve as imaging agents for very distinct, and potentially independent, tumorigenic pathways. In support of the independence between glucose and choline metabolism, one study has shown that RNA-interference mediated silencing of CK can terminate choline uptake by breast tumor cells without significantly altering radiolabeled FDG uptake [27]. Conversely, several tumor types known to be elusive to detection by FDG PET have proven detectable on the basis of radio-labeled choline uptake, most notably prostate cancer for which FCH PET/CT has shown significant promise for disease detection, staging, treatment planning, and measurement of therapeutic outcome [28-35]. However, while the high detection rate of prostate tumors by FCH PET/CT implies that there are significant alterations in choline metabolism in prostate cancer, the actual role of choline metabolism in the pathogenesis of this and other malignancies remains poorly understood.

Tumor Choline Metabolism May Not Correlate with Tumor Growth

Cell proliferation involves duplication of all cellular constituents, including DNA, proteins, and lipids. Given that the synthesis of phosphatidylcholine occurs primarily during S phase, the measurement of choline metabolism was originally thought to provide an assessment of cell proliferation. However, comparisons between tumor choline metabolism and cellular markers of proliferation have not uniformly confirmed this assertion, with several studies reporting a marked discordance between measures of choline metabolism and cellular proliferation [5, 6, 11, 36].

In one study, no significant correlations were noted between markers of cell proliferation (mitotic index, Ki-67 labeling, and S-phase fraction) and tissue levels of phosphocholine, GPC, phosphoethanolamine, and glycerophosphorylethanolamine as measured by ^{31}P-MRS in tumor tissues from patients with breast cancer [6]. Another study examining a range of normal and transformed cell lines found that rates of cell division measured *in vitro* were poorly correlated with cellular phosphocholine levels as well as the ratios of phosphocholine to GPC on ^{1}H- MRS [11]. And while the progression from normal to increasingly malignant cell phenotype in breast cancer was associated with a progressive increase in intracellular phosphocholine content, the changes in cellular metabolite levels themselves did not correlate significantly with cell doubling time [5]. And while one study of malignant breast tumor extracts found tissue CK activity to be associated with tumor grade, there were no significant correlations with tumor cell Ki-67 labeling, an immunohistochemical marker of cell proliferation [36].

The results of clinical research using PET and MRS to study cancer largely echo the results of these *in-vitro* studies. In one clinical feasibility study evaluating ^{11}C-choline PET in breast cancer, no significant correlation was noted between the levels of ^{11}C-choline uptake in breast tumors and estrogen and progesterone receptor status, HER-2/neu status, nodal status, or tumor Ki-67 labeling [37]. A clinical study of prostate cancer also found that tumor uptake of ^{11}C-choline correlated poorly with tumor Ki-67 labeling in the prostate specimen [38]. However, one study applying ^{1}H-NMR to post-surgical prostate specimens reported a moderate correlation between Ki-67 labeling and the ratio of total choline to creatine, although as with most *in vivo* MRS studies, individual spectral peaks reflecting the independent contributions of phosphocholine and GPC could not be resolved separately [13]. Conflicting results have also been reported in MRS studies of malignant gliomas, although some of the discrepancies may be related to variations in choline metabolism across the tumor grades examined in the different studies [10, 39, 40]. Nonetheless, with insufficient evidence supporting an association between choline metabolism and cell proliferation, one must consider the possibility that increases in choline metabolism found in cancer are driven by something other than the metabolic demand for phosphatidylcholine in support of cell membrane production and tumor cell proliferation.

A potential mechanism to explain how the upregulation of tumor choline metabolism may occur independently of cell proliferation was provided in a study by Glunde and colleagues [41]. In this study, hypoxic stress was shown to upregulate CK expression, leading to significantly increased levels of phosphocholine in prostate cancer cells. The mechanism leading to upregulated CK expression in this hypoxia model was found to involve increasing expression of hypoxia inducible factor 1 (HIF-1), which was shown to bind as a transcription factor to the putative promoter region of the CK-alpha gene in a human prostate cancer cell line. These findings suggest that the measurement of intracellular phosphocholine could potentially serve as an indicator of treatment-resistance related to tumor hypoxia, since hypoxia increases tumor cell resistance to radiation and chemotherapy.

Role of Choline Metabolites in Cell Signal Transduction

While not widely recognized, multiple lines of research have generated results suggesting that phosphocholine may act directly, or as a second messenger, in tumorigenic signaling. One of the earliest of these studies found that phosphocholine administration was sufficient to stimulate DNA synthesis in quiescent NIH3T3 fibroblasts, causing a five-fold increase in DNA synthesis, as well as restoring proliferative potential to cells treated with the CK inhibitor hemicholinium-3 [42]. Notably, other compounds similar to phosphocholine, including choline and phosphoethanolamine did not reproduce this mitogenic effect, which is compelling since CK also catalyzes the phosphorylation of ethanolamine.

In another early study, NIH3T3 fibroblasts stimulated by platelet derived growth factor or fibroblast growth factor demonstrated an increase in intracellular levels of phosphocholine that coincided with the activation of Raf-1 and the mitogen-activated protein kinase (MAPK) pathway [43]. Pathway activation was abrogated through direct inhibition of CK, implying that phosphocholine was necessry for growth factor mediated activation of Raf-1 and MAPK. CK inhibition in CK-overexpressing NIH3T3 cells was also shown to block insulin and insulin-like growth factor 1 stimulated DNA synthesis, further implicating phosphocholine as a mediator of mitogenic activity [44]. Again it was noted that, in contrast to phosphocholine, other phospholipid metabolites do not appear to be involved in activating these mitogenic pathways [45]. Furthermore, lymphocytes stimulated by IL-2 demonstrated a closely timed increase in phosphocholine and DNA synthesis that preceded the production of other choline metabolites and phospholipids, lending further support of phosphocholine as the metabolite responsible for initiating a mitogenic response [45]. Based on these *in-vitro* observations, it is worth speculating that the measurement of tissue phosphocholine synthesis, as made feasible *in vivo* by PET or MRS, may potentially provide a gauge for the activation of tumor signaling pathways.

REGULATION OF CHOLINE METABOLISM BY RAS AND RAS-LIKE ONCOGENES

Ras oncogenes encode for GTP-ase proteins that drive multiple tumorigenic pathways. Mutations leading to Ras activation, which have been found in the majority of human cancers, have been shown to cause partial or complete transformation along with activation of the CDP-choline pathway [46-48]. Teegarden et al. transfected mouse embryo fibroblast cells with H-ras and subsequently noted significant increases in the intracellular levels of phosphocholine, which are likely due to upregulated CK activity [48]. Ronen et al. also observed that overexpression of Ras led to an increase in the levels of phosphocholine in NIH3T3 cells, and further noted that this increase in phosphocholine synthesis did not correlate with changes in cell proliferation rate or cell cycle distribution [49]. Confirming that this was related to CDP-choline pathway metabolism, Macara et al. elucidated that the increased level of phosphocholine in Ras-transformed cells was primarily due to an enhancement of CK activity, and not hydrolysis of phosphatidylcholine by PLC [50].

Other GTPase proteins have also been shown affect on CK activity, particularly the Ras-homologous (Rho) GTPases, which is another family of GTPase proteins associated with tumorigenesis [51]. Since there is interest in the development of drugs that modulate GTP-ase activity as novel anti-cancer agents, PET and MRS-based measurement of choline metabolism may have potential pre-clinical and clinical value for monitoring the effects of these agents on tumors known to over-express Ras.

EFFECT OF MOLECULES DOWNSTREAM OF RAS ON CHOLINE METABOLISM

Ras proteins regulate a number of well-known effector molecules for tumor growth and survival, including the serine-threonine protein kinase Raf-1, the exchange factor for other GTPases Ral-GDS, and the lipid kinase PI3K. Activated Ras, bound to GTP, interacts with each of these effector molecules to initiate signaling cascades leading to tumor progression and metastasis. In a series of experiments, Ramirez de Molina et al. examined the independent role of each of these Ras effectors in regulating the activity of CK in Ras-transfected NIH3T3 cells [46]. Using mutants for Ras that selectively interact with the RAf-1,

Ral-GDS, or PI3K effector pathways, they found that Raf-1 activation led to only a small increase in CK activity, while Ral-GDS and PI3K activation exerted greater effects on CK activation. Incubation with PD98059, a specific inhibitor of MEK1, reduced MAPK pathway activation without significantly altering CK activity [46].

These observations suggest that Ras induced CK activation is more dependent on the Ral-GDS and PI3K pathways and less on the MAPK pathway. The requirement of phosphocholine to activate MAPK is compatible with these observations [26, 43]. Notably, activation of Ral-GDS or PI3K individually did not reproduce the full level of Ras-induced CK activation in these studies, suggesting that the recruitment of multiple signaling pathways may be required to fully activate CK. These results lend support for measuring *in vivo* tumor synthesis of phosphocholine with PET or MRS to ascertain the net activation status of these Ras effectors.

Effect of Mitogen Activated Protein Kinase Pathways on Choline Metabolism

MAPK proteins constitute a family of serine-threonine kinases involved in cell proliferation, differentiation, apoptosis, survival and stress response. Raf and ERK are among the most recognized upstream effectors of these proteins. The finding that Raf [47] and ERK-1/2 [52] can increase CK activity, suggests that the measurement of phosphocholine synthesis using PET or MRS could serve as a potential marker of MAPK activation. While MAPK itself appears to have a limited effect on CK activation [46], p42/p44 MAPK does appear to cause Sp3 transcription factor binding to the promoter region of the gene that encodes for CTP: phosphocholine citidylyltransferase (CTPT), the rate limiting enzyme in phosphatidylcholine synthesis [53]. Because phosphocholine serves as the primary substrate for CTPT, the measurement of phosphocholine levels by MRS will depend on both CK and CTPT activity.

In contrast, FCH is phosphorylated by CK but does not serve as a substrate of CTPT, allowing PET to be a more specific marker of tumor CK activity as a potential indicator of MAPK activation. The observation that the MAPK inhibitor U0126 causes a time dependent decrease in the levels of phosphocholine in breast cancer cells that precedes any change in cell-cycle distribution has led to the suggestion that measurement of phosphocholine levels can potentially serve as a marker for monitoring MAPK signaling blockade [54]. However, since MAPK activation has been shown to have little direct effect on CK activity [46], this effect of MAPK on phosphocholine levels may be related to PLC activation [55]. Further research is needed to consolidate the understanding of how phosphocholine synthesis can be used as a marker of activation along various levels of MAPK signaling pathway.

Interactions between the PI3K/Akt Pathway and Choline Metabolism

PI3K is another major effector in Ras-mediated transformation that has been proposed as a potential target for molecularly-targeted anti-cancer treatment. A study by Beloueche-

Babari et al. employed ^{31}P MRS to measure the effect of PI3K inhibition by the prototype PI3K inhibitor LY294002 on cellular phospholipid content [56]. In this study, treatment of MDA-MB-231, MCF-7, and Hs578T cell lines with LY294002 was shown to cause a 2-fold decrease in phosphocholine levels, as well as a 5-fold increase in GPC levels. Similar effects on phosphocholine and GPC metabolism have been reported as a consequence of more conventional anti-microtubule chemotherapy [14, 15]. CK has also been shown to be an important factor for the activation of Akt by PI3K. Akt, also known as protein kinase B, is a serine/threonine kinase involved in various cellular processes important in cell growth and survival. The phosphorylation of Akt at multiple sites is mediated by PI3K, and is required for its full activation [57]. However, inhibition of CK activity by small molecular inhibitors or siRNA has been shown to reduce Akt phosphorylation in a PI3K-independent manner, supporting a role for phosphocholine in of the activation of Akt along this pathway [58]. Based on these findings, molecular imaging assessments of tumoral phosphocholine synthesis using PET and MRS could potentially serve as indirect indicators of Akt/PI3K activation.

Conclusion

An increase in cellular choline metabolism is a common molecular trait of malignant tumors. Molecular imaging techniques to quantify phosphocholine production in living tissues are ready for use in the clinical setting. Mitogenic signal transduction appears to involve phosphocholine synthesis to a degree that cannot be fully explained on the basis of cell membrane turnover. Specifically, the activation of CK is required for growth-factor mediated activation of Raf-1 and MAPK, as well as for the activation of Akt by PI3K, raising the possibility that PET and MRS can be used to gauge the level of activation of these pathways. Furthermore, the activation of Ras and other GTPase proteins, as well as their downstream effectors, causes increased phosphocholine synthetic activity, suggesting that measuring phosphocholine synthesis with PET or MRS can potentially serve as a means for monitoring the effects of cancer treatments targeting these pathways.

References

[1] Zeisel, S. H. Choline: critical role during fetal development and dietary requirements in adults. *Annu. Rev. Nutr.* 2006;26:229-250.

[2] Nakagami, K., Uchida, T., Ohwada, S. et al. Increased choline kinase activity and elevated phosphocholine levels in human colon cancer. *Jpn. J. Cancer Res.* Apr. 1999; 90(4):419-424.

[3] Ramirez de Molina, A., Rodriguez-Gonzalez, A., Gutierrez, R. et al. Overexpression of choline kinase is a frequent feature in human tumor-derived cell lines and in lung, prostate, and colorectal human cancers. *Biochemical and biophysical research communications.* Aug. 23 2002;296(3):580-583.

[4] Ackerstaff, E., Glunde, K., Bhujwalla, Z. M. Choline phospholipid metabolism: a target in cancer cells? *J. Cell. Biochem.* Oct. 15 2003;90(3):525-533.

[5] Aboagye, E. O., Bhujwalla, Z. M. Malignant transformation alters membrane choline phospholipid metabolism of human mammary epithelial cells. *Cancer Res.* Jan. 1 1999; 59(1):80-84.

[6] Smith, T. A., Bush, C., Jameson, C. et al. Phospholipid metabolites, prognosis and proliferation in human breast carcinoma. *NMR Biomed.* Sep.-Oct.1993;6(5):318-323.

[7] Podo, F. Tumour phospholipid metabolism. *NMR Biomed.* Nov. 1999;12(7):413-439.

[8] Ackerstaff, E., Pflug, B. R., Nelson, J. B., Bhujwalla, Z. M. Detection of increased choline compounds with proton nuclear magnetic resonance spectroscopy subsequent to malignant transformation of human prostatic epithelial cells. *Cancer Res.* May 1 2001; 61(9):3599-3603.

[9] Glunde, K., Ackerstaff, E., Natarajan, K., Artemov, D., Bhujwalla, Z. M. Real-time changes in 1H and 31P NMR spectra of malignant human mammary epithelial cells during treatment with the anti-inflammatory agent indomethacin. *Magn. Reson. Med.* Nov. 2002;48(5):819-825.

[10] Righi, V., Roda, J. M., Paz, J. et al. 1H HR-MAS and genomic analysis of human tumor biopsies discriminate between high and low grade astrocytomas. *NMR Biomed.* Jul. 2009;22(6):629-637.

[11] Bhakoo, K. K., Williams, S. R., Florian, C. L., Land, H., Noble, M. D. Immortalization and transformation are associated with specific alterations in choline metabolism. *Cancer Res.* Oct. 15 1996;56(20):4630-4635.

[12] Glunde, K., Jie, C., Bhujwalla, Z. M. Molecular causes of the aberrant choline phospholipid metabolism in breast cancer. *Cancer research.* Jun. 15 2004;64(12):4270-4276.

[13] Swanson, M. G., Vigneron, D. B., Tabatabai, Z. L. et al. Proton HR-MAS spectroscopy and quantitative pathologic analysis of MRI/3D-MRSI-targeted postsurgical prostate tissues. *Magn. Reson. Med.* Nov. 2003;50(5):944-954.

[14] Sterin, M., Cohen, J. S., Mardor, Y., Berman, E., Ringel, I. Levels of phospholipid metabolites in breast cancer cells treated with antimitotic drugs: a 31P-magnetic resonance spectroscopy study. *Cancer Res.* Oct. 15 2001;61(20):7536-7543.

[15] Morse, D. L., Raghunand, N., Sadarangani, P. et al. Response of choline metabolites to docetaxel therapy is quantified *in vivo* by localized (31)P MRS of human breast cancer xenografts and *in vitro* by high-resolution (31)P NMR spectroscopy of cell extracts. *Magn. Reson. Med.* Aug. 2007;58(2):270-280.

[16] Miller, B. L., Chang, L., Booth, R. et al. *In vivo* 1H MRS choline: correlation with *in vitro* chemistry/histology. *Life sciences.* 1996;58(22):1929-1935.

[17] Baek, H. M., Chen, J. H., Nie, K. et al. Predicting pathologic response to neoadjuvant chemotherapy in breast cancer by using MR imaging and quantitative 1H MR spectroscopy. *Radiology.* Jun. 2009;251(3):653-662.

[18] Thomas, M. A., Lipnick, S., Velan, S. S. et al. Investigation of breast cancer using two-dimensional MRS. *NMR Biomed.* Jan. 2009;22(1):77-91.

[19] Hara, T., Kosaka, N., Kishi, H. Development of (18)F-fluoroethylcholine for cancer imaging with PET: synthesis, biochemistry, and prostate cancer imaging. *J. Nucl. Med.* Feb. 2002;43(2):187-199.

[20] Hara, T., Kosaka, N., Shinoura, N., Kondo, T. PET imaging of brain tumor with [methyl-11C]choline. *J. Nucl. Med.* Jun. 1997;38(6):842-847.

[21] Bansal, A., Shuyan, W., Hara, T., Harris, R. A., Degrado, T. R. Biodisposition and metabolism of [(18)F]fluorocholine in 9L glioma cells and 9L glioma-bearing fisher rats. *Eur. J. Nucl. Med. Mol. Imaging.* Feb. 9 2008.

[22] Kwee, S. A., Coel, M. N., Lim, J., Ko, J. P. Combined use of F-18 fluorocholine positron emission tomography and magnetic resonance spectroscopy for brain tumor evaluation. *Journal of neuroimaging: official journal of the American Society of Neuroimaging.* Jul. 2004;14(3):285-289.

[23] Vander Heiden, M. G., Cantley, L. C., Thompson, C. B. Understanding the Warburg effect: the metabolic requirements of cell proliferation. *Science.* May 22 2009;324 (5930):1029-1033.

[24] Ghosh, S., Strum, J. C., Bell, R. M. Lipid biochemistry: functions of glycerolipids and sphingolipids in cellular signaling. *Faseb J.* Jan. 1997;11(1):45-50.

[25] Ghosh, S., Strum, J. C., Sciorra, V. A., Daniel, L., Bell, R. M. Raf-1 kinase possesses distinct binding domains for phosphatidylserine and phosphatidic acid. Phosphatidic acid regulates the translocation of Raf-1 in 12-O-tetradecanoylphorbol-13-acetate-stimulated Madin-Darby canine kidney cells. *J. Biol. Chem.* Apr. 5 1996;271(14):8472-8480.

[26] Yalcin, A., Clem, B., Makoni, S. et al. Selective inhibition of choline kinase simultaneously attenuates MAPK and PI3K/AKT signaling. *Oncogene.* Jan. 7 2010;29 (1):139-149.

[27] Nimmagadda, S., Glunde, K., Pomper, M. G., Bhujwalla, Z. M. Pharmacodynamic markers for choline kinase down-regulation in breast cancer cells. *Neoplasia.* May 2009;11(5):477-484.

[28] Wang, H., Vees, H., Miralbell, R. et al. 18F-fluorocholine PET-guided target volume delineation techniques for partial prostate re-irradiation in local recurrent prostate cancer. *Radiother. Oncol.* Nov. 2009;93(2):220-225.

[29] Pinkawa, M., Attieh, C., Piroth, M. D. et al. Dose-escalation using intensity-modulated radiotherapy for prostate cancer--evaluation of the dose distribution with and without 18F-choline PET-CT detected simultaneous integrated boost. *Radiother. Oncol.* Nov. 2009;93(2):213-219.

[30] Kwee, S. A., Coel, M. N., Ly, B. H., Lim, J. (18)F-Choline PET/CT imaging of RECIST measurable lesions in hormone refractory prostate cancer. *Ann. Nucl. Med.* Aug. 2009;23(6):541-548.

[31] Pelosi, E., Arena, V., Skanjeti, A. et al. Role of whole-body 18F-choline PET/CT in disease detection in patients with biochemical relapse after radical treatment for prostate cancer. *Radiol. Med.* Sep. 2008;113(6):895-904.

[32] Igerc, I., Kohlfurst, S., Gallowitsch, H. J. et al. The value of 18F-choline PET/CT in patients with elevated PSA-level and negative prostate needle biopsy for localisation of prostate cancer. *Eur. J. Nucl. Med. Mol. Imaging.* May 2008;35(5):976-983.

[33] Beheshti, M., Vali, R., Waldenberger, P. et al. Detection of bone metastases in patients with prostate cancer by 18F fluorocholine and 18F fluoride PET-CT: a comparative study. *Eur. J. Nucl. Med. Mol. Imaging.* Oct. 2008;35(10):1766-1774.

[34] Price, D. T., Coleman, R. E., Liao, R. P., Robertson, C. N., Polascik, T. J., DeGrado, T. R. Comparison of [18 F]fluorocholine and [18 F]fluorodeoxyglucose for positron emission tomography of androgen dependent and androgen independent prostate cancer. *J. Urol.* Jul. 2002;168(1):273-280.

[35] Kwee, S. A., DeGrado, T. R., Talbot, J. N., Gutman, F., Coel, M. N. Cancer imaging with fluorine-18-labeled choline derivatives. *Semin. Nucl. Med.* Nov. 2007;37(6):420-428.

[36] Ramirez de Molina, A., Gutierrez, R., Ramos, M. A. et al. Increased choline kinase activity in human breast carcinomas: clinical evidence for a potential novel antitumor strategy. *Oncogene.* Jun. 20 2002;21(27):4317-4322.

[37] Contractor, K. B., Kenny, L. M., Stebbing, J. et al. [11C]choline positron emission tomography in estrogen receptor-positive breast cancer. *Clin. Cancer Res.* Sep. 1 2009; 15(17):5503-5510.

[38] Breeuwsma, A. J., Pruim, J., Jongen, M. M. et al. *In vivo* uptake of [11C]choline does not correlate with cell proliferation in human prostate cancer. *Eur. J. Nucl. Med. Mol. Imaging.* Jun. 2005;32(6):668-673.

[39] McKnight, T. R., Lamborn, K. R., Love, T. D. et al. Correlation of magnetic resonance spectroscopic and growth characteristics within Grades II and III gliomas. *J. Neurosurg.* Apr. 2007;106(4):660-666.

[40] Matsumura, A., Isobe, T., Anno, I., Takano, S., Kawamura, H. Correlation between choline and MIB-1 index in human gliomas. A quantitative in proton MR spectroscopy study. *J. Clin. Neurosci.* May 2005;12(4):416-420.

[41] Glunde, K., Shah, T., Winnard, P. T., Jr. et al. Hypoxia regulates choline kinase expression through hypoxia-inducible factor-1 alpha signaling in a human prostate cancer model. *Cancer Res.* Jan. 1 2008;68(1):172-180.

[42] Cuadrado, A., Carnero, A., Dolfi, F., Jimenez, B., Lacal, J. C. Phosphorylcholine: a novel second messenger essential for mitogenic activity of growth factors. *Oncogene.* Nov. 1993;8(11):2959-2968.

[43] Jimenez, B., del Peso, L., Montaner, S., Esteve, P., Lacal, J. C. Generation of phosphorylcholine as an essential event in the activation of Raf-1 and MAP-kinases in growth factors-induced mitogenic stimulation. *J. Cell. Biochem.* Jan. 1995;57(1):141-149.

[44] Chung, T., Huang, J. S., Mukherjee, J. J., Crilly, K. S., Kiss, Z. Expression of human choline kinase in NIH 3T3 fibroblasts increases the mitogenic potential of insulin and insulin-like growth factor I. *Cell Signal.* May 2000;12(5):279-288.

[45] Rodriguez-Gonzalez, A., Ramirez de Molina, A., Fernandez, F., Lacal, J. C. Choline kinase inhibition induces the increase in ceramides resulting in a highly specific and selective cytotoxic antitumoral strategy as a potential mechanism of action. *Oncogene.* Oct. 28 2004;23(50):8247-8259.

[46] Ramirez de Molina, A., Penalva, V., Lucas, L., Lacal, J. C. Regulation of choline kinase activity by Ras proteins involves Ral-GDS and PI3K. *Oncogene.* Jan. 31 2002; 21(6):937-946.

[47] Ratnam, S., Kent, C. Early increase in choline kinase activity upon induction of the H-ras oncogene in mouse fibroblast cell lines. *Arch. Biochem. Biophys.* Nov. 10 1995;323 (2):313-322.

[48] Teegarden, D., Taparowsky, E. J., Kent, C. Altered phosphatidylcholine metabolism in C3H10T1/2 cells transfected with the Harvey-ras oncogene. *J. Biol. Chem.* Apr. 15 1990;265(11):6042-6047.

[49] Ronen, S. M., Jackson, L. E., Beloueche, M., Leach, M. O. Magnetic resonance detects changes in phosphocholine associated with Ras activation and inhibition in NIH 3T3 cells. *Br. J. Cancer.* Mar. 2 2001;84(5):691-696.

[50] Macara, I. G. Elevated phosphocholine concentration in ras-transformed NIH 3T3 cells arises from increased choline kinase activity, not from phosphatidylcholine breakdown. *Mol. Cell. Biol.* Jan. 1989;9(1):325-328.

[51] Benitah, S. A., Valeron, P. F., van Aelst, L., Marshall, C. J., Lacal, J. C. Rho GTPases in human cancer: an unresolved link to upstream and downstream transcriptional regulation. *Biochim. Biophys. Acta.* Dec. 17 2004;1705(2):121-132.

[52] Liu, D., Hutchinson, O. C., Osman, S., Price, P., Workman, P., Aboagye, E. O. Use of radiolabelled choline as a pharmacodynamic marker for the signal transduction inhibitor geldanamycin. *Br. J. Cancer.* Sep. 23 2002;87(7):783-789.

[53] Bakovic, M., Waite, K., Vance, D. E. Oncogenic Ha-Ras transformation modulates the transcription of the CTP:phosphocholine cytidylyltransferase alpha gene via p42/44MAPK and transcription factor Sp3. *J. Biol. Chem.* Apr. 25 2003;278(17):14753-14761.

[54] Beloueche-Babari, M., Jackson, L. E., Al-Saffar, N. M., Workman, P., Leach, M. O., Ronen, S. M. Magnetic resonance spectroscopy monitoring of mitogen-activated protein kinase signaling inhibition. *Cancer Res.* Apr. 15 2005;65(8):3356-3363.

[55] Lopez-Barahona, M., Kaplan, P. L., Cornet, M. E. et al. Kinetic evidence of a rapid activation of phosphatidylcholine hydrolysis by Ki-ras oncogene. Possible involvement in late steps of the mitogenic cascade. *J. Biol. Chem.* Jun. 5 1990;265(16):9022-9026.

[56] Beloueche-Babari, M., Jackson, L. E., Al-Saffar, N. M. et al. Identification of magnetic resonance detectable metabolic changes associated with inhibition of phosphoinositide 3-kinase signaling in human breast cancer cells. *Mol. Cancer Ther.* Jan. 2006;5(1):187-196.

[57] Alessi, D. R., Deak, M., Casamayor, A. et al. 3-Phosphoinositide-dependent protein kinase-1 (PDK1): structural and functional homology with the Drosophila DSTPK61 kinase. *Curr. Biol.* Oct. 1 1997;7(10):776-789.

[58] Chua, B. T., Gallego-Ortega, D., Ramirez de Molina, A., Ullrich, A., Lacal, J. C., Downward, J. Regulation of Akt(ser473) phosphorylation by Choline kinase in breast carcinoma cells. *Mol. Cancer.* 2009;8:131.

In: Horizons in Cancer Research. Volume 61
Editor: Hiroto S. Watanabe
ISBN: 978-1-63484-503-8

Chapter 5

THE CORRELATION BETWEEN ANATOMIC SITES OF THE MELANOMA DISTRIBUTION ON THE UPPER BACK AREA AND LACK OF SUNSCREEN APPLICATION

Borut Poljšak, PhD, Martina Oder, Jure Polak, Andrej Starc, PhD, Tina Levec and Raja Dahmane*, MD, PhD
University of Ljubljana,
Faculty of Health Sciences, Ljubljana, Slovenia

ABSTRACT

Background/Objectives: The magnitude of sun exposure during childhood is a major risk factor in the development of skin cancer. Adolescents have the lowest skin protection rates of all age groups, especially in the time period of 10 to 18 years when children and teenagers do not allow their parents to cream them and they usually do not have partners who would apply sun cream on their back. The aim of our study was to investigate the possible correlation between anatomic melanoma distribution on the specific back area and lack of sunscreen application. Participants/Methods: 25 young adult volunteers in the age interval 19-35 years were randomly sampled and asked to apply the sunscreen on their back. In the second part of the study the visual observation of pictures from diverse studies showing malignant melanoma anatomical distributions were compared in order to assess the possible correlation between the observed lack of sun protection on the upper back areas and upper back malignant melanoma incidence. Results and conclusions: The results revealed that the sunscreen is not optimally applied on the back. This often missed and hard-to-see area is a common location of the increased melanoma skin cancer incidence. It is important to remember that one needs help to apply sunscreen appropriately and fully cover one's back, especially its upper part.

* Corresponding author: Raja Dahmane, MD, PhD, Faculty of Health Sciences, Zdravstvena pot 5, 1000 Ljubljana, Slovenia, Phone: + 386 40 900 878, Fax: +386 1 300 11 19, E-mail: raja.dahmane@guest.arnes.si.

Keywords: malignant melanoma; anatomic site distribution of malignant melanoma; sunscreen

INTRODUCTION

Skin cancer remains a major public health problem. Its incidence is increasing more rapidly than that of all other kinds of cancer. Approximately 130,000 malignant melanomas (MM) occur globally each year, substantially contributing to the mortality rates in fair-skinned populations. It is estimated that 66,000 deaths occur annually from MM and other skin cancers [1]. It is necessary to slow down this trend through preventive steps in order to reduce morbidity and mortality rates and to decrease the financial burden on the health systems [2]. In the United States, primary prevention of melanoma and nonmelanoma skin cancer has focused on encouraging sensible sun-exposure behaviors, while secondary prevention consists of a yearly national campaign that promotes skin awareness, self-examination and free examinations to detect evolving tumors, sponsored by the American Academy of Dermatology and the American Cancer Society [3]. The longing of our western society for a "healthy tanning" as well as the unbroken trend to spend the holidays in sunny regions lead to the fact that human skin is increasingly exposed to ultraviolet radiation (UV) and its detrimental effects [4]. Regular sunscreen use prevents cutaneous squamous cell carcinoma in long term, but the effect on MM is highly controversial [5]. Several epidemiological studies suggested that an increase in skin lesions among sunscreen users is probably due to compensatory changes in risk behaviors (e.g., prolonged exposure to the sun). On the other hand, the results could be related to the earlier use of sunscreens of low Sun Protecting Factor (SPF) lacking the efficient UVB and UVA filters [6]. Contrary to the above, trial data have shown that incidence of benign melanocytic nevi or dysplastic nevi, the strongest markers of melanoma risk, is reduced in children by sunscreen use [7]. Additionally, in several short-term trials [8], regular sunscreen use has been shown to reduce the occurrence of solar keratoses, the benign squamous cell tumors that strongly determine not only the risk of squamous cell carcinoma but also of basal cell carcinoma [9] and MM [10]. A recent study of Green et al., (2011) concluded that melanoma may be preventable by regular sunscreen use in adults [11]. Several other authors concluded that regular applications of a broad-spectrum SPF-16 sunscreen in white adults aged 25 to 75 years can decrease the incidence of MM. On the other hand, Goldenhersh and Koslowsky (2011) believe that the data generated from the study by Green et al. (2011) is not sufficiently convincing to justify acceptance by the medical community as proof or even reassurance that sunscreen use prevents MM [12]. The evidence from epidemiologic studies regarding sunscreen use and MM incidence are thus inconclusive and controversial. While the correlational relationship between sunscreen and MM was observed by some studies, it is hard to establish a causal relationship between sunscreen and MM. Besides, US Environmental Protection Agency (2006) states that, "there is no evidence that sunscreens protect you from MM" [13]. Although the use of sunscreens has a limited or a controversial effect on MM prevention [14] (further studies are needed), this does not imply that sunscreens are not advisable, but stresses the importance of correct use of sunscreens along with other sun protective measures [15].

The magnitude of sun exposure during childhood is a major risk factor in the development of skin cancer [16], especially in the age group from 10 to 18 years. This population of preadolescents and adolescents often refuse to be sunscreened by their parents and usually do not have partners who would apply sun cream on their back. Besides, children's skin is thinner than that of adults and has lower melanin concentrations. Thus, UV penetrates more deeply into the skin that is less able to absorb UV radiation [17, 18]. Dusza et al., (2012) have identified a crucial period of preadolescence in which students increase time spent in the sun to get a tan and strengthen tan-promoting attitudes. Dusza et al., (2012) have also shown that the time between ages 11 and 14 is one of volatility, as more than 50% of at-risk children increase or decrease their use of sun protection, obtain sunburns, or change their tan-promoting attitudes. Bulliard et al., (2007) observed that at younger age, the relative melanoma density was highest on the intermittently sun-exposed back and shoulder. This supports the apparently greater impact of intermittent exposure in producing MM. An intermittent pattern of sun exposure over many years appears to significantly increase MM risk. It could be summarized that both chronic sun damage and intermittent sun exposure are important risk factors for skin cancer formation.

The aim of our study was to investigate the possible correlation between anatomic melanoma distribution on the specific back area and lack of sunscreen application.

Participants and Methods

25 young adult volunteers in the age interval 19-35 years were randomly sampled and asked to apply the sunscreen on their back as if they were going to the beach. To the commercial sunscreen blue or brown color was added. The color was obtained from the food shop for coloring the cakes. After the sunscreen application, the pictures of the back of individuals participating in the research were taken with an 8 megapic camera. All the participants declared that "their entire back surface is covered with the sun protection cream." In the second part of the study, the visual observation of pictures from diverse studies showing MM anatomical distributions were compared in order to assess the possible correlation between the observed lack of sun protection on the upper back areas and upper back MM incidence and thus provide a tentative proof that lack of sunscreen application and the incidence of MM of the back are related.

Results

From the obtained results, it can be seen that only three participants totally covered their back with sunscreen (Figure 4). While six participants left small parts of the back uncovered (Figure 3), 19 participants left significant area of their back uncovered by the sunscreen (Figure 1 and 2).

It can be concluded that the majority of participants applied insufficient amount or no sunscreen at all on the specific part of the back, specifically on the area between their scapula bones. The purpose of our study was to discuss the question whether there is a correlation between the lack of sunscreen application between the scapula bones area of the back and the incidence of MM in this area of the back.

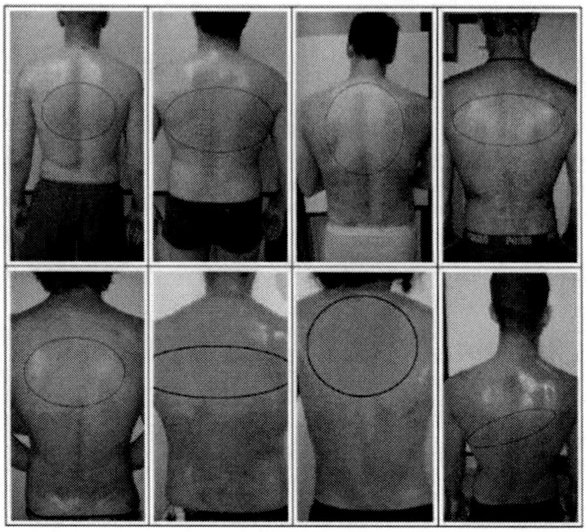

Figure 1. Male participants: examples of insufficiently applied sun cream on the back (circled areas show the lack of sunscreen application).

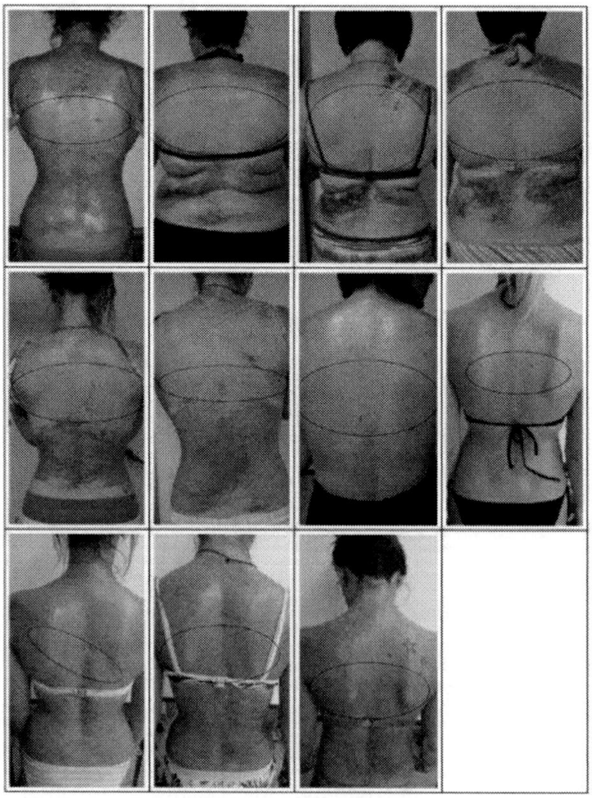

Figure 2. Female participants: examples of insufficiently applied sun cream on the back (circled areas show the lack of sunscreen application).

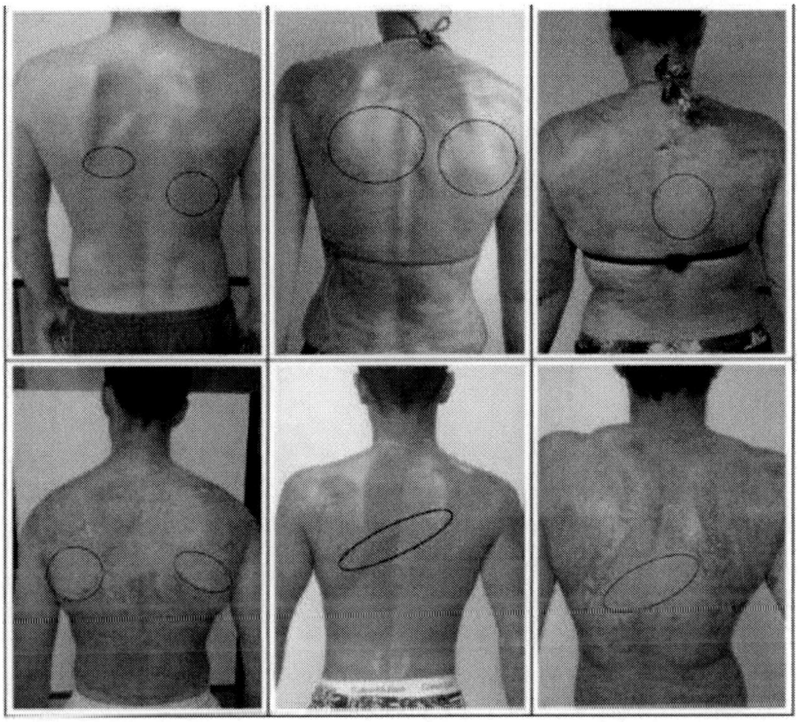

Figure 3. Examples of sites with partially omitted sunscreen application on the upper back.

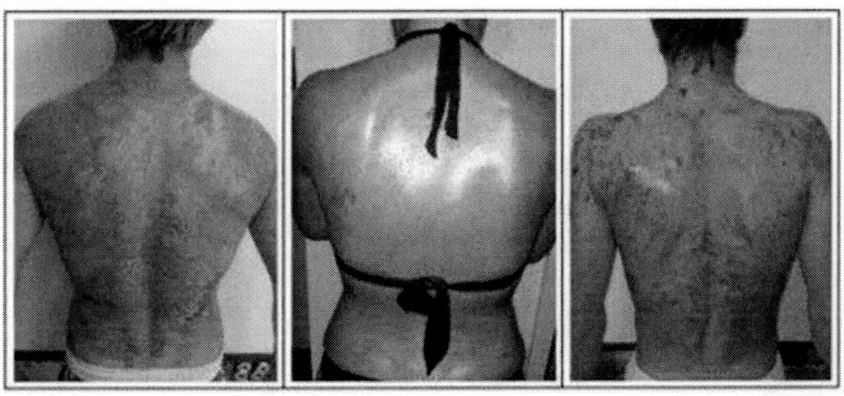

Figure 4. Example of sufficiently applied sun cream on the back.

In order to answer this question, the distribution of MM on the back area of the body should be established. Pictures obtained from studies showing anatomic MM distribution are presented (Table 1) in order to investigate possible increase in MM appearance on the upper back (marked with circles). Relative MM density on the back area was assessed visually by the authors and information was obtained by pictorial support with the possibility of the selection bias (Table1). It should be stressed, however, that the only purpose is to point to the possible correlation between lack of sun protection on the upper back and increased upper back MM distribution.

Table 1. Malignant melanoma distribution on the back

Picture showing melanoma distribution on the back	Comment	Study
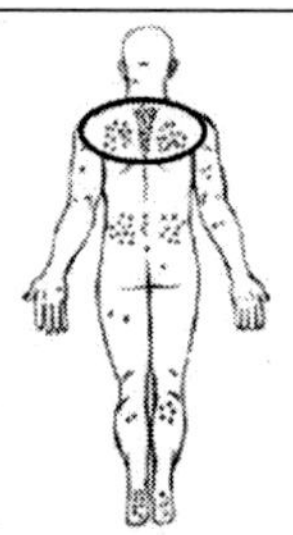	Anatomical sites of cutaneous melanoma lesions in male patients in the western region of Santa Clara, Brazil, (2002 – 2009) (n=205).	Moreno M, Schmitt RL, Lang MG, Gheno V. Clinical Study, Epidemiological Profile of Patients with Cutaneous Melanoma in a Region of Southern Brazil. Journal of Skin Cancer 2012: 917346.
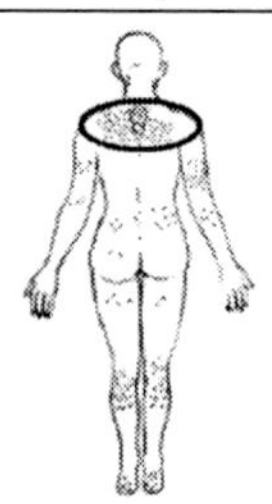	Anatomical sites of cutaneous melanoma lesions in female patients in the western region of Santa Catarina, Brazil, (2002 – 2009) (n= 292).	Moreno M, Schmitt RL, Lang MG, Gheno V. Clinical Study, Epidemiological Profile of Patients with Cutaneous Melanoma in a Region of Southern Brazil. Journal of Skin Cancer 2012: 917346.
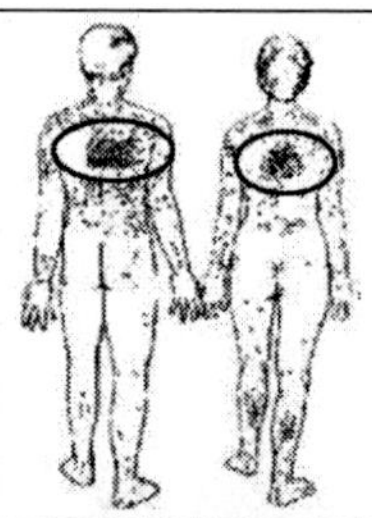	Anatomic distribution of melanoma for pigmented lesion group patients seen in 2004.	http://www.aboutcancer.com/melanoma_basic.htm
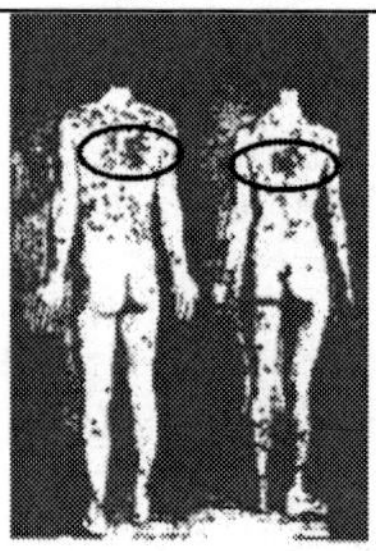	Anatomical distribution of melanomas in man and women.	Diffey B L. Solar ultraviolet radiation effects on biological systems. Review in Physics Medicine and Biology 1991; 36 (3): 299-328.
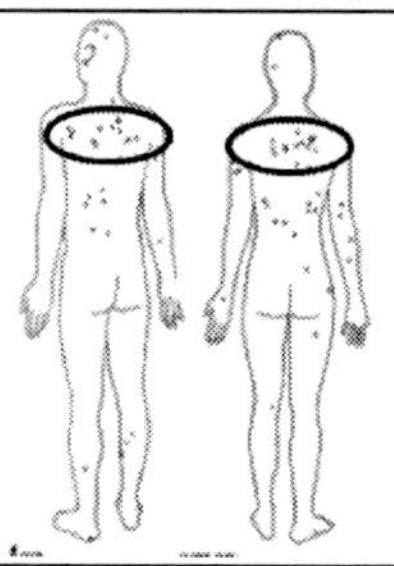	Anatomic distribution of Melanoma for pigmented lesion group patients (2004).	Clark LN, Shin DB, Troxel AB, et al. Association between the anatomic distribution of melanoma and sex. J Am Acad Dermatol 2007; 56: 768-73.

Picture showing melanoma distribution on the back	Comment	Study
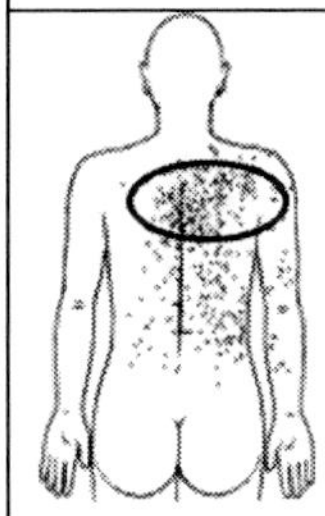	Melanoma sites on the posterior trunk and arm that drained to the right axilla. Note the wide distribution of sites to the left of the midline that included right axillary drainage. Similar drainage from the right back across the midline to the left axilla was observed. From: Location of sentinel lymph nodes in patients with cutaneous melanoma: new insights into lymphatic anatomy).	Pruthi DK, Guilfoyle R, Nugent Z, et al. Incidence and anatomic presentation of cutaneous malignant melanoma in central Canada during a 50- year period: 1956 to 2005. Journal of the American Academy of Dermatology 2009; 61(1): 44-50.
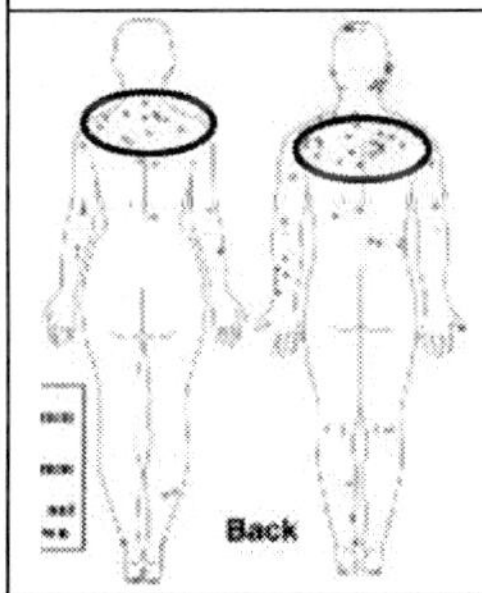	Anatomic location for 257 melanomas in situ in 4 private practice clinics (2005 – 2009).	Private practice clinics in Plantation Florida, Columbia and Rolla MO, and Stanford CT.

DISCUSSION

Based on literature review, the body site distribution of MM shows lower rates per unit area on sites usually unexposed to the sun than on usually or regularly exposed ones. When expressed as lesions per unit area, MM are 10- to 20-fold more frequent on the face and male ears than on intermittently exposed sites such as the lower legs in women, shoulders, back, or neck [9]. In men, the incidence of invasive MM on the ears, a chronically sun-exposed site, was extraordinarily high, with annual rates of over 200 per 10(5) units of surface area in the Queensland population. Next highest rates of over 100 MM per 10(5) units were found on the face, neck, shoulders and back in men and on the face and shoulders in women. Comparison with site-specific incidence rates in the same population 7½ years previously showed that incidence of invasive disease had significantly increased for all these sites, though the largest relative increase in this period occurred on the forearm in both men and women [9]. Changes have been observed in the anatomic distribution of MM by different authors [19, 20; 21; 22; 23]. The changes of MM distribution found in different studies might be due to different time period, different populations, increased awareness, increased sun-protective practices, and differences in sun-exposure behaviors (either recreational or occupational) [24]. For example, Pruthi et al., (2009) observed that among male and female patients, MM of the head and of the lower extremities have become proportionally less frequent. However, MM of the trunk and of the upper extremities has proportionally increased. Cho et al., (2005) showed divergent etiologic pathways of MM development by anatomic sites. Results from their study indicate that history of severe and painful sunburn was most strongly related to MM of the upper extremity. Number of moles was most strongly related to MM of the trunk. Anatomic site of the cancer was not statistically significantly influenced by age, family history of MM, and hair color. Sites of highest MM risks were in the study of Bulliard et al. (2007) the face, shoulder and upper arm for both sexes, the back for men and leg for women [19].

Green et al. (1993) reported that in contrast to predictions based on apparent frequency of sun exposure at subsites on the upper limbs, the relative concentration of MM on the shoulder suggests that wearing sleeveless garments outdoors in the sun should be avoided whenever possible [9]. Also, the similar densities of leg and forearm MM seem inconsistent with the relative degree of exposure of each and further suggest that women's adoption of ankle-length skirts or trousers, in preference to knee-length skirts, would be a worthwhile modern control measure. Increases in MM have been greatest in intermittently sun-exposed sites such as the trunk and limbs. Many studies have observed an increase of melanoma incidence of the trunk and limbs, and thus indicated a behavioral genesis (Table 1). Dal et al. (2007) observed in the Swedish population that the shift of MM from the head to the trunk with mostly intermittent UV exposure coincides with behavioral and societal changes with regard to sun exposure [24]. Whiteman et al., (2006) also observed that MM of the head and neck are associated with chronic patterns of sun exposure whereas trunk MM are associated with intermittent patterns of sun exposure, supporting the hypothesis that MM may arise through divergent causal pathways [10].

It has been observed that sunscreen users are using sunscreen lotions inconsistently. Our results revealed that participants applied insufficient amount of sunscreen to the upper parts of the back - the common areas of melanoma skin cancer incidence. Promoting sunscreen use is an integral part of prevention programs aimed at reducing ultraviolet (UV) radiation-induced skin damage and skin cancers. Protection against both UVB and UVA radiation is advocated. It should be emphasized that an individual cannot fully cover their back with the sunscreen unaided, especially the upper back part as shown in the pictures (figure 1 and 2). Sunscreen should be applied uniformly to the skin at a thickness of 2 mg/cm^2.

The properly evaluated long-term sunscreen effectiveness in humans is lacking. Evidence from randomized controlled trials is required, principally because observational studies of sunscreen use and skin cancer are compromised by intractable confounding. Further research is needed before the optimal sunscreen is developed. In the meantime, people using sunscreens should use the products with the highest SPF and be aware that the products are used for protective and not for tanning purposes. Increased distribution of MM on the upper back cannot be explained by lack of sun cream protection alone. Melanocytes, the cells of origin for melanoma, which are unequally distributed on the skin surface might differ in their response to UV insults and susceptibility to malignant transformation according to anatomical region [25]. A significant benefit from regular sunscreen use has not yet been confirmed for primary prevention of basal cell carcinoma and MM. Thus, primary MM incidence prevention efforts should not be limited only to using sunscreen, but should also focus on decreasing exposure to the sun's UV rays. Isaksson Vogel et al., (2014) reported relatively lower MM incidence in individuals who use more sunscreen. The same results were obtained in individuals who take advantage of the shade and wear protective clothing. The first line of protection is to avoid sunburn or excessive exposure by staying out of direct sunlight. When possible, avoidance of outdoor activities during peak sun hours between 10 AM and 4 PM is recommended.

In conclusion, the sunscreens should be used to reduce exposure rather than prolong the period of exposure to the sun, as it is wrongly believed by many sunscreen users. When used improperly, sunscreen can potentially increase the risk for MM development by conferring a false sense of protection against sunburn.

References

[1] World Health Organization, World Meteorological Organization, United Nations Environment Program, International Commission on Non-Ionizing Radiation Protection (2002). Global Solar UV Index: A Practical Guide. Geneva: WHO. http://www.who.int/uv/publications/en/ (30.6.2013).

[2] Greinert R, Volkmer B, Wende A et al. Prevention of skin cancer. Necessity, implementation and success. *Hautarzt.* 2003; 54(12): 1152-63.

[3] Rhodes AR. Public education and cancer of the skin. What do people need to know about melanoma and nonmelanoma skin cancer? *Cancer.* 1995; 15(75): 613-36.

[4] Mang R, Krutmann J. Sun protection during holidays. *Hautarzt.* 2003; 54(6): 498-505.

[5] Vainio H, Bianchini F. Cancer-preventive effects of sunscreens are uncertain. *Scand J. Work Environ. Health.* 2000; 26 (6): 529–31.

[6] Westerdahl J, Ingvar C, Masbäck A, Olsson H. Sunscreen use and malignant melanoma. *Int. J. Cancer.* 2000; 87 (1): 145–50.

[7] Gallagher RP, Rivers JK, Lee TK, et al. Broad-spectrum sunscreen use and the development of new nevi in white children: a randomized controlled trial. *JAMA.* 2000; 283: 2955–60.

[8] Darlington S, Williams G, Neale R, et al. A randomized controlled trial to assess sunscreen application and betacarotene supplementation in the prevention of solar keratoses. *Arch. Dermatol.* 2003; 139: 451–5.

[9] Green A, Battistutta D, Hart V, et al. Study Group. Skin cancer in a subtropical Australian population: incidence and lack of association with occupation. *Am. J. Epidemiol.* 1993; 144: 1034–40.

[10] Whiteman DC, Stickley M, Watt P, et al. Melanomas of the head and trunk have different associations with chronic and intermittent patterns of sun exposure. *J. Clin. Onco.* 2006; 24: 3172–7.

[11] Green AC, Williams GM, Logan V, Strutton GM. Reduced melanoma after regular sunscreen use: randomized trial follow-up. *J. Clin. Oncol.* 2011; 29(3): 257-63.

[12] Goldenhersh MA, Koslowsky M. Increased melanoma after regular sunscreen use? *J. Clin. Oncol.* 2011; 29(18): 557-8.

[13] United States Environmental Protection Agency. Sunscreen: The Burning Facts. Available at: http://www.epa.gov/sunwise/doc/sunscreen.pdf. Accessed 26.5.2013.

[14] Bastuji-Garin S, Diepgen TL. Cutaneous malignant melanoma, sun exposure, and sunscreen use: epidemiological evidence. *Br. J. Dermatol.* 2002; 61: 24-30.

[15] Weismann K, Lorentzen HF. Sunbathing habits and risk of melanoma. Ugeskr Laeger. 2000; 162(23): 3307-10.

[16] Whiteman DC, Whiteman CA, Green AC. Childhood sun exposure as a risk factor for melanoma: a systematic review of epidemiologic studies. *Cancer Causes Control.* 2001; 12: 69-82.

[17] Jou PC, Feldman RJ, Tomecki KJ. UV protection and sunscreens: what to tell patients. *Cleve Clin. J. Med.* 2012; 79(6): 427-36.

[18] Dusza SW, Halpern AC, Satagopan JM, et al. Prospective study of sunburn and sun behavior patterns during adolescence. *Pediatrics.* 2012; 129(2): 309-17.

[19] Bulliard JL, De Weck D, Fisch T, et al. Detailed site distribution of melanoma and sunlight exposure: etiological patterns from a Swiss series. *Ann. Oncol.* 2007; 18(4): 789-94.

[20] Pruthi DK, Guilfoyle R, Nugent Z, et al. Incidence and anatomic presentation of cutaneous malignant melanoma in central Canada during a 50- year period: 1956 to 2005. *Journal of the American Academy of Dermatology.* 2009; 61(1): 44-50.

[21] Cho E, Rosner BA, Colditz GA. Risk factors for melanoma by body site. *Cancer Epidemiol. Biomarkers Prev.* 2005; 14(5): 1241-4.

[22] Bulliard JL, Cox B. Cutaneous malignant melanoma in New Zealand: trends by anatomical site, 1969-1993. *Int. J. Epidemiol.* 2000; 29(3): 416-23.

[23] Stang A, Stabenow R, Eisinger B, Jöckel KH. Site and gender specific time trend analyses of the incidence of skin melanomas in the former German Democratic Republic (GDR) including 19351 cases. *Eur. J. Cancer.* 2003; 39(11): 1610-8.

[24] Dal H, Boldemann C, Lindelöf B. Does relative melanoma distribution by body site reflect changes in intermittent exposure and intentional tanning in the Swedish population? *Eur. J. Dermatol.* 2007; 17(5): 428-34.

[25] Green A. A theory of site distribution of melanoma: Queensland, Australia. *Cancer Causes Control.* 1992; 3: 513-516.

[26] Isaksson Vogel R, Ahmed RL, Nelson HH, Berwick M, Weinstock MA, Lazovich D. Exposure to Indoor Tanning Without Burning and Melanoma Risk by Sunburn History. *J. Natl. Cancer Inst.* 2014; 106(7).

In: Horizons in Cancer Research. Volume 61
Editor: Hiroto S. Watanabe
ISBN: 978-1-63484-503-8

Chapter 6

ANTI-CANCER ACTIVITIES OF THE GREEN TEA POLYPHENOLS EGC AND EGCG IN HUMAN MALIGNANT NEUROBLASTOMA

Mrinmay Chakrabarti and Swapan K. Ray*
Department of Pathology, Microbiology, and Immunology,
University of South Carolina School of Medicine, Columbia, SC, US

ABSTRACT

Malignant neuroblastoma, which is a solid tumor in children, is responsible for more than 15% of all childhood cancer deaths. Epidemiological data show that Asian populations who consume significant quantities of green tea have a low risk of cancer. Green tea contains anti-cancer compounds such as epigallocatechin (EGC) and epigallocatechin-3-gallate (EGCG), which are polyphenols endowed with various anti-cancer activities. Many investigations have shown that these green tea polyphenols (EGC and EGCG) inhibit tumor cell proliferation and induce tumor cell apoptosis *in vitro* and *in vivo*. Although the direct mechanisms of action of EGC and EGCG have not yet been clarified, it has been proposed that these green tea polyphenols modulate key molecular drivers of cell proliferation and survival. EGCG, which shows much better anti-cancer efficacy than EGC, modulates expression of fatty acid synthase (FAS), a key metabolic enzyme for catalyzing the synthesis of long chain fatty acids. Expression of FAS is highly increased in various human cancers including malignant neuroblastoma. A green tea catechin can vary its structural conformation, thus allowing it to behave as a chemical chaperone that is able to interact with other biomolecules including DNA, RNA, lipids, and proteins in the cancer cells. The anti-cancer mechanisms of EGC and EGCG in cell culture model are due to modulation of expression of key molecules in cell cycle progression, inhibition of inflammatory molecules, binding to FAS, and activation of

* Corresponding author: Swapan K. Ray, PhD, Professor, Department of Pathology, Microbiology, and Immunology, University of South Carolina School of Medicine, Building 2, Room C11, 6439 Garners Ferry Road, Columbia, SC 29209, US. Phone: 803-216-3420; Fax: 803-216-3428; Email: swapan.ray@uscmed.sc.edu.

mitogen-activated protein kinase cascade. When used in combination with another appropriate therapeutic agent, the anti-cancer activities of EGC or EGCG can be increased synergistically in malignant neuroblastoma. This chapter will describe the known molecular mechanisms of EGC and EGCG in malignant neuroblastoma that can help find new directions for future research.

INTRODUCTION

Malignant neuroblastoma, an extracranial solid tumor in children, is originated from primitive neural cells of the sympathetic nervous system and it accounts for 6-10% of all childhood cancers, and 15% of cancer deaths in children (Chen and Stallings, 2007). Malignant neuroblastoma is heterogeneous in nature and it is known to demonstrate relapse even after aggressive chemotherapeutic treatments.

Common phytochemicals are well known for their anti-cancer effects on various human cancers, including malignant neuroblastoma (Chakrabarti et al., 2013). Green tea is enriched with several anti-cancer catechins such as epigallocatechin (EGC), epigallocatechin-3-gallate (EGCG), epicatechin gallate (ECG), gallocatechin (GC), epicatechin (EC), and catechin (C) (Ninomiya et al., 1997). The chemoprotective actions of green tea catechins are due to their opposing activities on cyclooxygenase and lipoxygenase enzymes (Hong et al., 2001). Green tea catechins can modulate the release of hormones from endocrine system (Murase et al., 2002) and also hinder the release of some allergic factors like leukotrienes and prostaglandins in human body (Jose et al., 2014). Catechins have also been observed to regulate many signaling molecules in different biochemical pathways that are involved in cancer progression. EGCG is the most potent catechin for chemopreventive and anti-cancer activities. Efficacy of EGCG has been investigated in several animal models of cancers, including neuroblastoma (Golden et al., 2009). EGCG can alter its structural conformation and function as a chemical chaperone. Thus, EGCG is able to interact with other biomolecules like DNA, RNA, lipids, and proteins (Chakrabarti et al., 2013). Hossain and co-workers recently showed that EGCG could alter the expression of key signaling molecules involved in tumor cell proliferation, inflammation, and activation of fatty acid synthase (FAS), a key metabolic enzyme for catalyzing the synthesis of long chain fatty acids, in cell culture model of neuroblastoma (Hossain et al., 2012). EGCG could also promote anti-oxidant response element (ARE)-mediated gene expression through activation of mitogen-activated protein kinase (MAPK) pathway signaling molecules such as p38, JNK, and ERK (Chen et al., 2000).

Beside these, EGCG could significantly decrease food uptake, body weight, and concentration of steroid hormones such as estradiol and testosterone (Kao et al., 2000; Gramza et al., 2005).

MALIGNANT NEUROBLASTOMA AND ITS TREATMENT STRATEGIES

The stages of the neuroblastoma are determined by physical examinations, X-ray analysis, bone scans, computerized tomography (CT) scan, magnetic resonance imaging

(MRI), and biopsies of the main tumor and other tissues. Surgical removal of tumors is generally performed for stage I and II neuroblastoma patients. For malignant neuroblastoma or advanced stage neuroblastoma, multiple chemotherapeutic drugs like cisplatin, doxorubicin, cyclophosphamide, teniposide, and etoposide are used. Beside these, plasmapheresis and gamma globulin are also used for selected patients suffering from malignant neuroblastoma. Adrenocorticotropin hormone (ACTH) is supposed to be effective against neuroblastoma (Babié et al., 2012). Therapeutic strategies with combination of different dugs are also beneficial due to lower toxicity, drug synergism, and less adverse side effects. Topotecan, which is a topoisomerase I inhibitor, alone or in combination with cyclophosphamide has been observed to be very much effective against recurrent neuroblastoma (Saulnier et al., 2015). Several *in vitro* studies suggest that natural and synthetic retinoids can inhibit cell proliferation in human malignant neuroblastoma by inhibiting expression of N-myc mRNA (Janardhanan et al., 2009). Thus, clinical trials are now underway to observe the efficacy of 13-*cis*-retinoic acid (13-CRA) in children with relapsed neuroblastoma. United States Food and Drug Administration (FDA) has permitted Unituxin™ (dinutuximab) in combination with granulocyte-macrophage colony-stimulating factor (GM-CSF), interleukin-2 (IL-2), and 13-CRA for the treatment of high-risk neuroblastoma patients (Dhillon, 2015). Therapeutic strategies with recombinant IC-2, modified dendritic cells, and cytotoxic T lymphocytes are also found to be effective against neuroblastoma (Babié et al., 2012). Although many *in vitro* studies suggest that neuroblastoma is radiosensitive, but most clinical trials show varying and indecisive outcomes. Beside these, several chemotherapeutic drugs effectively decrease the volume of the primary tumor and sometimes alter the neuroblastoma into benign ganglioneuroma, but the cure rate has not yet been improved notably.

PROPERTIES AND OCCURRENCE OF GREEN TEA POLYPHENOLS

Green tea, made from unfermented leaves, contains high levels of polyphenolic compounds (Ho et al., 1997). Green tea leaves contain flavanols, flavadiols, flavonoids, and phenolic acids that constitute almost 30% of fresh leaves dry weight (Wang et al., 2000). Several research findings suggested that tea polyphenols could act as anti-fungal, anti-oxidative, anti-carcinogenic, and anti-tumor agents in several systems (Al-Attar et al., 2010; 2013). The most important polyphenolic compounds in green tea leaves are found to be catechins (flavan-3-ols) (Balentine, 1997). Catechins are hydrophilic compounds with the highest oxidation degree of the heterocyclic rings (Gramza et al., 2005). The key components of green tea catechins are catechin (C), epicatechin (EC), gallocatechin (GC), epicatechin gallate (ECG), epigallocatechin (EGC), and epigallocatechin-3-gallate (EGCG) (Montague et al., 2012).

Age of the tea leaves is a crucial factor that determines the content of catechins in tea leaves. It has been observed that tea produced from the young leaves contains larger amount of catechins than the older ones. Several analytical studies suggest that EGCG, which is the most potent catechin with eight –OH groups, is only found in green tea leaves among various plant derived food products (Chu and Juneja, 1997). Green teas have higher percentage of catechins than the black teas (Khokhar and Magnusdottir, 2002). However, black teas have

Table 1. Combination of EGCG and anti-cancer agent for synergistic therapeutic effects in human malignant neuroblastoma

Combination therapy	Effects	Neuroblastoma Cells	Anti-cancer mechanisms	References
EGCG + ATRA, 13-CRA, or 4-HPR	Synergistic	SH-SY5Y	Increase in apoptosis, down regulation of telomerase activity, induction of neuronal differentiation, and overexpression of NFP	Das et al., 2009
EGCG + SU5416	Synergistic	SH-SY5Y and SK-N-BE2	Inhibition of cell survival, induction of apoptosis, suppression of VEGFR-2 gene expression, and cell migration	Mohan et al., 2011
EGCG + 4-HPR	Synergistic	SK-N-BE2 and IMR-32	Inhibition of oncogenic miRs, upregulation of tumor suppressor miRs (TSmiRs), and induction of mitochondria and death receptor mediated apoptosis	Chakrabarti et al., 2012
EGCG + survivin shRNA	Synergistic	SK-N-BE2 and SH-SY5Y	Inhibition of migration, suppression of p-Akt, NF-κB, MMPs, VEGF, and b-FGF, and induction of apoptosis	Hossain et al., 2012
EGC or EGCG + TSmiR-7-1	Synergistic	SH-SY5Y and SK-N-DZ	Inhibition of oncogenic miRs (miR-92, miR-93, and miR-106b), upregulation of TSmiRs (miR-7-1, miR-34a, miR-99a), and induction of apoptosis	Chakrabarti et al., 2013

These studies showed that EGCG was more potent than EGC in inducing apoptosis in human malignant neuroblastoma cells. Also, apoptotic potential of EGCG could be enhanced following overexpression of the tumor suppressor microRNA miR-7-1 in human malignant neuroblastoma SH-SY5Y and SK-N-DZ cells (Chakrabarti et al., 2013) (Table 1).

Green Tea Polyphenols Act Synergistically with Natural and Synthetic Compounds for Inhibition of Growth of Malignant Neuroblastoma

The most favorable strategy for the treatment of all cancers including human malignant neuroblastoma is the use of combination of two or more drugs to enhance therapeutic efficacy. The main reasoning for combination therapy is the choice of drugs with different mechanisms of action, thus yielding additive or synergistic anti-cancer activities. Recent studies showed that the green tea catechins EGC and EGCG were effective in inhibiting growth of human malignant neuroblastoma and most importantly combination of EGCG with a chemotherapeutic drug could act synergistically for better efficacy than monotherapy in controlling the growth of different human malignant neuroblastoma cells (Mohan et al., 2011). There are several advantages of using combination therapy: (1) different drugs may modulate diverse signaling pathways and thus show additive or synergistic effects; (2)

different drugs help to overcome the drug resistance in tumor cells; and (3) drugs in combination reduce the undesirable side effects and toxicity of a particular agent at higher dose. Synergistic or additive efficacy of EGCG and other anti-cancer agents such as celecoxib, retinoids, sulindac, and tamoxifen has been explored in many studies (Suganuma et al., 2011). Combination of EGCG and an anti-cancer drug synergistically augmented apoptosis 10 – 15 times more than the anti-cancer drug alone in PC-9 cells (Suganuma et al., 2006). Green tea extract could promote the potential of sulindac synergistically to block intestinal tumor growth in mice (Suganuma et al., 2001). Similarly, combination of EGCG and the COX-2 selective inhibitor NS398 significantly prevented cell proliferation and induced apoptosis in LNCaP, PC-3, and CWR22Rv1 cells (Adhami et al., 2007). The same group of investigators also showed that green tea catechins and celecoxib could inhibit tumor growth in athymic nude mice implanted with CWR22Rv1 cells (Adhami et al., 2007). An earlier study demonstrated that EGC or EGCG treatment could induce mitochondria and death receptor mediated apoptotic pathways in malignant neuroblastoma SH-SY5Y cells (Das et al., 2006). A later study reported that combination of EGCG and a retinoid inhibited expression of pro-angiogenic factor (VEGF) and survival factor (NF-κB), and also induced apoptosis in human malignant neuroblastoma SH-SY5Y cells (Das et al., 2009) (Table 1). A more recent study indicated that combination of EGCG and SU5416, an inhibitor of the vascular endothelial growth factor receptor-2 (VEGFR-2), promoted cell cycle arrest and apoptosis through down regulation of Bcl-2 and activation of caspase-3 in human malignant neuroblastoma SH-SY5Y and SK-N-BE2 cells (Mohan et al., 2011) (Table 1).

CONCLUSION

Several preclinical investigations documented the crucial roles of green tea polyphenols in inhibition of many human cancers. Although the health benefits of green tea were known before, basic research with the key catechins like EGC and EGCG has recently shown their extremely promising anti-cancer activities for the treatment of various cancers including human malignant neuroblastoma. Most chemotherapeutic agents are wasteful as they show severe adverse side effects due to modulation in several vital molecular routes. Since the earliest time, green tea is broadly used as traditional anti-cancer medicine due to its low-cost, effectiveness, and low side effects. Many *in vitro* and *in vivo* investigations have now clearly shown that anti-cancer activities of green tea catechins include modulation of cell signaling pathways linked to angiogenesis, apoptosis, and production of transcription factors in malignant neuroblastoma. But, bioavailability of the ingested EGCG is very poor. After absorption it undergoes a lot of degradation and modification in human body. Thus, it can be hypothesized that contradictory therapeutic conclusions between cell culture and animal studies may be due to unpredictable bioavailability of green tea polyphenols. Current clinical trials with green tea catechins for exploring their anti-cancer activities in malignant neuroblastoma should concentrate on bioavailability, therapeutic dose, administration frequency, and potential side effects. Widespread animal model studies may also contribute to understanding the exact mechanism of action and toxicity levels/side effects without alteration of therapeutic potential. Additionally, the detailed study of green tea and its constituents based on clinical trials may be very helpful in designing of novel combination therapy for controlling the growth of malignant neuroblastoma in pediatric patients in the near future.

Acknowledgments

This work was supported in part by the SC SCIRF-2015-I-01 and USC SOM RDF grants.

References

Adhami, VM; Malik, A; Zaman, N; Sarfaraz, S; Siddiqui, IA; Syed, DN; Afaq, F; Pasha, FS; Saleem, M; Mukhtar, H. Combined inhibitory effects of green tea polyphenols and selective cyclooxygenase-2 inhibitors on the growth of human prostate cancer cells both *in vitro* and *in vivo*. *Clin. Cancer Res.,* 2007, 13, 1611-1619.

Al-Attar, AM; Abu Zeid, IM. Effect of tea (*Camellia sinensis*) and olive (*Olea europaea* L.) leaves extracts on male mice exposed to diazinon. *Biomed. Res. Int.,* 2013, 2013, 461415.

Al-Attar, AM; Zari, TA. Influences of crude extract of tea leaves, Camellia sinensis, on streptozotocin diabetic male albino mice. *Saudi J. Biol. Sci.,* 2010, 17, 295-301.

Babié, PT; Toirac, RJR; Renó, JS; Derich, SP. *Neuroblastoma – Molecular Basis for Diagnosis and Staging System, Contemporary Pediatrics,* Ö. Özdemir (Ed.), InTech, 2012.

Balentine, D. Tea and health. *Crit. Rev. Food Sci. Nutr.,* 1997, 37, 691-692.

Chakrabarti, M; Ai, W; Banik, NL; Ray, SK. Overexpression of miR-7-1 increases efficacy of green tea polyphenols for induction of apoptosis in human malignant neuroblastoma SH-SY5Y and SK-N-DZ cells. *Neurochem. Res.,* 2013, 38, 420-432.

Chakrabarti, M; Khandkar, M; Banik, NL; Ray, SK. Alterations in expression of specific microRNAs by combination of 4-HPR and EGCG inhibited growth of human malignant neuroblastoma cells. *Brain Res.,* 2012, 1454, 1-13.

Chen, C; Yu, R; Owuor, ED; Kong, AN. Activation of antioxidant response element (ARE), mitogen-activated protein kinases (MAPKs) and caspases by major green tea polyphenol components during cell survival and death. *Arch. Pharm. Res.,* 2000, 23, 605-612.

Chen, Y; Stallings, RL. Differential patterns of microRNA expression in neuroblastoma are correlated with prognosis, differentiation, and apoptosis. *Cancer Res.,* 2007, 67, 976-983.

Chu, DC; Juneja, LR. General chemical composition of green tea and its infusion. In: Yamamoto, T; Juneja LR; Chu, DC; Kim, M. (Eds.). *Chemistry and Applications of Green Tea.* NY, CRC, 1997, pp. 13-22.

Das, A; Banik, NL; Ray, SK. Mechanism of apoptosis with the involvement of calpain and caspase cascades in human malignant neuroblastoma SH-SY5Y cells exposed to flavonoids. *Int. J. Cancer,* 2006, 119, 2575-2585.

Das, A; Banik, NL; Ray, SK. Retinoids induce differentiation and down regulate telomerase activity and N-Myc to increase sensitivity to flavonoids for apoptosis in human malignant neuroblastoma SH-SY5Y cells. *Int. J. Oncol.,* 2009, 34, 757-765.

Dhillon, S. Dinutuximab: first global approval. Drugs, 2015, 75, 923-927.

Golden, EB; Lam, PY; Kardosh, A; Gaffney, KJ; Cadenas, E; Louie, SG; Petasis, NA; Chen, TC; Schönthal, AH. Green tea polyphenols block the anticancer effects of bortezomib and other boronic acid-based proteasome inhibitors. *Blood,* 2009, 113, 5927-5937.

Graham, HN. Green tea composition, consumption and polyphenol chemistry. *Prev. Med.,* 1992, 21, 334-350.

Gramza, A; Korczak, J; Amarowicz, R. Tea polyphenols – their antioxidant properties and biological activity. *Pol. J. Food Nutr. Sci.,* 2005, 14, 219-235.

Halder, J; Tamuli, P; Bhaduri, AN. Isolation and characterization of polyphenoloxidase from Indian tea leaf (*Camellia sinensis*). *J. Nutr. Biochem.,* 1998, 9, 75-80.

Harada, M; Kan, Y; Naoki, H; Fukui, Y; Kageyama, N; Nakai, M; Miki, W; Kiso, Y. Identification of the major antioxidative metabolites in biological fluids of the rat with ingested (+)-catechin and (-)-epicatechin. *Biosci. Biotechnol. Biochem.,* 1999, 63, 973-977.

Ho, CT; Chen, CW; Wanasundara, UN; Shahidi, F. Natural antioxidant from tea. In: Shahidi F. (Ed), Natural Antioxidants. Chemistry. Health Effects and Applications. Illinois, *AOCS Press Champaign,* 1997, pp. 213-223.

Hong, J; Smith, TJ; Ho, CT; August, DA; Yang, CS. Effects of purified green and black tea polyphenols on cyclooxygenase- and lipoxygenase-dependent metabolism of arachidonic acid in human colon mucosa and colon tumor tissues. *Biochem. Pharmacol.,* 2001, 62, 1175-1183.

Hossain, MM; Banik, NL; Ray, SK. Survivin knockdown increased anti-cancer effects of (-)-epigallocatechin-3-gallate in human malignant neuroblastoma SK-N-BE2 and SH-SY5Y cells. *Exp. Cell Res.,* 2012, 318, 1597-1610.

Janardhanan, R; Banik, NL; Ray, SK. N-Myc down regulation induced differentiation, early cell cycle exit, and apoptosis in human malignant neuroblastoma cells having wild type or mutant p53. *Biochem. Pharmacol.,* 2009, 78, 1105-1114.

Jeong, JH; Kim, HJ; Lee, TJ; Kim, MK; Park, ES; Choi, BS. Epigallocatechin 3-gallate attenuates neuronal damage induced by 3-hydroxykynurenine. *Toxicology,* 2004, 195, 53-60.

Jose, R; Sajitha, GR; Augusti, KT. A review on the role of nutraceuticals as simple as Se^{2+} to complex organic molecules such as glycyrrhizin that prevent as well as cure diseases. *Indian J. Clin. Biochem.,* 2014, 29, 119-132.

Kao, YH; Hiipakka, RA; Liao, S. Modulation of endocrine systems and food intake by green tea epigallocatechin gallate. *Endocrinology,* 2000, 141, 980-987.

Kashima, M. Effects of catechins on superoxide and hydroxyl radical. *Chem. Pharm. Bull.,* (Tokyo), 1999, 47, 279-283.

Kelly, MR; Geigerman, CM; Loo, G. Epigallocatechin gallate protects U937 cells against nitric oxide-induced cell cycle arrest and apoptosis. *J. Cell Biochem.,* 2001, 81, 647–658.

Khalatbary, AR; Ahmadvand, H. Anti-inflammatory effect of the epigallocatechin gallate following spinal cord trauma in rat. *Iran Biomed. J.,* 2011, 15, 31-37.

Khokhar, S; Magnusdottir, SGM. Total phenol, catechins and caffeine contents of teas commonly consumed in the United Kingdom. *J. Agric. Food Chem.,* 2002, 50, 565-570.

Koh, SH; Kim, SH; Kwon, H; Park, Y; Kim, KS; Song, CW; Kim, J; Kim, MH; Yu, HJ; Henkel, JS; Jung, HK. Epigallocatechin gallate protects nerve growth factor differentiated PC12 cells from oxidative-radical-stress-induced apoptosis through its effect on phosphoinositide 3-kinase/Akt and glycogen synthase kinase-3. *Brain Res. Mol. Brain Res.,* 2003, 118, 72-81.

Kuo, KL; Weng, MS; Chiang, CT; Tsai, YJ; Lin-Shiau, SY; Lin, JK. Comparative studies on the hypolipidemic and growth suppressive effects of oolong, black, puerh, and green tea leaves in rats. *J. Agric. Food Chem.,* 2005, 53, 480-489.

Lee, LS; Kim, SH; Kim, YB; Kim, YC. Quantitative analysis of major constituents in green tea with different plucking periods and their antioxidant activity. *Molecules,* 2014, 19, 9173-9186.

Levites, Y; Amit, T; Youdim, MB; Mandel, S. Involvement of protein kinase C activation and cell survival/cell cycle genes in green tea polyphenol (-)-epigallocatechin 3-gallate neuroprotective action. *J. Biol. Chem.,* 2002, 277, 30574-30580.

Mohan, N; Karmakar, S; Banik, NL; Ray, SK. SU5416 and EGCG work synergistically and inhibit angiogenic and survival factors and induce cell cycle arrest to promote apoptosis in human malignant neuroblastoma SH-SY5Y and SK-N-BE2 cells. *Neurochem. Res.,* 2011, 36, 1383-1396.

Montague, JA; Butler, LM; Wu, AH; Genkinger, JM; Koh, WP; Wong, AS; Wang, R; Yuan, JM; Yu, MC. Green and black tea intake in relation to prostate cancer risk among Singapore Chinese. *Cancer Causes Control,* 2012, 23, 1635-1641.

Mukhtar, H; Ahmad, N. Green tea in chemoprevention of cancer. *Toxicol. Sci.,* 1999, 52, 117-117.

Murase, T; Nagasawa, A; Suzuki, J; Hase, T; Tokimitsu, I. Beneficial effects of tea catechins on diet-induced obesity: stimulation of lipid catabolism in the liver. *Int. J. Obes. Relat. Metab. Disord.,* 2002, 26, 1459-1464.

Ninomiya, M; Unten, L; Kim, M. Chemical and physicochemical properties of green tea polyphenols. In: Yamamoto, T; Juneja, LR; Chu, DC; Kim, M. (Eds.). *Chemistry and Applications of Green Tea.* NY, CRC, 1997, pp. 23-35.

Price, WE; Spitzer, JC. Variation in the amounts of individual flavanols in a range of green tea. *Food Chem.,* 1993, 47, 271-276.

Sang, S; Tian, S; Wang, H; Stark, RE; Rosen, RT; Yang, CS; Ho, CT. Chemical studies of the antioxidant mechanism of tea catechins: radical reaction products of epicatechin with peroxyl radicals. *Bioorg. Med. Chem.,* 2003, 11, 3371-3378.

Saulnier Sholler, GL; Gerner, EW; Bergendahl, G; MacArthur, RB; Vander Werff, A; Ashikaga, T; Bond, JP; Ferguson, W; Roberts, W; Wada, RK; Eslin, D; Kraveka, JM; Kaplan, J; Mitchell, D; Parikh, NS; Neville, K; Sender, L; Higgins, T; Kawakita, M; Hiramatsu, K; Moriya, SS; Bachmann, AS. A phase I trial of DFMO targeting polyamine addiction in patients with relapsed/refractory neuroblastoma. *PLoS One,* 2015, 10, e0127246.

Schroeter, H; Spencer, JP; Rice-Evans, C; Williams, RJ. Flavonoids protect neurons from oxidized low-density-lipoprotein-induced apoptosis involving c-Jun N-terminal kinase (JNK), c-Jun and caspase-3. *J. Biochem.,* 2001, 358, 547-557.

Suganuma, M; Kurusu, M; Suzuki, K; Tasaki, E; Fujiki, H. Green tea polyphenol stimulates cancer preventive effects of celecoxib in human lung cancer cells by upregulation of GADD153 gene. *Int. J. Cancer,* 2006, 119, 33-40.

Suganuma, M; Ohkura, Y; Okabe, S; Fujiki, H. Combination cancer chemoprevention with green tea extract and sulindac shown in intestinal tumor formation in Min mice. *J. Cancer Res. Clin. Oncol.,* 2001, 127, 69-72.

Suganuma, M; Saha, A; Fujiki, H. New cancer treatment strategy using combination of green tea catechins and anticancer drugs. *Cancer Sci.,* 2011, 102, 317-323.

Sutherland, BA; Rahman, RM; Appleton, I. Mechanisms of action of green tea catechins, with a focus on ischemia-induced neurodegeneration. *J. Nutr. Biochem.,* 2006, 17, 291-306.

Wang, H; Provan, GJ; Helliwell, K. Tea flavonoids, their functions, utilization and analysis. *Trends Food Sci. Tech.,* 2000, 11, 152-160.

Weinreb, O; Amit, T; Mandel, S; Youdim, MB. Neuroprotective molecular mechanisms of (-)-epigallocatechin-3-gallate: a reflective outcome of its antioxidant, iron chelating and neuritogenic properties. *Genes. Nutr.,* 2009, 4, 283-296.

In: Horizons in Cancer Research. Volume 61
Editor: Hiroto S. Watanabe
ISBN: 978-1-63484-503-8

Chapter 7

The Effects and Long-Term Outlook of Cancer Therapies on Cardiovascular Structure and Function in Childhood Cancer Survivors

Donald R. Dengel[1,2,*], Kara L. Marlatt[3] and Christiana J. Raymond[1]
[1]School of Kinesiology, University of Minnesota, Minneapolis, Minnesota, US
[2]Department of Pediatrics, University of Minnesota, Minneapolis, Minnesota, US
[3]Pennington Biomedical Research Center, Baton Rouge, Louisiana, US

Abstract

Cancer is the leading cause of death by disease among United States children and adolescents. Although cancer incidence among children and adolescents has remained relatively constant over the last few decades, enhanced technological innovation, diagnostic techniques, and improved treatment approaches have led to an improvement in overall survival rate for all cancers. Moreover, the increase in childhood cancer survivorship has resulted in a new area of concern among healthcare professionals. Childhood and adolescent cancer survivors are more likely to develop cardiovascular and metabolic diseases than have a reoccurrence of cancer. Therefore, healthcare professionals need to be aware of the long-term consequences of cancer treatments to ensure a cancer survivor is free of future disease for years to come. While the exact mechanisms by which these cancer treatments cause cardiovascular and metabolic dysfunction are largely unknown, vascular dysfunction and its modulation of cardiovascular disease (CVD) progression among childhood cancer survivors is an avenue of research that has gained increased attention.

Current cancer regimens typically employ multi-modal treatments, which can include surgery, radiation therapy, and/or multi-agent chemotherapy. Certain

* Corresponding author: Donald R. Dengel, Ph.D., University of Minnesota 1900 University Avenue S.E. 110 Cooke Hall Minneapolis, MN 55455, Phone Number: (612) 626-9701, Fax Number: (612) 625-8867, E-mail: denge001@umn.edu.

chemotherapeutic agents have been implicated in both early onset cardiotoxicity and the late development of cardiac abnormalities. In particular, repetitive administration of anthracyclines, as well as cyclophosphamides, has been shown to have cardiotoxic effects. Indeed, abnormalities in left ventricular structure and function have been observed with cumulative doses of these agents, leading to cardiac-related diseases such as cardiomyopathy and congestive heart failure. Cancer patients who undergo irradiation of the head and neck have been found to have a higher risk of developing significant carotid stenosis and increased carotid intima-media thickness. In addition, cancer patients who undergo thoracic irradiation have been found to develop inflammation and fibrotic lesions within the heart, increasing the risk of CVD.

Research from our laboratory in young adult survivors of childhood acute lymphoblastic leukemia has demonstrated that vascular function is reduced some 25 years after these individuals had undergone chemotherapy. Additional studies in children who survived central nervous system tumors, solid tumors or leukemia, demonstrated that individuals who received chemotherapy had reductions in brachial artery function. In addition, leukemia survivors who received chemotherapy also had reduced carotid compliance and distensibility compared to healthy controls. Time since diagnosis was found to have no effect on endothelial dysfunction, suggesting the declines in vascular structure and function may be present early on in survivorship. Thus, monitoring cardiovascular risk factors in childhood cancer survivors of all ages is critical to ensuring long-term survival. In the following chapter we will discuss the burdens of childhood cancer survivorship and the consequences of different treatment therapies on the incidence of CVD. In addtion, this chapter will explore potential monitoring methods and the need for consistent cardiovascular monitoring of childhood cancer survivors regarding their cardiovascular health.

Cancer is the second most common cause of death in the United States, exceeded only by heart disease, and accounts for nearly one quarter of all annual deaths (U.S. Mortality Public Use Data Tape, 2003; Cancer Facts & Figures 2015). Approximately 50% of men and 33% of women will develop cancer during their lifetime (Ehrman et al., 2009), with cancer mortality being higher in men compared to women for every racial and ethnic group. In 2015, it is expected that there will be approximately 1.6 million newly diagnosed cancer cases and over half a million cancer deaths (roughly 1,620 people per day) in the United States alone, of which approximately 1,250 cancer deaths are expected to occur in children aged 0 to 14 years (Cancer Facts & Figures, 2015) At this rate, cancer is set to become the leading cause of death in the United States within the next 25 years. The economic burden of cancer-related medical costs, including hospital outpatient doctor office visits, hospital inpatient stays, and prescription drugs, in the United States in 2011 alone was $88.7 billion, and it has been estimated that these costs could increase to $158 billion by the year 2020 (Cancer Facts & Figures, 2015; Mariotto et al., 2010).

Although the rate of diagnosed cancer cases is growing, there is some good news. Improvements in technological innovation, diagnostic techniques, and treatment approaches over the past few decades have led to an improved 5-year relative survival rate for all cancers diagnosed (Cancer Facts & Figures, 2015). This increase in cancer survivors, however, has resulted in a new area of concern among healthcare professionals. Specifically, childhood and adolescent cancer survivors are more likely to develop cardiovascular and metabolic diseases than have a reoccurrence of cancer (Mertens et al., 2001; Mertens, 2007). The long-term consequences of cancer treatment, often referred to as "late effects," (greater than 1 year post cancer treatment) are critical to be aware of and to monitor to ensure a survivor is free of future disease for years to come. While the exact mechanisms by which these treatments cause cardiovascular and metabolic dysfunction are largely unknown, vascular dysfunction and its modulation of cardiovascular disease (CVD) progression among childhood cancer survivors is an avenue of research that has gained increased attention.

The following chapter will also discuss the burdens of cancer survivorship and the consequences of different treatment therapies on the central and peripheral vasculature. We will examine the physiology and function as they relate to both central and peripheral endothelium, cardiac myocyte cells and cardiac electrical conduction. Understanding the effect of cancer therapies on the vascular endothelium is vital to assessing the damage these therapies have on overall vascular health. Further, changes in cardiac structure and function resulting from treatment therapies can cause dysfunction within any region of the heart, including the pericardium, chambers, valves, and conduction system. These changes in the heart lead to cardiac hypertrophy, the development of fibrotic lesions, and excess wall stress (Lipshultz et al., 2013). Ultimately these cardiac abnormalities may lead to the development of cardiac-related diseases such as cardiomyopathy and congestive heart failure (Adams and Lipshultz, 2005). Finally, this chapter will examine the therapeutic approaches to readily and cost-effectively evaluate cardiac and vascular function and structure among childhood cancer survivors. These assessment techniques may help healthcare professionals' better monitor CVD progression and the presence of related abnormalities among this population of cancer survivors.

Cancer Diagnosis and Treatment Consequences

Cancer Diagnosis

Since the risk of being diagnosed with cancer increases with age, most cancer diagnoses occur in adults who are middle-aged or older. According to 2015 statistics reported by the American Cancer Society, 78% of all cancers are diagnosed in individuals 55 years of age and older, with only 4% diagnosed between the ages of 20 and 39 years (Cancer Facts & Figures, 2015). Still, among children and adolescents in the United States, cancer is the leading cause of death by disease and the second leading cause of all childhood fatalities, exceeded only by accidents (Cancer Facts & Figures, 2015). In 2007 alone, approximately 10,400 children under 15 years of age were diagnosed with cancer in the United States (ACS 2007 Report), and estimates of 10,380 new cases of childhood cancer are expected to occur in the year 2015 (Cancer Facts & Figures, 2015). More than half of these newly diagnosed cases are leukemia and cancers of the brain and central nervous system (CNS). Indeed, a 2015 report by the American Cancer Society revealed that acute lymphoblastic leukemia (30%), brain and CNS (26%), neuroblastoma (6%), and non-Hodgkin's lymphoma (5%) are the most common cancers in children 0 to 14 years of age, while Hodgkin's lymphoma (15%), thyroid carcinoma (11%), brain and CNS (10%) and testicular germ cell tumors (8%) are the most common among adolescents ages 15 to 19 years.

Although the incidence of children diagnosed with all forms of invasive cancer increased slightly from 11.5 cases in 1975 to 16.4 cases per 100,000 children in 2010 and has increased by 0.6% per year from 2007 to 2011, the mortality rate due to childhood cancer has decreased 67% in the past few decades, from 6.3 deaths in 1970 to 2.1 deaths per 100,000 children in 2011 (Cancer Facts & Figures, 2015). At the same time, the survival rate has increased dramatically for most childhood cancers (Cancer Facts & Figures, 2015). In fact, the 5-year survival rates for childhood cancers altogether increased from 58.1 percent in 1975-1977 to 83.1 percent in 2003-2009 (Howlader et al., 2013). In the United States alone, this success translates into more than 325,000 survivors of childhood cancer, of whom 24% are now 30 years or more from diagnosis and are now young to middle-aged adults (Mariotto et al., 2009). This dramatic improvement in survival rates for many childhood cancers is due to more effective diagnosis of certain cancers at an earlier stage, as well as improvements in multi-modal treatment techniques such as surgical interventions, risk-stratified, multi-agent chemotherapeutic and radiation approaches, as well as hematopoietic stem cell transplantation (i.e., bone marrow transplantation) (Smith & Ries, 2002). Yet while these cancer treatments dramatically improve survival rates, various cancer therapies and administering techniques may cause particular health complications later in life. As a result, there is an expanding and aging population of childhood cancer survivors in need of continual healthcare and monitoring to ensure longevity.

Treatment Consequences

One of the growing challenges in oncology is providing appropriate healthcare for these childhood and adolescent cancer survivors due to increased risks of early mortality often associated with the treatment-induced development of secondary malignancies and cardiac or pulmonary disease (Mertens et al., 2001). These extremely effective cancer treatments are designed to limit cell growth and eliminate the offending malignancy, and as such, have the potential to damage or interfere with function in essential organ systems that are otherwise healthy (Ness & Gurney, 2007). Since no organ system functions independently, it is clear that long-term complications are usually interrelated and rarely limited to one system. Indeed, childhood cancer survivors have a 7 to 8 times greater risk of dying from CVD and experiencing related metabolic abnormalities as a result of these therapeutic approaches compared to the general population (Mertens et al., 2001; Mertens, 2007). Studies estimate that two-thirds of childhood and adolescent survivors have at least one chronic or late-occurring complication of their cancer therapy, with about one-third having serious or life-threatening complications (Oeffinger & Hudson, 2004). Nearly one-half of young adult survivors of childhood cancer have at least one major adverse outcome of their health status as a result of their cancer therapy (Hudson et al., 2003). Additionally, the time lapse since therapy completion often exacerbates these late effects (Lipshultz et al., 1991; Yeung et al., 1991).

The late effects commonly observed among children and adolescents are different than those observed among adults. Whereas adult cancers are more strongly related to lifestyle and environmental risk factor exposure (e.g., radiation and chemical exposure, hormones, unhealthy diet, or lack of physical activity), childhood cancers are often the result of cellular DNA mutations that take place in the first few years of life (fetal or neonatal) when cells are dividing at a faster rate. Furthermore, adults have the added complexity of a longer medical history prior to treatment that makes it difficult to assess the independent contribution of these treatments to the observed late-effects. Indeed, the vascular endothelium is negatively affected by a number of lifestyle choices (i.e., smoking, obesity, physical inactivity, elevated lipids, etc.,) as well as aging (Dengel et al., 2014; Juonala et al., 2004; Kotsis et al., 2006; Burke et al., 2008; Steinberg et al., 1996; Williams et al., 2005; Olson et al., 2006; DeSouza et al., 2000). As a result, the vast majority of adult research has focused on decreasing future event rates (e.g., heart attack, stroke, coronary plaque) (Greve et al., 2010; Andersen et al., 2010; Oh et al., 2007; Hooning et al., 2006; Hooning et al., 2007; Jagsi et al., 2006; Hull et al., 2003).

Children and adolescents, on the other hand, are often diagnosed and treated for cancer at an age at which pubertal maturation is not yet complete, making it possible to more easily identify subclinical outcomes of their cancer treatment. Treatment in these early years of development can result in compromised cardiovascular and organ-specific developments that may delay or even halt sexual maturation, as well as compromise musculoskeletal (i.e., bone, joint), respiratory, and sensory (e.g., hearing, vision) development, if treated before or during these critical development years. Similarly, these therapies likely cause damage to both the cardiac and vascular endothelium leading to the induction of atherosclerosis and eventual CVD progression over time. And because childhood cancer survivors are still very young following treatment cessation, the impact of these cancer therapies on the endothelium over time is critical to understand.

The Vascular Endothelium

Even though the human vascular system extends continuously throughout the body, there is one structural component that commonly extends throughout the entire vascular system – the endothelial cell. Throughout the vascular system, these endothelial cells form a single-celled layer commonly referred to as the endothelium. Although capillaries consist only of the endothelium, the large conduit arteries of the body (aorta, carotid, iliac, femoral, and brachial) consist of an outer cylinder composed of smooth muscle surrounding the inner layer of endothelial cells that provide a low resistance path for the blood supply to travel from the heart to the visceral organs and limbs. The ability of an artery to dilate or constrict is controlled by both the ability of the endothelium to dilate the artery known as endothelial-dependent dilation, as well as the ability of the endothelial cells in commanding the smooth muscle to relax and dilate the artery often referred to as endothelial-independent dilation.

The endothelium not only serves as a semipermeable barrier between the vessel wall and the bloodstream, but also functions as a highly active autocrine, paracrine, and endocrine organ that plays a crucial role in regulating blood flow, vascular tone, and vascular repair (Smith et al, 2000; Liebermann et al., 2006). A primary function of all vascular endothelial cells is the secretion of a wide variety of active molecules in the regulation of vascular homeostasis. One such molecule secreted by the vascular endothelium is nitric oxide (NO), which is responsible for endogenous vasodilation (Stamler et al., 1994; Vallance et al., 1989; Furchgott & Zawadzki, 1980). Nitric oxide has also been shown to possess many potent antiatherogenic properties such as inhibition of leukocyte adhesion (Kubes et al., 1991), platelet aggregation (Randomski et al., 1990), vascular smooth muscle proliferation (Garg & Hassid, 1989; Halcox & Deanfield, 2004), and thrombosis, thereby conferring a protective effect on the human vasculature (Anderson et al., 1995; Cines et al., 1998; Yoshida et al., 2006). Perturbations, such as those caused by inflammation or high hydrodynamic shear stress, can disrupt these homeostatic activities and induce endothelial cells to create a prothrombotic and anti-fibrinolytic microenvironment. Therefore, avoiding damage to the endothelium is imperative to maintain cardiovascular health due to the prominent role the endothelium plays in maintaining basal and dynamic vascular tone, as well as normal vascular function.

Measuring Arterial Structure and Function

Given atherosclerosis begins early in life and likely develops at a faster rate in childhood cancer survivors, there is strong evidence to suggest that endothelial function should be evaluated among childhood cancer survivors to better understand the risk of CVD and metabolic abnormalities throughout life. In addition, evaluating vascular structure and function may be used as a monitoring tool for the early detection of CVD. The following are techniques used to assess vascular structure and function for detecting potential subclinical atherosclerosis.

Endothelial-Dependent Dilation

The most widely used non-invasive technique for measuring endothelial-dependent dilation (EDD) is high-resolution ultrasound imaging of the brachial artery in response to reactive hyperemia (Agewall et al., 2001; Corretti et al., 2002). Prior to the initiation of reactive hyperemia a resting ultrasound image is captured. The hyperemic stimulus is then created by inflating a blood pressure cuff placed on the forearm or calf to approximately 50 mmHg or greater above systolic pressure, for 5 minutes. The cuff is rapidly deflated, creating an increase in blood flow, which causes the endothelium to release NO, resulting in dilation of the artery through communication with the vascular smooth muscle. The artery is imaged for approximately 2 to 5 minutes after the release of the blood pressure cuff and evaluated for the peak dilation of the artery above the baseline measure.

This technique is the preferred means of providing a non-invasive index of endothelial health in both healthy and diseased populations (Celermajer et al., 1992; Celermajer et al., 1993; Chowienczyk et al., 1992; Corretti et al., 1995; Corretti et al., 2002; Lieberman et al., 1996; Raitakari & Celermajer, 2000; Roman et al., 2006; Williams et al., 1996) given its ability to suitably assess early preclinical stages of atherosclerosis or in instances of repeated measurement. Additionally, EDD of the brachial arteries is highly correlated with vascular function in the coronary arteries (Anderson et al., 1995). The main drawback for this method is the clarity of the brachial images is dependent to a large degree on the skill of the ultrasound sonographer. Poor image quality often leads to low reproducibility of this technique and decreases the clinical usefulness of this methodology.

Endothelial-Independent Dilation via Nitroglycerin

Endothelial-independent dilation (EID) can also be determined via high-resolution imaging of arterial response to sublingual nitroglycerin administration. Using this technique, a resting ultrasound image is made and sublingual nitroglycerin is administered. Artery images are collected for 5 to 10 minutes after nitroglycerin administration. The typical EID response is often 3-4 times greater than EDD (Thelen et al., 2008), and helps ensure that abnormalities of EDD are due truly to endothelial dysfunction and the result of abnormal NO-bioavailability, not necessarily smooth muscle insensitivity to NO (Bressler et al., 2000; Ducharme et al., 1999; Pepe et al., 2004; Roman et al., 2006). Specifically, nitroglycerin is converted to NO in the body by mitochondrial aldehyde dehydrogenase and does not require the endothelium to generate NO. Thus, smooth muscle relaxation will occur regardless of any endothelial dysfunction present. Similar to EDD, this non-invasive method has proven to be both cost-effective and reliable and has been used successfully in children (>6 years of age) and vulnerable populations. However, like EDD this method is again dependent on image quality and a skilled ultrasound sonographer. In addition, the use of sublingual nitroglycerin makes some researchers and clinicians hesitant to measure EID using this technique.

EDD and EID via Pulse Wave Amplitude

A newer method of determining EDD and EID involves measuring changes in the pulse wave amplitude in response to reactive hyperemia or sublingual nitroglycerin. Changes in the pulse wave amplitude are typically registered at the finger, so this method is sometimes referred to as finger-pulse plethysmography (Munzel et al., 2008). Although the method is simple to use and is less dependent on technical skill than high-resolution ultrasound imaging, it is limited to the finger and does not allow one to measure other vascular beds. It should also be noted that this method measures a resistance vessel (microvasculature) rather than a conduit vessel (e.g., brachial and carotid arties). In addition, in has been reported that in young children, using digital reactive hyperemia is not a completely valid method to quantify microvascular function and often leads to uninterpretable values (Kelly et al., 2014). Part of the issue of using finger-pulse plethysmography may be the finger probes used were designed for the adult finger and may not fit a child's smaller fingers properly.

Arterial Compliance

Another way to determine vascular function is to measure the change in lumen diameter in response to diastole and systole (e.g., arterial compliance) (Fernhall et al., 2008). Similar to EDD and EID, arterial compliance can be measured using high-resolution ultrasound imaging. These high-resolution ultrasound images are typically captured at the carotid artery or the aorta, but they can also be made at other arteries (brachial and femoral). Although this measure is reasonably accurate, it is limited somewhat by the fact that it is best to have a direct measure of blood pressure at the artery where compliance is actually being determined (Fernhall et al., 2008).

Pulse Wave Velocity

Measuring the arterial pulse wave velocity (PWV) is another way to determine arterial function. The arterial PWV can be measured using either Doppler ultrasound or a pressure-sensitive transducer. Both central (aortic and carotid to femoral artery) and peripheral (femoral to dorsalis pedis artery) PWV can be determined. This method involves measuring the time for the pulse wave to travel the length of a particular arterial pathway; the higher the PWV, the stiffer or less compliant the vessel. The methodology used to measure pulse wave velocity is both simple to use and cost-effective (Huck et al., 2007; Dengel & Bronas, 2010).

Carotid Intima-Media Thickness

High-resolution ultrasound imaging of the right and left common carotid artery wall is the most widely used method to evaluate the structure of the artery (Dengel & Bronas, 2010). Determining carotid intima-media thickness (IMT) often involves collecting a series of images of the far vessel wall, approximately 1 cm in length and 1 to 2 cm proximal to the bifurcation of the carotid. A mean value for these images of the IMT is then calculated (Dengel & Bronas, 2010). Measures of IMT can also be made of both the internal and external carotid artery as well as the bifurcation of the carotid artery. In addition, the IMT of other arteries (i.e., abdominal aorta, femoral, brachial, etc.) can also be used to determine the IMT because other arteries may actually demonstrate thickening of the IMT earlier than the carotid artery (Dawson et al., 2009).

Brachial or Femoral Artery Infusions

While intra-arterial infusion methods are considered the gold standard to measure endothelial-dependent and independent dilation, the invasive nature of this technique makes it impractical for measurement of endothelial function in children and adolescents, as well as other populations for voluntary, sub-clinical assessment. Indeed, EDD can be assessed using brachial artery infusions of endothelium-dependent vasodilation agents such as acetylcholine, bradykinin, substance P, and adenosine (Munzel et al., 2008). Similarly, EID can be evaluated via intra-arterial infusions of sodium nitroprusside, which bypasses the endothelium and works directly on the smooth muscle of the artery. The response of the artery to these vasodilatory agents is monitored by high-resolution ultrasound imaging or strain gauge plethysmography. The latter method involves placing an elastic strain gauge around the forearm or calf that will record the change in the volume.

Echocardiography

Non-invasive monitoring of myocardial toxicity from radiation therapy, anthracyclines and other chemotherapeutic agents can be performed via the assessment of left ventricular systolic function, with either radionuclide ventriculography or echocardiography. Fractional shortening and left ventricular ejection fraction are the most commonly used measurements (Lipshultz et al., 2008) yet often depend on preload and afterload.

Positron Emission, Computed Tomography and Magnetic Resonance Imaging

Positron emission (PET), computed tomography (CT), and magnetic resonance imaging (MRI) scans provide another method of assessing not only cardiac responsiveness but also cerebrovascular responsiveness post-treatment. Although not as cost effective or easily administered due to movement error (especially cardiac), these techniques can provide insight pertaining to both cardiac and cerebral perfusion rates following radiotracer administration, as well as presence of cortical atrophy, calcification, and white matter hypodensity following treatment (Kahkonen et al., 1999; Bouwers et al., 1985). Of these techniques, MRI imaging is preferred given the level of emitted radiation via PET and CT scanning.

Treatment Consequences on the Endothelium

Although atherosclerosis takes many years to develop, the initial process begins early in life and is likely accelerated in childhood cancer survivors as a result of the chemotherapy and radiation used to treat the cancer. While often having differing effects when used alone or in combination with one another, many of these cancer treatments are thought to promote an internal environment favorable to obesity, atherosclerosis, impaired glucose metabolism, as well as other cardiovascular and metabolic risk factors that promote the development of CVD (Shankar et al., 2008).

Research from our laboratory (Dengel et al., 2008; Dengel et al., 2014) and others (Chow et al., 2006; Heinkens et al., 2000; Herceg-Cavrak et al., 2011; Jarvela et al., 2013; Jenei et al., 2013; Meeske et al., 2009; Oeffinger et al., 2009) on young adult survivors of childhood cancer has demonstrated that vascular function and structure are reduced following completion of chemotherapy and radiation, as well as stem cell transplantation. Table 1 summarizes the existing literature on the current cancer treatment modalities, and their impact on the vasculature is discussed.

Surgical Intervention

Surgery has a very limited role in the treatment of childhood cancer, usually reserved for those individuals diagnosed with benign or malignant neoplasms. While the type of cancer and regional location within the body dictates the extent in which surgery is performed, oncologists and surgeons do their best to limit the effects of surgery by striking a balance between removing all the cancer and taking out as little healthy tissue as possible. Indeed, surgical removal of such neoplasms is often prescribed in combination with radiation therapy. However, research has demonstrated that surgical treatment (in combination with or without radiation therapy) has little effect on vascular reactivity, EDD, and EID (Dengel et al., 2014).

Table 1. Vascular Function and Structure in Childhood Cancer Survivors (CCS)

Participants	Vascular Function	Vascular Structure	Arterial Stiffness	Reference
26 survivors of childhood brain cancer vs. healthy controls		cIMT ↑		Heikens et al. (2000)
14 child and adolescent CCS who received anthracycline treatment vs. 14 healthy controls	EDD ↓			Chow et al. (2006)
75 adults ALL survivors; 3 groups examined: chemo only, chemo+radiation, and healthy controls	EDD ↓ EID ↔			Dengel et al. (2008)
30 CCS who received neck radiation vs. healthy controls		cIMT ↑		Meeske et al. (2009)
53 Youth CCS vs. healthy controls			PWV ↑	Herceg-Cavrak et al. (2011)
96 Youth CCS vs. 72 controls; 3 Groups Examined: anthracycline treated, chemo only, and healthy controls	EDD ↑			Jenei et al. (2013)
21 ALL survivors (age 16-30 y) vs. 21 healthy controls	EDD ↓			Jarvela et al. (2013)
319 youth CCS vs. 208 sibling controls	EDD ↓ EID ↑	cIMT ↔	IEM ↓ DD ↓ CSD ↓	Dengel et al. (2014)

Abbreviation (in order of appearance): cIMT = carotid intima-media thickness, EDD = endothelium-dependent dilation, EID = endothelium-independent dilation, PWV = pulse wave velocity, IEM = incremental elastic modulus, DD = carotid diameter distensibility, CSD = carotid cross-sectional distensibility.

Radiation Therapy

Radiation therapy is also an effective tool for the treatment of malignant neoplasms, as well as suppressing the immune system prior to transplant. However, unlike surgical interventions, radiation has been demonstrated to alter the vascular endothelium as well as introduce related cardiovascular and metabolic risk factors. Interestingly, radiation therapy has been shown to affect the structural integrity of the endothelium yet has little effect on endothelial cell responsiveness compared to chemotherapy. Two factors (e.g., location, dosage) are important in determining the impact of radiation therapy on the vascular endothelium.

Location

The impact of radiation therapy on the vasculature is greatly affected by the direct path and region of therapy administration. Indeed, cranial radiation therapy (CRT), which targets the head and neck, has been shown to affect the structure of the vessel wall. For instance, carotid IMT is often thicker in those cancer survivors who have received CRT (Heikens et al.,

2000; Dengel et al., 2014; Meeske et al., 2009). Similar findings have also been reported in CNS brain tumor survivors (Dengel et al., 2014).

Head and neck radiation has also been shown to affect both the thyroid and pituitary gland and thereby alter metabolism. CRT may also lead to delayed pubertal development or halt it altogether. Indeed, survivors of acute lymphoblastic leukemia (ALL) who received CRT have higher triglyceride, low-density lipoprotein cholesterol (LDL-C), total cholesterol, blood pressure, and body mass index (BMI) values in comparison with those individuals treated with only chemotherapy (Oeffinger et al., 2001; Dengel et al., 2008). Furthermore, CRT has also been shown to increase risk of developing the metabolic syndrome in childhood survivors of ALL compared with survivors not treated with CRT (van Waas et al., 2010; Talvensaari et al., 1996; Dvorak et al., 2011). Similar findings on increased risk of developing the metabolic syndrome have also been observed in childhood brain tumor survivors (Pietilä et al., 2009).

Radiation to the mediastinum region has been shown to have multiple effects on the heart such as the development of fibrotic lesions in the myocardium; pericardial fibrosis; valvular dysfunction; electrical conduction abnormalities (i.e., arrhythmias); heart failure; and premature coronary artery disease (CAD) (Lipshultz et al., 1993; Adams et al., 2003; Adams and Lipshultz, 2005; Mulrooney et al., 2009; Schellong et al., 2010). Mediastinal radiation therapy also causes inflammation in the heart, which leads to an increase in and accumulation of platelets and fibrin to the affected region. Consequently, the lumen diameter of the affected myocardial blood vessel decreases, while platelet- and fibrin-containing thrombi develop; the blood vessel may therefore become completely blocked, eventually causing myocardial cell death and infarction (Adams et al., 2003; Lipshultz et al., 2013). Mediastinal radiation has been reported to increase the relative risk of death from a cardiac-related event anywhere from 2.2 to 7.2-fold compared with the general population, approximately two-thirds of which are caused by myocardial infarction (Adams et al., 2003). In addition, research has indicated that those who receive mediastinal radiation therapy alone (i.e., with no concurrent chemotherapy) are at a greater risk of developing restrictive cardiomyopathy as a result of diastolic dysfunction. Conversely, those who receive radiation therapy in combination with chemotherapeutic agents, or chemotherapeutic agents alone, are at a greater risk of developing dilated cardiomyopathy as a result of systolic dysfunction (Adams & Lipshultz, 2005).

Dosage

Therapeutic dosage is another important factor when considering cardiovascular consequences due to radiation treatment. Indeed, CRT dosage greater than or equal to 20 Gy has been shown to be associated with an increased prevalence of obesity, especially in females treated at a young age (Oeffinger et al., 2003). High doses of radiation to the head and neck can cause increased risk of stroke. In fact, survivors of childhood leukemia and brain tumors, particularly those treated with CRT at doses of >30 Gy, are also at an increased risk of stroke and are associated with increased carotid IMT at doses as low as 1,800 cGY (Bowers et al., 2006; Meeske et al., 2009).

Similarly, high doses of radiation to the thoracic region of the body can increase the risk of serious conditions affecting the cardiovascular system, including CVD, cardiomyopathy, and congestive heart failure, as well as the development of additional neoplasms. Specifically, the risk of mortality increases in those treated with a mediastinal radiation dose >30 Gy

(Castellino et al., 2011; Schellong et al., 2010). Further, radiation doses of 35 Gy or greater are associated with an increased risk of myocardial infarction (Mulrooney et al., 2009). These study results can be found in Table 2. Additional studies have shown that death due to CAD and other cardiac-related diseases is significantly increased following a cumulative mediastinal radiation dose between 40 and 45 Gy (Hancock et al., 1993). Recently, however, efforts have been made to reduce and modify radiation dosage in the treatment of childhood cancers based on a patient's risk factors of disease. When those diagnosed with early-stage Hodgkin's lymphoma have been treated with chemotherapeutic agents alone, tumor growth has been successfully limited (Ruhl et al., 2001; Behrendt et al., 1987; Yaniv et al., 1993); however, negative outcomes have resulted when radiation therapy was completely withheld from those patients diagnosed with late-stage Hodgkin's lymphoma and who were therefore given greater doses of chemotherapeutic treatment as compensation (Ekert et al., 1988). Essentially, patients exposed to any dosage of radiation therapy are susceptible to cardiotoxic late effects; however, the ability to diagnose the patient in the early stages of cancer—thereby limiting the radiation and anthracycline dosages received—may allow for improved five-year survival rates and decrease the cardiotoxic late effects of treatment.

Chemotherapeutic Agents

Chemotherapy is the primary offender in the initiation and acceleration of endothelial dysfunction and atherosclerosis in survivors of childhood and adolescent cancers. While the exact mechanisms by which chemotherapy causes vascular dysfunction is not clear, several chemotherapeutic agents (i.e., alkylators, antimetabolites, alkaloids, anthracyclines, cyclophosphamide, cisplatin, and methotrexate) have been shown to elicit endothelial damage (Oeffinger et al., 2008; Murata et al., 2001; Wu et al., 2002; Nuver et al., 2005). Anthracyclines are one of the most widely used and effective cancer therapies that have been studied extensively, yet they cause the greatest amount of cardiotoxicity in children and adults than other chemotherapeutic agents (Lipshultz et al., 1999; Lipshultz et al., 2013; Kremer et al., 2001). Anthracycline-induced cardiotoxicity studies have revealed that doxorubicin administered both *in vitro* and *in vivo* cause apoptosis of vascular endothelial cells (Murata, Yamawaki, & Yoshimoto, 2001; Wu, Ko, & Teng, 2002; Shankar et al., 2008). Furthermore, apoptosis is associated with reduced endothelial cell density, decreased NO bioavailability, and a decrease in endothelial function as determined by acetylcholine infusions (Asai et al., 2000). Therefore, it is possible that administration of these chemotherapeutic agents increases apoptosis that causes permanent damage to the vasculature.

Limited research exists about the effects of chemotherapy on endothelial function (Table 1). Dengel et al. (Dengel et al., 2008) observed that young adult survivors of childhood ALL are at risk for reduced EDD regardless of whether or not they received CRT, yet did not find differences in EID; similar EDD findings were reported by Chow et al. (2006). Jenei et al. (2013) also observed decreased EDD, distensibilty, and increased aortic stiffness in survivors examined more than 10 years post-treatment. Specifically, brachial artery EDD, distensibilty, and stiffness index were all significantly reduced in survivors who received chemotherapy or chemotherapy plus anthracycline compared to healthy controls. No differences in EID were reported. These findings demonstrate that chemotherapy likely leads to endothelial-mediated decrements, with anthracyclines often exacerbating these decrements, yet display little effect on endothelial-smooth muscle communication.

Table 2. Cardiac Function and Structure in Childhood Cancer Survivors (CCS)

Reference	Participants	Measure of Cardiac Structure, Function, or Disease Incidence	Results
Nysom et al. (1998)	189 survivors of childhood ALL: • 3 levels of anthracycline treatment (mg/m^2): • 0-23, 45, 73-301, 244-550	• LVEDD • LV fractional shortening	• Significantly ↑ mean LVEDD & ↓ mean LV fractional shortening in highest dose group compared to other 3 • Significantly ↑ LV fractional shortening in the other 3 groups; declined with increasing anthracycline dose
Adams et al. (2004)	48 childhood HL survivors (~14.3 years after diagnosis); median dose of 40.0 Gy mRT	• Valvular function • Conduction • LVWT; LVEDD; LVM; LVC	• ↔ LVWT; ↓ LVEDD; ↓ LVM; only 1 with ↓ LVC • 42% with mitral & aortic valvular defects (>30 Gy) • 75% with conduction defects
Lipshultz et al. (2005)	115 survivors of childhood ALL: • 3 levels of doxorubicin treatment (mg/m^2) <300; 300-400, >400	• LVC; LVWT; LVD; LV mass:volume ratio	• ↓ LVC ≥12 years post-diagnosis in moderate and high groups • ↓ LVWT relative to BSA • ↓ LVD with increasing follow-up • ↓ LV mass:volume ratio
Hudson et al. (2007)	278 CCS: 223 at-risk for cardiotoxicity after treatment: • Anthracyclines (mean dose 202±109mg/m^2) • Thoracic irradiation	• LVC (LV fractional shortening, afterload)	• ↓ mean LV fractional shortening for at-risk (0.33 ± 0.06) compared with not at-risk (0.36 ± 0.05) and healthy controls (0.36 ± 0.04) • ↑ mean afterload for at-risk (58 g/cm^2) than not at-risk (46 g/cm2) and healthy controls (48 g/cm^2)
Schellong et al. (2010)	1,132 HL CCS treated <18 years of age: • 834 with mRT: 5 subgroups by dose (36, 30, 25, 20, 0 Gy; median dose 25.0 Gy) • 298 with no mRT	• Valvular function • Conduction • Coronary artery function	• 898 survivors (80% of study group) • 50 with CD; 28/50 with dyspnea and/or angina • VD (33/50); CAD & MD (14/50); conduction abnormalities (10/50); pericardial injury (8/50) • Highest probabilities for CD and VD in 36 Gy group, lowest in 20 Gy & 0 Gy groups.

Table 2. (Continued)

Reference	Participants	Measure of Cardiac Structure, Function, or Disease Incidence	Results
Rathe et al. (2007)	63 ALL CCS with multi-drug chemotherapy including anthracyclines – cumulative dose <300mg/m^2 vs. healthy age- and BSA-matched controls	• IVS; LVEDD; EF; LVEDS; LVM	• ↓ IVS & ↑ LVEDD compared with controls • 9/63 with EF <60%; 7/9 given cumulative dose >200mg/m^2 • Risk Factors: Young age for ↑ LVEDD; ↑ age for ↓ EF; male sex for ↑ LVEDD, LVEDS; female sex for ↓ LVM; length of follow up for ↑ LVEDD, ↓ EF; cumulative dose >200mg/m^2 for ↓ EF
Mulrooney et al. (2009)	14,358 5-year CCS aged <21 years, 4 treatment, 1 control: Chemo+radiation; RT & surgery alone; Chemo & surgery alone; RT only	• Incidence of and risk factors for: • CHF; MI; PD • Valvular abnormalities	• CCSs: greater likelihood of all measures • Chemo dose ≥250mg/m^2: ↑ relative hazard of CHF, PD, and valve dysfunction 2-5 times that of non-chemo; treated CCS • RT dose ≥15 Gy: ↑ relative hazard of all measures 2-6 times that of non-irradiated CCS; ↑ risk with higher dose (>35 Gy)

ALL: acute lymphoblastic leukemia; HL: Hodgkins Lymphoma; mRT: mediastinal radiation therapy; CD: cardiac disease; VD: valvular disease; CAD: coronary artery disease; MD: myocardial disease; LVD: left ventricular dimension; LVM: left ventricular mass; LVC: left ventricular contractility; LVWT: left ventricular wall thickness; LVPW: left ventricular posterior wall thickness at end systole; LVEDS: left ventricular dimensions at end systole; IVS: thickness of interventricular septum at end systole; LVEDD: left ventricular dimensions at end diastole; EF: ejection fraction; LVM: left ventricular mass; BSA: body surface area; CHF: congestive heart failure; MI: myocardial infarction; PD: pericardial disease.

Chemotherapy dose is also an important factor in determining the degree of cardiac and vascular dysfunction as a result of treatment. Lipshultz and colleagues (2005) conducted a study in which serial echocardiograms were performed on 115 doxorubicin-treated long-term survivors of childhood ALL. These survivors were given median individual doses of 30 mg/m^2 per dose and a median cumulative dose of 352 mg/m^2 and were subsequently grouped into three cumulative dosage categories: low, <300 mg/m^2; moderate, 300-400 mg/m^2; and high, >400 mg/m^2. At least twelve years after diagnosis, depressions in left ventricular contractility were observed, with statistical significance in the moderate and high dosage groups, in addition to significantly reduced left ventricular wall thickness relative to body surface area at treatment completion. Further, left ventricular wall thickness became thinner over time and was significantly less than normal beyond 6-year follow-up. Two other studies reported similar left ventricular wall thinning (Ness & Gurney, 2007; Shan et al., 1996).

Anthracycline therapy has also been implicated in higher incidence of subclinical dysfunction (Shankar et al., 2008; Kremer et al., 2002; Lipshultz et al., 2005; Mulrooney et al., 2009; Steinherz et al., 1991). We define subclinical dysfunction as cardiovascular or metabolic dysfunction that is not detectable via common medical diagnosis techniques. Among childhood cancer survivors, subclinical dysfunction in 11%, 23%, 47%, and 100% of patients treated with cumulative anthracycline doses of <400, 400 to 599, 600 to 799, and >800 mg/m^2, respectively, have been reported (Steinherz et al., 1991). Similar findings appear to be related to dose and time from treatment cessation (Kremer et al., 2002; Lipshultz et al., 2005; Mulrooney et al., 2009). Other cohort studies have reported development of subclinical cardiac dysfunction in survivors of ALL treated with doses of anthracyclines between 90 and 270 mg/m^2 (Sorensen et al., 1997), with longer cohort follow-up demonstrating patients receiving <240 mg/m^2 exhibit improved cardiac performance, yet those with higher doses had progressive deterioration in function as assessed by echocardiography (Sorensen et al., 2003). Indeed, an association between exposure to cumulative anthracycline doses of 250 mg/m^2 or greater, along with an increased risk for cardiac-related diseases such as pericardial disease, has been reported (Mulrooney et al., 2009).

While the use of anthracyclines, specifically doxorubicin and daunorubicin, have contributed significantly to the increased cancer survival rates observed in children, these drugs have been found to cause cardiac-related abnormalities; these include congestive heart failure and dilated cardiomyopathy (Mulrooney et al., 2009; Lipshultz, 2006). The heart is one of the most susceptible organs to the cardiotoxic effects of anthracyclines due to the limited ability of the endothelial cells of the myocardium to regenerate following myocardial cell death (Lipshultz et al., 2013). This fact is especially critical in the pediatric population, in which physical growth is not yet completed. In particular, doxorubicin acts to reduce the number of progenitor cells within the myocardium as a result of its production of oxygen-free radicals, which inhibits the differentiation and regeneration of these cells. As a direct result of this inhibition, myocardial structure (e.g., left ventricular wall thickness, left ventricular dimension and mass) and function (e.g., left ventricular contractility) are compromised (Lipshultz et al., 2013; Krischer et al., 1997). Anthracycline treatment has been shown to lead to both diastolic and systolic dysfunction and ultimately heart failure (Mulrooney et al., 2009; Lipshultz et al., 2013). In addition to these late effects, further susceptibility to this type of treatment is seen within the peripheral vascular system of cancer patients. Explicitly, blood flow is altered in the vascular system, affecting the overall health and function of endothelial cells in the cardiovascular system.

Additional studies (Table 2) have assessed the incidence of cardiac abnormalities and cardiac-related disease observed more than 20 years after diagnosis and cessation of treatment. In a sub-study comparing a subgroup of childhood cancer survivors from the Childhood Cancer Survivor Study to a sibling control group, Mulrooney and colleagues (2009) found that the most prevalent cardiac diseases associated with anthracycline plus mediastinal radiation treatment were heart failure, pericardial disease, valvular abnormalities, and myocardial infarction. Notably, the relative hazard of heart failure was increased in cancer survivors compared with sibling controls. In detail, risk of congestive heart failure was associated with the female sex, higher cumulative anthracycline and/or radiation dosage, less than 10 years of age at diagnosis, and treatment during the 1980s (Mulrooney et al., 2009). Moreover, this relative hazard increased more than 5-fold for anthracycline doses greater than 250 mg/m^2 and more than 2-fold for doses less than 250 mg/m^2 compared to sibling controls.

Similar findings by Steinherz and colleagues (1991) reported that 23% of CCSs were diagnosed with CVD more than 20 years following diagnosis. Nearly half of these individuals (11%) had developed heart failure following cumulative anthracycline doses <400 mg/m^2 and all experienced heart failure with anthracycline dosage >800 mg/m^2 (Steinherz et al., 1991). In summary, although a greater number of late effects have been observed among childhood cancer survivors that received higher dosages of anthracyclines, exposure to chemotherapeutic agents at any dosage can be cardiotoxic and should be carefully monitored.

Various other cardiovascular and metabolic abnormalities exist among survivors treated with chemotherapeutic agents. Increased body weight, body fat mass, fasting plasma glucose, and insulin levels, as well as decreased serum high-density lipoprotein cholesterol (HDL-C) and reduced ratio of HDL-C to total cholesterol have also been reported in childhood cancer survivors compared to healthy controls (Talvensaari et al., 1996). Other studies have reported increased body mass index z-scores between diagnosis and therapy completion among ALL survivors (mean age at diagnosis: 4.8 years); the highest level of corticosteroid exposure being associated with both obesity as well as hypertension, and females being more likely to have increased body mass index and elevated blood pressure compared to males (Chow et al., 2007).

Bone Marrow Transplantation

Hematopoietic stem cell transplantation, commonly referred to as bone marrow transplantation (BMT), is thought of as the ultimate form of treatment intensification and is often associated with the highest risk patients who fail to benefit from traditional chemotherapy and/or radiation. This particular treatment has a high curative rate for numerous types of leukemia, including ALL (Socié et al., 1999). Higher relative doses of chemotherapy and radiation are commonly administered prior to BMT, resulting in both vascular and organ damage intensification. Indeed, the endocrine system is highly susceptible to damage following chemotherapy and/or radiation in addition to BMT. Specifically, the thyroid gland, the pituitary, and the gonads are heavily influenced by BMT treatment and can lead to delayed pubertal development or halt it altogether (Dvorak et al., 2011; Berger et al., 2005; Bailey et al., 2008; Sanders et al., 2009). Bone mineral density may also be affected (Dvorak et al., 2011; Kaste et al., 2004). However, since the pathogenesis of the development of these disorders is multi-factorial, it is often difficult to implicate BMT as an independent cause of these disorders given high relative doses of chemotherapy and/or radiation prior to BMT administration.

Outlook and Monitoring in Childhood Cancer Survivors

Currently, long-term monitoring of childhood cancer survivors is inconsistent due to the fact that standardized clinical guidelines for the frequency and timing of follow-up have not been established. Lack of follow-up guidelines is evident when observing that the number of childhood cancer survivors that return for follow-up visits significantly decreases five years following the end of cancer treatment, especially among those who are asymptomatic (Lipshultz et al., 2013). Childhood cancer survivors treated with anthracyclines, however, are more likely to return for long-term follow-up than are those who received radiation therapy due to the greater likelihood of the presentation of symptoms in the anthracycline-treated patients. Additionally, non-oncologic community health care providers and physicians may be unaware of the extent of the incidence or severity of cardiovascular complications occurring as a result of late effects of cancer therapy. Consequently, less emphasis may be placed on the importance of consistent follow-up, especially among those treated with radiation therapy. Therefore, it is important that a standardized follow-up regimen be established and implemented to monitor and mediate the late effects of cancer therapy.

In an attempt to limit the extent of late effect severity in the pediatric population, particularly for patients who received anthracycline, radiation therapy, or a combination of the two treatments, pediatric oncology clinics have developed programs for the purpose of monitoring cardiotoxic late effects and providing interventions for various childhood cancer survivor populations (Lipshultz & Sallan, 1993). Currently, the two most commonly used methods to examine cardiovascular structure and function in cancer survivors are transthoracic echocardiography and radionuclide angiography. Transthoracic echocardiography is more convenient due to its non-invasive nature and its capability of imaging particular structures of the heart (e.g., pericardium) as well as measuring load-dependent (e.g., left ventricular fractional shortening) and load-independent variables (e.g., left ventricular contractility and wall stress).

In contrast with echocardiography, radionuclide angiography is an invasive technique used to assess left ventricular structure and function and does not allow for the assessment of load-independent measurements like echocardiography. This modality is, however, most useful for assessing left ventricular ejection fraction—the difference in the amount of blood in the left ventricle between end-diastole and end-systole due to its high reproducibility (Shankar et al., 2008). It is recommended that this modality be used every five years of follow-up in childhood cancer survivors, especially among childhood cancer survivors who are asymptomatic, for early detection of potential CAD and CVD risk due to cancer treatment (Adams and Lipshultz, 2005).

The extent of long-term monitoring and follow-up of childhood cancer survivors is dependent upon, but not limited to, the type of treatment (e.g., anthracyclines, mediastinal radiation therapy, etc.), age at diagnosis, cumulative dose of chemotherapeutic agent or radiation received, and the presence of symptoms and abnormalities (Children's Oncology Group, 2013; Lipshultz et al., 1993). Previous research has demonstrated that anthracyclines are often associated with systolic dysfunction, and therefore dilated cardiomyopathy, whereas treatment with radiation is associated with diastolic dysfunction and possible systolic dysfunction, and therefore restrictive cardiomyopathy; however, systolic dysfunction is more easily assessed due to the presence of symptoms than is diastolic dysfunction (Adams and Lipshultz, 2005).

Recently, the Children's Oncology Group established clinically based survivorship guidelines for children, adolescents, and young adults for the purpose of tracking late effects following cancer treatment and monitoring the long-term follow-up of childhood cancer survivors (Children's Oncology Group, 2013). Though not mandated, it is of utmost importance that symptomatic and asymptomatic childhood cancer survivors alike follow a consistent, regimented monitoring program with physical examinations and cardiovascular assessments. Immediately following treatment, a baseline echocardiography screening should be implemented in order to track any myocardial structural and functional changes (Shankar et al., 2008). Generally, childhood cancer survivors treated with anthracyclines, mediastinal radiation, or a combination of the two should have an annual follow-up visit with a physician beginning two years after the completion of cancer treatment. Further, childhood cancer survivors should be administered echocardiography-based screenings at least once every one to five years depending on the following: age at diagnosis and treatment, radiation and/or anthracycline dose, time since treatment, and the presence of CVD symptoms such as dyspnea and angina (Shankar et al., 2008; Lipshultz et al., 2013; Children's Oncology Group, 2013).

Specifically, the survivorship guidelines established by Children's Oncology Group are stratified based on age at treatment: less than one year of age, between one and four years of age, and older than five years of age. These guidelines recommend that those treated for cancer younger than five years of age and who received radiation treatment alone should have consistent echocardiography screenings once every two years, or annually if treated with a combination of radiation and anthracyclines. More specifically, those one to four years of age should be echocardiogram-screened every one, two, or five years if treated with a cumulative anthracycline dose ≥300 mg/m^2, ≥100 mg/m^2 to <300 mg/m^2, or <100 mg/m^2, respectively. Conversely, those who were treated at age five years or older with ≥30 Gy of therapeutic irradiation alone or in combination with an anthracycline dose <300 mg/m^2 should be given an echocardiogram every two years, and those with the same dose of therapeutic irradiation but a higher dose of anthracyclines (≥300 mg/m^2) should be administered an echocardiogram annually (Children's Oncology Group, 2013). Following these recommendations will improve assurance that any changes in cardiovascular structure or function can be closely monitored in an attempt to prevent a cardiac event or cardiac-related disease.

Finally, for those childhood cancer survivors who are asymptomatic at rest, exercise stress testing is recommended during follow-up visits to assess risk or signs of cardiac-related diseases. Indeed, this type of testing has been found to reveal abnormalities in cardiac structure and function, including signs of ischemia, coronary artery disease, and heart failure. For example, exercise stress testing in survivors of Hodgkin's Lymphoma who received mediastinal radiation treatment ≥35 Gy revealed indices of ischemia and CAD (Heidenreich et al., 2007). Further, severely reduced cardiac function with a resulting oxygen consumption of <20 ml/kg/min—indicative of heart failure—has been observed previously in 30% of Hodgkin's Lymphoma survivors (Adams et al., 2004). Therefore, exercise stress testing provides yet another modality allowing physicians and health care professionals to assess any changes in cardiovascular functioning in childhood cancer survivors who may be symptomatic or asymptomatic.

CONCLUSION

To date, research studies suggest that early in life, childhood cancer survivors have cardiovascular changes indicative of increased risk of cardiovascular-related diseases. While atherosclerosis takes many decades to develop, yet is thought to be accelerated in childhood cancer survivors, cost-effective techniques for routinely assessing cardiac and vascular dysfunction in this population may provide a useful step in the early diagnosis of sub-clinical CVD or accelerated atherosclerotic progression that may decrease future or long-term complications. Furthermore, the detrimental impact that cancer therapies, particularly chemotherapeutic agents and radiation therapy, have on the cardiac myocyte and endothelial cells within the body necessitates consistent follow-up and screening to prevent the progression and incidence of cardiac-related diseases, such as cardiomyopathy or congestive heart failure. Therefore, it is reasonable to advocate that efforts should be directed at monitoring and managing cardiovascular risk factors in childhood cancer survivors. In addition, future studies are needed to determine the exact mechanism by which chemotherapy causes endothelial dysfunction, as well as potential therapies aimed at reducing the decline in cardiovascular function in cancer survivors.

REFERENCES

Adams, M. J., Lipshultz, S. E., Schwartz, C., Fajardo, L. F., Coen, V. & Constine, L. S. (2003). Radiation-associated cardiovascular disease: manifestations and management. *Seminars in Radiation Oncology*, *13*(3), 346-356.

Adams, M. J., Lipsitz, S. R., Colan, S. D., Tarbell, N. J., Treves, S. T., Diller, L. & Lipshultz, S. E. (2004). Cardiovascular status in long-term survivors of Hodgkin's disease treated with chest radiotherapy. *Journal of Clinical Oncology*, *22*(15), 3139-3148.

Adams, M. J. & Lipshultz, S. E. (2005). Pathophysiology of anthracycline-and radiation-associated cardiomyopathies: Implications for screening and prevention. *Pediatric Blood & Cancer*, *44*(7), 600-606.

Agewall, S., Doughty, R.N., Bagg, W., Whalley, G.A., Braatvedt, G. & Sharpe, N. (2001). Comparison of ultrasound assessment of flow-mediated dilatation in the radial and brachial artery with upper and forearm cuff positions. *Clinical Physiology*, *21*(1), 9-14.

American Cancer Society. *Cancer Facts and Figures 2007*. Atlanta, GA: American Cancer Society. Retrieved December 26, 2007. Available from: http://www.cancer.org/downloads/STT/CAFF2007PWSecured.pdf. Retrieved April 10, 2014.

American Cancer Society (ACS). (2015). *Cancer Facts & Figures 2015*. Atlanta, GA: American Cancer Society. Retrieved September 29, 2015.

Anderson, T. J., Uehata, A., Gerhard, M. D., Meredith, I. T., Knab, S., Delagrange, D., Lieberman, E. H., Ganz, P., Creager, M. A., Yeung, A. C. & Selwyn, S. (1995). Close relation of endothelial function in human coronary and peripheral circulations. *Journal of the American College of Cardiology*, *26*, 1235-1241.

Andersen, R., Wethal, T., Gunther, A., Fossa, A., Edvardsen, T., Fossa, S. D. & Kjekshus, J. (2010). Relation of coronary artery calcium score to premature coronary artery disease in survivors >15 years of Hodgkin's lymphoma. *The American Journal of Cardiology*, *105*(2), 149-152.

Bailey, H., Kappy, M., Giller, R. & Gralla, J. (2008). Time-course and risk factors of hypothyroidism following allogeneic hematopoietic stem cell transplantation (HSCT) in children conditioned with fractionated total body irradiation. *Pediatric Blood & Cancer*, *51*, 405-409.

Beckman, J. A., Thakore, A., Kalinowski, B. H., Harris, J. R. & Creager, M. A. (2001). Radiation therapy impairs endothelium-dependent vasodilation in humans. *Journal of the American College of Cardiology*, *37*(3), 761-765.

Behrendt, H., van Bunningen, B. & van Leeuwen, E. F. (1987). Treatment of Hodgkin's disease in children without radiotherapy. *Cancer*, *59*, 1870–1873.

Berger, C., Le-Gallo, B., Donadieu, J., Richard, O., Devergie, A., Galambrun, C., Bordigoni, C., Vilmer, E., Plouvier, E., Perel, Y., Michel, G. & Stephan, J. L. (2005). Late thyroid toxicity in 153 long-term survivors of allogeneic bone marrow transplantation for acute lymphoblastic leukemia. *Bone Marrow Transplant*, *35*, 991-995.

Bilora, F., Pietrogrande, F., Petrobelli, F., Polato, G., Pomerri, F. & Muzzio, P. C. (2006). Is radiation a risk factor for atherosclerosis? An echo-color Doppler study on Hodgkin and non-Hodgkin patients. *Tumor*, *92*(4), 295-298.

Black, M. A., Cable, N. T., Thijssen, D. H. & Green, D. J. (2008). Importance of measuring the time course of flow-mediated dilatation in humans. *Hypertension*, *51*, 203-210.

Bowers, D., Liu, Y., Leisenring, W., McNeil, E., Stovall, M., Gurney, J. G., Robison, L. L., Packer, R. J. & Oeffinger, K. C. (2006). Late-occurring stroke among long-term survivors of childhood leukemia and brain tumors: a report from the Childhood Cancer Survivor Study. *Journal of Clinical Oncology*, *24*, 5277-5282.

Bouwers, P., Riccardi, R., Fedio, P. & Poplack, D. G. (1985). Long-term neuropsychologic sequelae of childhood leukemia: correlations with CT brain scan abnormalities. *Journal of Pediatrics*, *106*, 723-728.

Bressler, B., Chan, S. & Mancini, G. (2000). Temporal response of brachial artery dilation after occlusion and nitroglycerin. *American Journal of Cardiology*, *85*(3), 396-400.

Bristow, M. R., Thompson, P. D., Martin, R. P., Mason, J. W., Billingham, M. E. & Harrison, D. C. (1978a). Early anthracycline cardiotoxicity. *American Journal of Medicine*, *65*, 823-832.

Bristow, M. R, Billingham, M. E., Mason, J. W. & Daniels, J. R. (1978b). Clinical spectrum of anthracycline cardiotoxicity. *Cancer Treatment Reports*, *62*, 873-879.

Burke, G. L., Bertoni, A. G., Shea, S., Tracey, R., Watson, K. E., Blumenthal, R. S., Chung, H. & Carnethon, M. R. (2008). The impact of obesity on cardiovascular disease risk factors and subclinical vascular disease: the Multi-Ethnic Study of Atherosclerosis. *Archives of Internal Medicine*, *168*, 928-935.

Castellino, S. M., Geiger, A. M., Mertens, A. C., Leisenring, W. M., Tooze, J. A., Goodman, P. & Hudson, M. M. (2011). Morbidity and mortality in long-term survivors of Hodgkin's lymphoma: a report from the Childhood Cancer Survivor Study. *Blood*, *117*(6), 1806-1816.

Celermajer, D., Sorensen, K., Gooch, V., Spielgelhalter, D., Miller, O., Sullivan, I., Lloyd, J. & Deanfield, J. (1992). Non-invasive detection of endothelial dysfunction in children and adults at risk of atherosclerosis. *Lancet*, *340*, 1111-1115.

Celermajer, D., Sorensen, K., Spiegelhalter, D., Georgakopoulos, D. & Deanfield, J. (1993). Aging is associated with endothelial dysfunction in healthy men years before the age-related decline in women (Abstract). *Circulation*, *88*, I-78.

Cheitlin, M. D., Armstrong, W. F., Aurigemma, G. P., Beller, G. A., Bierman, F. Z., Davis, J. L. & Russell, R. O. (2003). ACC/AHA/ASE 2003 guideline update for the clinical application of echocardiography: summary article: a report of the American College of Cardiology/American Heart Association Task Force on Practice Guidelines (ACC/AHA/ASE Committee to Update the 1997 Guidelines for the Clinical Application of Echocardiography). *Journal of the American College of Cardiology*, *42*(5), 954-970.

Children's Oncology Group (2013). Long-term follow-up guidelines for survivors of childhood, adolescent, and young adult cancers. Version 4.0. http://www.survivorshipguidelines.org/pdf/LTFUGuidelines_40.pdf. (electronic citation).

Chow, A. Y., Chin, C., Dahl, G. & Rosenthal, D. N. (2006). Anthracyclines cause endothelial injury in pediatric cancer patients: a pilot study. *Journal of Clinical Oncology*, *24*(6), 925-928.

Chow, E. J., Pihoker, C., Hunt, K., Wilkinson, K. & Friedman, D. L. (2007). Obesity and hypertension among children after treatment for acute lymphoblastic leukemia. *Cancer*, *110*(10), 2313-2320.

Chowienczyk, P., Watts, G., Cockcroft, J. & Ritter, J. (1992). Impaired endothelium-dependent vasodilatation of forearm resistance vessels in hypercholesterolemia. *Lancet*, *340*, 1430-1432.

Cines, D. B., Pollak, E. S., Buck, C. A., Loscalzo, J., Zimmerman, G. A., McEver, R. P., Pober, J. S., Wick, T. M., Konkle, B. A., Schwartz, B. S., Barnathan, E. S., McCrae, K. R., Hug, B. A., Schmidt, A. M. & Stern, D. M. (1998). Endothelial cells in physiology and in the pathophysiology of vascular disorders. *Blood*, *91*, 3527-3561.

Corretti, M., Plotnick, G. & Vogel, R. (1995). Technical aspects of evaluating brachial artery vasodilation using high-frequency ultrasound. *American Journal of Physiology*, *268*, H1397-H1404.

Corretti, M., Anderson, T., Benjamin, E., Celermajer, D., Charbonneau, F., Creager, M., Deanfield, J., Drexler, H., Gerhard-Herman, M., Herrington, D., Vallance, P., Vita, J. & Vogel, R. (2002). International Brachial Artery Reactivity Task Force. Guidelines for the ultrasound assessment of endothelial-dependent flow mediated vasodilation of the brachial artery. *Journal of the American College of Cardiology*, *39*(2), 257-265.

Dawson, J. D., Sonka, M., Blecha, M. B., Lin, W. & Davis, P. H. (2009). Risk factors associated with aortic and carotid intima-media thickness in adolescents and young adults. *Journal of the American College of Cardiology*, *53*, 2273-2279.

Dengel, D. R. & Bronas, U. G. (2010). The role of endothelial dysfunction on development and progression of atherosclerosis and methods to assess vascular function and structure. *American Journal of Lifestyle Medicine*, *4*(6), 445-456.

Dengel, D. R., Ness, K. K., Glasser, S. P., Williamson, E. B., Baker, K. S. & Gurney, J. G. (2008). Endothelial function in young adult survivors of childhood acute lymphoblastic leukemia. *Journal of Pediatric Hematology/Oncology*, *30*(1), 20-25.

Dengel, D. R., Kelly, A. S., Zhang, L., Hodges, J. S., Baker, K. S. & Steinberger, J. (2014). Signs of early sub-clinical atherosclerosis in childhood cancer survivors. *Pediatric Blood & Cancer*, *61*, 532-537.

DeSouza, C. A., Shapiro, L. F., Clevenger, C. M., Dinenno, F. A., Monahan, K. D., Tanaka, H. & Seals, D. R. (2000). Regular aerobic exercise prevents and restores age-related declines in endothelium-dependent vasodilation in healthy men. *Circulation*, *102*, 1351-1357.

Drafts, B. C., Twomley, K. M., D'Agostino, R., Jr. Lawrence, J., Avis, N., Ellis, L. R., Thohan, V., Jordan, J., Melin, S. A., Torti, F. M., Little, W. C., Hamilton, C. A. & Hudley, W. G. (2013). Low to moderate dose anthracycline-based chemotherapy is associated with early noninvasive imaging evidence of subclinical cardiovascular disease. *JACC Cardiovascular Imaging*, *6*(8), 877-885.

Doll, R. & Peto, R. (1981). *The Causes of Cancer*. New York, NY: Oxford Press.

Ducharme, A., Dupuis, J., McNicoll, S., Harel, F. & Tardif, J. (1999). Comparison of nitroglycerin lingual spray and sublingual tablet on time of onset and duration of brachial artery vasodilation in normal subjects. *American Journal of Cardiology*, *84*(8), 952-954.

Dvorak, C., Gracia, C. R., Sanders, J. E., Cheng, E. Y., Baker, S. K., Pulsipher M. A. & Petryk A. (2011). NCI, NHLBI/PBMC first international conference on late effects after pediatric hematopoietic cell transplantation: Endocrine challenges-thyroid dysfunction, growth impairment, bone health, & reproductive risks. *Biology of Blood and Marrow Transplantation*, *17*(12), 1725-1738.

Ehrman, J. K., Gordon, P. M., Visich, P. S. & Keteyian, S. J. Clinical exercise physiology (2nd ed.). In J. Schairer and S. Keteyian, *Cancer*, (pp. 425-442). Champaign, IL: Human Kinetics: 2009.

Ekert, H., Waters, K. D., Smith, P. J., Toogood, I. & Mauger, D. (1988). Treatment with MOPP or ChlVPP chemotherapy only for all stages of childhood Hodgkin's disease. *Journal of Clinical Oncology*, *6*(12), 1845-1850.

Fajardo, L. F., Stewart, J. R. & Cohn, K. E. (1968). Morphology of radiation-induced heart disease. *Archives of Pathology*, *86*(5), 512.

Fajardo, L. F. & Stewart, J. R. (1973). Pathogenesis of radiation-induced myocardial fibrosis. *Laboratory Investigation; A Journal of Technical Methods and Pathology.*, *29*(2), 244.

Fernhall, B. & Agiovlasitis, S. (2008). Arterial function in youth: window into cardiovascular risk. *Journal of Applied Physiology*, *105*, 325-333.

Ford, E. S., Giles, W. H. & Mokdad, A. H. (2004). Increasing prevalence of the metabolic syndrome among U. S. adults. *Diabetes Care*, *27*(10), 2444-2449.

Furchgott, R. & Zawadzki, J. (1980). The obligatory role of endothelial cells in the relaxation of arterial smooth muscle by acetylcholine. *Nature*, *288*, 373-376.

Garg, U. & Hassid, A. (1989). Nitric oxide-generating vasodilators and 8-bromocyclic guanosine monophosphate inhibit mitogenesis and proliferation of cultured rat vascular smooth muscle cells. *Journal of Clinical Investigation*, *83*, 1774-1777.

Greve, J., Bas, M., Schuler, P., Turowski, B., Scheckenbach, K., Budach, W., Bolke, E., Bergmann, C., Lang, S., Arweiler-Harbeck, D., Lehnerdt, G., Mettheis, S., Bier, H. & Hoffman, T. K. (2010). Acute arterial hemorrhage following radiotherapy of oropharyngeal squamous cell carcinoma. *Strahlentherapie und Onkologie*, *186*(5), 269-273.

Halcox, J. P. J. & Deanfield, J. E. (2004). Endothelial cell function testing: how does the method help us in evaluating vascular status? *Acta Paediatrica Supplement*, *446*, 48-54.

Hancock, S. L., Donaldson, S. S. & Hoppe, R. T. (1993). Cardiac disease following treatment of Hodgkin's disease in children and adolescents. *Journal of Clinical Oncology*, *11*(7), 1208-1215.

Heidenreich, P. A., Schnittger, I., Strauss, H. W., et al. (2007). Screening for coronary artery disease after mediastinal irradiation for Hodgkin's disease. *Journal of Clinical Oncology*, *25*(1), 43-49.

Heikens, J., Ubbink. M., van der Pal H., Bakker, P. J., Fliers, E., Smilde, T. J., Kastelein, J. J. & Trip, M.D. (2000). Long term survivors of childhood brain cancer have an increased risk for cardiovascular disease. *Cancer*, *88*, 2116-2121.

Hochster, H., Wasserheit, C. & Speyer, J. (1995). Cardiotoxicity and cardioprotection during chemotherapy. *Current Opinion in Oncology*, *7*, 304-309.

Howlader, N., Noone, A. M., Krapcho, M., Garshell, J., Neyman, N., Altekruse, S. F., Kosary, C. L., Yu, M., Ruhl, J., Tatalovich, Z., Cho, H., Mariotto, A., Lewis, D. R., Chen, H. S., Feuer, E. J. & Cronin, K. A. (eds). SEER Cancer Statistics Review, 1975-2010, National Cancer Institute. Bethesda, MD, http://seer.cancer.gov/csr/1975_2010/, based on November 2012 SEER data submission, posted to the SEER web site, April 2013.

Hudson, M. M., Mertens, A. C., Yasui, Y., Hobbie, W., Chen, H., Gurney, J. G., Yeazel, M., Recklitis, C. J., Marina, N., Robison, L. R. & Oeffinger, K. C. (2003). Health status of adult long-term survivors of childhood cancer: a report from the Childhood Cancer Survivor Study. *Journal of the American Medical Association*, *290*, 1583-1592.

Hudson, M. M., Rai, S. N., Nunez, C., Merchant, T. E., Marina, N. M., Zalamea, N. & Rosenthal, D. (2007). Noninvasive evaluation of late anthracycline cardiac toxicity in childhood cancer survivors. *Journal of Clinical Oncology*, *25*(24), 3635-3643.

Herceg-Cavak, V., Ahel, V., Batinica, M., Matec, L. & Kardos, D. (2011). Increased arterial stiffness in children treated with anthracyclines for malignant disease. *Collegium Antropologicum*, *35*, 389-395.

Hooning, M. J., Dorresteijn, L. D., Aleman, B. M., Kappelle, A. C., Klijn, J. G., Boogerd, W. & van Leeuwen, F. E. (2006). Decreased risk of stroke among 10-year survivors of breast cancer. *Journal of Clinical Oncology*, *24*(34), 5388-5394.

Hooning, M. J., Botma, A., Aleman, B. M., Baaijens, M. H., Bertelink, H., Klijn, J. G., Taylor, C. W. & van Leeuwen, F. E. (2007). Long-term risk of cardiovascular disease in 10-year survivors of breast cancer. *Journal of the National Cancer Institute*, *99*(5), 365-375.

Huck, C. J., Bronas, U. G., Williamson, E. B., Draheim, C. C., Duprez, D. A. & Dengel, D. R. (2007). Noninvasive measurements of arterial stiffness: repeatability and interrelationships with endothelial function and arterial morphology measures. *Journal of Vascular Health & Risk Management*, *3*(3), 343-349.

Hull, M. C., Morris, C. G., Pepine, C. J. & Mendenhall, N. P. (2003). Valvular dysfunction and carotid, subclavian, and coronary artery disease in survivors of Hodgkin lymphoma treated with radiation therapy. *Journal of the American Medical Association*, *290*(21), 2831-2837.

Jagsi, R., Griffith, K. A., Koelling, T., Roberts, R. & Pierce, L. J. (2006). Stroke rates and risk factors in patients treated with radiation therapy for early-stage breast cancer. *Journal of Clinical Oncology*, *24*(18), 2779-2785.

Jarvela, L., Niinikoski, H., Heinonen, O., Lahteenmaki, P. M., Arola, M. & Kemppainen, J. (2013). Endothelial function in long-term survivors of childhood acute lymphoblastic leukemia: Effects of a home-based exercise program. *Pediatric Blood & Cancer*, *60*, 1546-1551.

Jenei, Z., Bardi, E., Magyar, M., Horvath, A., Paragh, G. & Kiss, C. (2013). Anthracycline causes impaired vascular endothelial function and aortic stiffness in long term survivors of childhood cancer. *Pathology and Oncology Research*, *19*, 375-383.

Juonala, M., Viikari, J. S. A., Laitinen, T., Marniemi, J., Helenius, H., Ronnemaa, T. & Raitakari, O. T. (2004). Interrelations between brachial endothelial function and carotid intima-media thickness in young adults: the Cardiovascular Risk in Young Finns Study. *Circulation*, *110*, 2918-2923.

Kahkonen, M., Harila-Saari, A., Metsahonkala, L., Korhonen, T., Norvasuo-Heila, M. K., Utriainen, T., Ahonen, A., Bergman, J., Salmi, T. T. & Minn, H. (1999). Cerebral blood flow and glucose metabolism in long-term survivors of childhood acute lymphoblastic leukaemia. *European Journal of Cancer*, *35*(7), 1102-1108.

Kaste, S. C., Shidler, T. J., Tong, X., Srivastava, D. K., Rochester, R., Hudson, M. M., Shearer, P. D. & Hale, G. A. (2004). Bone mineral density and osteonecrosis in survivors of childhood allogeneic bone marrow transplantation. *Bone Marrow Transplant*, *33*(4), 435-441.

Kelly, A. S., Marlatt, K. L., Steinberger, J. & Dengel, D. R. (2014). Younger age is associated with lower reactive hyperemic index but not lower flow-mediated dilation among children and adolescents. *Atherosclerosis*, *234*(2), 410-414.

Kotsis, V. T., Stabouli, S. V., Papamichael, C. M. & Zakopoulos, N. A. (2006). Impact of obesity in intima media thickness of carotid arteries. *Obesity*, *14*, 1708-1715.

Kremer, L. C., van Dalen, E. C., Offringa, M., Ottenkamp, J. & Voute, P. A. (2001). Anthracycline-induced clinical heart failure in a cohort of 607 children: long-term follow-up study. *Journal of Clinical Oncology*, *19*(1), 191-196.

Kremer, L. C., van der Pal, H. J., Offringa, M. & Voute, P. A. (2002). Frequency and risk factors of subclinical cardiotoxicity after anthracycline therapy in children: a systematic review. *Annals of Oncology*, *13*(6), 819-829.

Krischer, J. P., Epstein, S., Cuthbertson, D. D., Goorin, A. M., Epstein, M. L. & Lipshultz, S. E. (1997). Clinical cardiotoxicity following anthracycline treatment for childhood cancer: the Pediatric Oncology Group experience. *Journal of Clinical Oncology*, *15*(4), 1544-1552.

Kubes, P., Suzuki, M. & Granger, D. (1991). Nitric oxide: an endogenous modulator of leukocyte adhesion. Proceedings of the National Academy of Sciences of the United States of America, *88*, 4651-4655.

Kunsch, C. & Medford, R. M. (2000). Oxidation sensitive transcription and gene expression in atherosclerosis. In: Keaney, J.F., ed. *Oxidative Stress and Vascular Disease*., 135-154. Boston: Kluwer Academic.

Libby, P. (2002). Atherosclerosis: the new view. *Scientific American*, *286*, 47-55.

Lieberman, E. H., Gerhard, M. D., Uehata, A., Selwyn, A. P., Ganz, P., Yeung, A. C. & Creager, M. A. (1996). Flow-induced vasodilation of the human brachial artery is impaired in patients <40 years of age with coronary artery disease. *American Journal of Cardiology*, *78*, 1210-1214.

Liebermann, E. H., Garces, M. R. & Lopez-Jimenez, T. (2006). Endothelial function and insights into prevention. In: Fody JM, ed. *Preventive Cardiology Insights Into the Prevention and Treatment of Cardiovascular Disease*., pp. 19-28. Totowa, NJ: Humana.

Lipshultz, S., Colan, S., Gelber, R., Perez-Atayde, A. R., Sallan, S. E. & Sanders, S. P. (1991). Late cardiac effects of doxorubicin therapy for acute lymphoblastic leukemia in childhood. *New England Journal of Medicine*, *324*, 808-815.

Lipshultz, S. E., Sanders, S. P., Colan, S. D., Goorin, A. M., Sallan, S. E. & Krischer, J. P. (1994). Monitoring for anthracycline cardiotoxicity. *Pediatrics*, *93*(3), 433-437.

Lipshultz, S. E., Grenier, M. A. & Colan, S. D. (1999). Doxorubicin-induced cardiomyopathy. The *New England Journal of Medicine*, *340*(8), 653-654.

Lipshultz, S. E. & Sallan, S. E. (1993). Cardiovascular abnormalities in long-term survivors of childhood malignancies. *Journal of Clinical Oncology*, *11*(7), 1199-1203.

Lipshultz, S. E., Lipsitz, S. R., Sallan, S. E., Dalton, V. M., Mone, S. M., Gelber, R. D. & Colan, S. D. (2005). Chronic progressive cardiac dysfunction years after doxorubicin therapy for childhood acute lymphoblastic leukemia. *Journal of Clinical Oncology*, *23*(12), 2629-2636.

Lipshultz, S. E. (2006). Exposure to anthracyclines during childhood cancer causes cardiac injury. *Seminars in Oncology*, *33*, S8-S14.

Lipshultz, S. E., Alvarez, J. A. & Scully, R. E. (2008). Clinical pharmacology: anthracycline associated cardiotoxicity in survivors of childhood cancer. *Heart*, *94*, 525-533.

Lipshultz, S. E., Adams, M. J., Colan, S. D., Constine, L. S., Herman, E. H., Hsu, D. T. Hudson, M. M., Kremer, L. C., Landy, D. C., Miller, T. L., Oeffinger, K. C., Rosenthal, D. N., Sable, C. A., Sallan, S. E., Singh, G. K., Steinberger, J., Cochran, T. R. & Wilkinson, J. D. (2013). Long-term cardiovascular toxicity in children, adolescents, and young adults who receive cancer therapy: Pathophysiology, course, monitoring, management, prevention, and research directions – A scientific statement from the American Heart Association. *Circulation*, *128*, 1927-1995.

Ludmer, P. L., Selwyn, A. P., Shook, T. L., Wayne, R. R., Mudge, G. H., Alexander, R. W. & Ganz, P. (1986). Paradoxical vasoconstriction induced by acetylcholine in atherosclerotic coronary arteries. *New England Journal of Medicine*, *315*(17), 1046-1051.

Mariotto, A. B., Rowland, J. H., Yabroff, K. R., Scoppa, S., Hachey, M., Ries, L. & Feuer, E. J. (2009). Long-term survivors of childhood cancers in the United States. *Cancer Epidemiology, Biomarkers & Prevention*, *18*(4), 1033-1040.

Mariotto, A. B., Yabroff, R., Shao, Y., Feuer, E. J. & Brown, M. L. (2010). Projections of the cost of cancer care in the United States 2010-2020. *Journal of the National Cancer Institute*, *103*, 1-12.

Meeske, K., Siegel, S., Gilsanz V., Bernstein, L., Nelson, M. B., Sposto, R., Weaver, F. A., Lavey, R. S., Mack, M. P. & Nelson, M. D. Jr. (2009). Premature carotid artery disease in pediatric cancer survivors treated with neck irradiation. *Pediatric Blood & Cancer*, *53*, 615-621.

Mertens, A. C. (2007). Cause of mortality in 5-year survivors of childhood cancer. *Pediatric Blood & Cancer*, *48*(7), 723-726.

Mertens, A. C., Yasui, Y., Neglia, J. P., Potter, J. D., Nesbit, M. E., Jr. Ruccione, K., Smithson, W. A. & Robison, L. L. (2001). Late mortality experience in five-year survivors of childhood and adolescent cancer: the Childhood Cancer Survivor Study. *Journal of Clinical Oncology*, *19*(13), 3163-3172.

Mulrooney, D. A., Yeazel, M. W., Kawashima, T., Mertens, A. C., Mitby, P., Stovall, M., Donaldson, S. S., Green, D. M., Sklar, C. A., Robison, L. L. & Leisenring, W. M. (2009). Cardiac outcomes in a cohort of adult survivors of childhood and adolescent cancer: retrospective analysis of the Childhood Cancer Survivor Study cohort. *British Medical Journal*, *339*, b4606.

Mulrooney, D. A., Kelly, A. S., Baker, K. S., Steffen, L. M., Lunsford-Lee, J., Petryk, A., Sinaiko, A. R., Dengel, D. R., Perkins, J., Messinger, Y., Zhou, X. & Steinberger, J. (2009). Cardiometabolic risks among survivors of childhood hematologic malignancies (Abstract). *Blood*, *114*, pp. 4113.

Munzel, T., Sinning, C., Post, F., Warnholtz, A. & Schultz, E. (2008). Pathophysiology, diagnosis and prognostic implications of endothelial dysfunction. *Annals of Medicine*, *40*, 180-196.

Murata, T., Yamawaki, H. & Yoshimoto, R. (2001). Chronic effects of doxorubicin on vascular endothelium assess by organ culture study. *Life Sciences*, *69*, 2685-2695.

Ness, K. K. & Gurney, J. G. (2007). Adverse late effects of childhood cancer and its treatment on health and performance. *The Annual Review of Public Health*, *28*, 279-302.

Nuver, J., Smit, A. J., van der Meer, J., van den Berg, M. P., van der Graaf, W. T., Meinardi, M. T., Sleijfer, D. T., Hoekstra, H. J., van Gessel, A. I., van Roon, A. M. & Gietema, J. A. (2005). Acute chemotherapy-induced cardiovascular changes in patients with testicular cancer. *Journal of Clinical Oncology*, *23*, 9130-9137.

Nysom, K., Holm, K., Lipsitz, S. R., Mone, S. M., Colan, S. D., Orav, E. J. & Lipshultz, S. E. (1998). Relationship between cumulative anthracycline dose and late cardiotoxicity in childhood acute lymphoblastic leukemia. *Journal of Clinical Oncology*, *16*(2), 545-550.

Oeffinger, K., Buchanan, G., Eshelman, D., Denke, M., Andrews, T., Germak, J., Tomlinson, G., Snell, L. & Foster, B. (2001). Cardiovascular risk factors in young adult survivors of childhood acute lymphoblastic leukemia. *Journal of Pediatric Hematology/Oncology*, *23*(7), 424-430.

Oeffinger, K., Mertens, A., Sklar, C., Yasui, Y., Fears, T., Stovall, M., Vik, T., Inskip, P. & Robison, L. (2003). Obesity in adult survivors of childhood acute lymphoblastic leukemia: a report from the Childhood Cancer Survivor Study. *Journal of Clinical Oncology*, *21*, 1359-1365.

Oeffinger, K. C. & Hudson, M. M. (2004). Long-term complications following childhood and adolescent cancer: foundations for providing risk-based health care for survivors. *CA: A Cancer Journal for Clinicians*, *54*, 208-236.

Oeffinger, K. (2008). Are survivors of acute lymphoblastic leukemia (ALL) at increased risk of cardiovascular disease? *Pediatric Blood & Cancer*, *50*, 462-467, Discussion 468.

Oeffinger, K. C., Adams-Huet, B., Victor, R. G., Church, T. S., Snell, P. G., Dunn, A. L., Eshelman-Kent, D. A., Ross, R., Janiszewski, P. M., Turoff, A. J., Brooks, S. & Vega, G. L. (2009). Insulin resistance and risk factors for cardiovascular disease in young adult survivors of childhood acute lymphoblastic leukemia. *Journal of Clinical Oncology*, *27*(22), 3698-3704.

Oh, J. H., Baum, D. D., Pham, S., Cox, M., Nguyen, S., Ensor, J. & Chen, I. (2007). Long-term complications of platinum-based chemotherapy in testicular cancer survivors. *Medical Oncology*, *24*(2), 175-181.

Olson, T. P., Schmitz, K. H., Leon, A. S. & Dengel, D. R. (2006). Vascular structure and function in women: relationship with body mass index. *American Journal of Preventive Medicine*, *30*, 487-492.

Pepe, A., Lombardi, M., Takacs, I., Positano, V., Panzarella, G. & Picano, E. (2004). Nitrate-induced coronary vasodilation by stress-magnetic resonance imaging: a novel noninvasive test of coronary vasomotion. *Journal Magnetic Resonance Imaging*, *20*, 390-394.

Pietilä, S., Mäkipernaa, A., Sievänen, H., Koivisto, A. M., Wigren, T. & Lenko, H. (2009). Obesity and metabolic changes are common in young childhood brain tumor survivors. *Pediatric Blood & Cancer*, *52*, 853-859.

Pyke, K. E. & Tschakovsky, M. E. (2005). The relationship between shear stress and flow mediated dilation: implications for the assessment of endothelial function. *Journal of Physiology*, *568*, 357-369.

Raitakari, O. & Celermajer, D. (2000). Flow-mediated dilatation. *British Journal of Clinical Pharmacology*, *50*, 397-404.

Randomski, M., Palmer, R. & Moncada, S. (1990). An L-arginine/nitric oxide pathway present in human platelets regulated aggregation. Proceedings of the National Academy of Sciences of the United States of America, *87*, 5193-5197.

Rathe, M., Carlsen, N. L. & Oxhøj, H. (2007). Late cardiac effects of anthracycline containing therapy for childhood acute lymphoblastic leukemia. *Pediatric Blood & Cancer, 48*(7), 663-667.

Roman, M., Naqvi, T., Gardin, J., Gerhard-Herman, M., Jaff, M. & Mohler, E. (2006). Clinical application of noninvasive ultrasound in cardiovascular risk stratification: A report from the American Society of Echocardiography and the Society of Vascular Medicine and Biology. *Journal of the American Society of Echocardiography, 19*, 943-954.

Sanders, J. E., Hoffmeister, P. A., Woolfrey, A. E., Carpenter, P. A., Storer, B. E., Storb, R. F. & Appelbaum, F. R. (2009). Thyroid function following hematopoietic cell transplantation in children: 30 years' experience. *Blood, 113*, 306-308.

Schellong, G., Riepenhausen, M., Bruch, C., Kotthoff, S., Vogt, J., Bolling, T., Dieckmann, K., Potter, R., Heinecke, A., Bramswig, J. & Dorffel, W. (2010). Late valvular and other cardiac diseases after different doses of mediastinal radiotherapy for Hodgkin disease in children and adolescents: Report form the longitudinal GPOH follow-up project of the German-Austrian DAL-HD studies. *Pediatric Blood & Cancer, 55*, 1145-1152.

Shan, K., Lincoff, A. & Young, J. (1996). Anthracycline-induced cardiotoxicity. *Annals of Internal Medicine, 125*, 47-58.

Shankar, S., Marina, N., Hudson, M., Hodgson, D., Adams, M., Landier, W., Bhatia, S., Meeske, K., Chen, M., Kinahan, K., Steinberger, J. & Rosenthal, D. (2008). Monitoring for cardiovascular disease in survivors of childhood cancer: report from the Cardiovascular Disease Task Force of the Children's Oncology Group. *Pediatrics, 121*, e387-e396.

Smith, S. C. Jr. Greenland, P. & Grundy, S. M. (2000). AHA Conference Proceedings. Beyond secondary prevention: identifying the high-risk patient for primary prevention. Executive Summary. *Circulation, 1001*, 111-116.

Smith, M. A. & Ries, L. A. G. (2002). Childhood Cancer: Incidence, Survival, and Mortality. In: Pizzo, P. A. I., Poplack, D. G., eds. Principles and Practice of Pediatric Oncology (ed Fourth Edition). *Philadelphia, PA: Lippincott Williams & Wilkins*, 1-12.

Socié, G., Stone, J. V., Wingard, J. R., Weisdorf, D., Henslee-Downey, P. J., Bredeson, C., Cahn, J. Y., Passweg, J. R., Rowlings, P. A., Schouten, H. C., Kolb, H. J. & Klein, J. P. (1999). Long-term survival and late deaths after allogeneic bone marrow transplantation. *The New England Journal of Medicine, 341*, 14-21.

Sorensen, K., Levitt, G., Bull, C., Chessells, J. & Sullivan, I. (1997). Anthracycline dose in childhood acute lymphoblastic leukemia: issues of early survival versus late cardiotoxicity. *Journal of Clinical Oncology, 15*, 61-68.

Stamler, J., Loh, E., Roddy, M., Currie, K. & Creager, M. (1994). Nitric oxide regulates basal systemic and pulmonary vascular resistance in healthy humans. *Circulation, 89*, 2035-2040.

Steinberg, H. O., Chaker, H., Leaming, R., Johnson, A., Brechtel, G. & Baron, A. D. (1996). Obesity/insulin resistance is associated with endothelial dysfunction. *Journal of Clinical Investigation, 97*, 2601-2610.

Steinherz, L. J., Steinherz, P. G., Tan, C. T., Heller, G. & Murphy, M. L. (1991). Cardiac toxicity 4 to 20 years after completing anthracycline therapy. *Journal of the American Medical Association, 266*(12), 1672-1677.

Sugihara, T., Hattori, Y., Yamamoto, Y., Qi, F., Ickikawa, R., Sato, A., Liu, M. Y., Abe, K. & Kanno, M. (1999). Preferential impairment of nitric oxide-mediated endothelium-dependent relaxation in human cervical arteries after irradiation. *Circulation*, *100*(6), 635-641.

Talvensaari, K., Lanning, M., Tapanainen, P. & Knip, M. (1996). Long-term survivors of childhood cancer have an increased risk of manifesting the metabolic syndrome. *Journal of Clinical Endocrinology & Metabolism*, *81*, 3051-3055.

Thelen, M. A., Kelly, A. S., Williamson, E. B. & Dengel, D. R. (2008). Examining the time course of endothelium-independent dilation by nitroglycerin. *Ultrasound in Medicine & Biology*, *34*, 1217-1220.

U.S. Mortality Public Use Data Tape 2001, National Center for Health Statistics, Centers for Disease Control and Prevention. 2003.

Vallance, P., Collier, J. & Moncada, S. (1989). Effects of endothelium-derived nitric oxide on peripheral arteriolar tone in man. *Lancet*, *2*, 997-1000.

Vander, A., Sherman, J. & Luciano, D. (2001). *Human Physiology: The Mechanisms of Body Function*. 8th ed. New York: McGraw-Hill.

van Waas, M., Neggers, S., Pieters, R. & van den Heuvel-Eibrink, M. (2010). Components of the metabolic syndrome in 500 adult long-term survivors of childhood cancer. *Annals of Oncology*, *21*, 1121-1126.

Vaughn, D. J., Palmer, S. C., Carver, J. R., Jacobs, L. A. & Mohler, E. R. (2008). Cardiovascular risk in long-term survivors of testicular cancer. *Cancer*, *112*(9), 1949-1953.

Williams, S. B., Cusco, J. A., Roddy, M. A., Johnstone, M. T. & Craeger, M. A. (1996). Impaired nitric oxide in the local regulation of pulmonary vascular resistance in humans. *Journal of the American College of Cardiology*, *27*, 567-574.

Williams, I. L., Chowienczyk, P. J., Wheatcroft, S. B., Patel, A. G., Sherwood, R. A., Momin, A., Shah, A. M. & Kearney, M. T. (2005). Endothelial function and weight loss in obese humans. *Obesity Surgery*, *15*, 1055-1060.

World Cancer Research Fund and American Institute for Cancer Research. *Policy and Action for Cancer Prevention*. Washington, DC, 2009.

Wu, S., Ko, Y. & Teng, M. (2002). Adriamycin-induced cardiomyocyte and endothelial cell apoptosis: *In vitro* and *in vivo* studies. *Journal of Molecular Cell Cardiology*, *34*, 1595-1607.

Yaniv, I., Saab, A., Cohen, I. J., Goshen, Y., Loven, D., Stark, B. & Zaizov, R. (1996). Hodgkin disease in children: reduced tailored chemotherapy for stage I-II disease. *Journal of Pediatric Hematology/Oncology*, *18*(1), 76-80.

Yeung, S., Yoong, C., Spink, J., Galbraith, A. & Smith, P. J. (1991). Functional myocardial impairment in children treated with anthracyclines for cancer. *Lancet*, *337*, 816-818.

Yoshida, T., Kawano, H., Miyamoto, S., Motoyama, T., Fukushima, H., Hirai, N. & Ogawa, H. (2006). Prognostic value of flow-mediated dilation of the brachial artery in patients with cardiovascular disease. *Internal Medicine*, *45*(9), 575-579.

In: Horizons in Cancer Research. Volume 61
Editor: Hiroto S. Watanabe
ISBN: 978-1-63484-503-8

Chapter 8

THE BROAD END OF THE STICK: CONSENSUS CONFERENCE POLICY DEVELOPMENT OF A PUBLIC HEALTH APPROACH TO LYNCH SYNDROME

Stephen M. Modell[1,2,*], Sharon L. R. Kardia[2] and Toby Citrin[1]
[1]Department of Health Management and Policy,
[2]Department of Epidemiology
University of Michigan School of Public Health, Ann Arbor, MI, US

ABSTRACT

Lynch syndrome (LS) is one of several heritable colorectal cancer (CRC) conditions clinicians diagnose in the course of standard practice, others being familial adenomatous polyposis, juvenile polyposis, and Peutz-Jeghers syndrome. Also known as hereditary nonpolyposis colorectal cancer (HNPCC), polyps in LS are sparse, occurring with the same frequency as in the general population, a feature distinguishing HNPCC from the other, polyp-bearing cancers. The epidemiology is also noteworthy -- Lynch syndrome is the most common inherited endometrial cancer and CRC susceptibility syndrome, occurring on the average 3 decades before most forms of CRC in the general population. It has received considerable attention in public health as well as medical circles.

In September of 2012, the U.S. Centers for Disease Control and Prevention Office of Public Health Genomics, in collaboration with the University of Michigan Center for Public Health and Community Genomics, and Genetic Alliance convened a 74-person multi-sectoral (medicine, public health, genetics, nursing, disease advocacy) meeting in Atlanta, Georgia to develop evidence-based strategies to reduce the burden posed by three familial conditions, the first being Lynch syndrome. The gathering utilized a participatory approach to yield recommendations involving condition-related working groups and consensus building. The literature suggests that the use of molecular screening and germline genetic testing for LS has achieved clinical validity and utility.

* Corresponding author: Stephen M. Modell, Center for Public Health and Community Genomics, University of Michigan School of Public Health, 4628 SPH Tower, 1415 Washington Heights, Ann Arbor, MI, US 48109-2029, E-mail: mod@umich.edu.

Participants concluded sufficient evidence exists to move forward with universal screening for Lynch syndrome among those diagnosed with CRC. Recommendations pertained to both clinically- and population-oriented policy.

Participants covered criteria for the screening of individuals found to be at-risk for LS, the use of electronic systems for alerting clinicians to the need for LS screening and genetic testing, electronic medical record tracking, and reimbursement issues for mutation testing. Cascade screening is recommended for family members of all confirmed CRC patients. Coordinated action should occur between the medical and public health communities. State health departments currently engaged in surveillance of LS clinical data and cancer registries can act as models for other states. To promote universal screening of at-risk individuals and families, public health departments should engage in partnership building with relevant stakeholders, and educational programs for providers engaged in referral and test interpretation. Conference outcomes touched on both clinical guidelines and broader, population-oriented perspectives such as Healthy People 2020, incorporating the use of family history and genetic testing for Lynch syndrome.

Keywords: Lynch syndrome, colorectal cancer, endometrial cancer, genetic testing, cascade screening, universal screening, surveillance, electronic medical records, public health policy, clinical guidelines, consensus building

INTRODUCTION: A CONDITION AT THE CROSSROADS

Consideration of a major public health condition such as colorectal cancer invites several levels of approach, one being the investigation of the pathophysiology and epidemiology of the condition, another being its individual management, yet a third being its handling for groups of people who are at risk.

Lynch syndrome, the most common heritable cause of colorectal cancer, sits at the intersection of medical and public health concern. It demonstrates the continuity between what must take place at the individual and group levels to make a dent in colorectal cancer. The recognition of screening interventions for Lynch syndrome by bodies like the U.S. Department of Health and Human Service's *Healthy People 2020* [1] indicates that the technology is at hand to tackle the condition in an effective way, in essence showing that the time is ripe to grant attention and resources to the condition. Policy questions come into play because alternative solutions exist to proposed efforts to expand screening initiatives for Lynch syndrome.

In what follows we describe the process used by participants in a conference – *New Strategies in Public Health Genomics: Actions to Save Lives Now* – aimed at policy formulation for three major heritable conditions, the first being Lynch syndrome, the other two being hereditary breast and ovarian cancer and familial hypercholesterolemia – and the recommendations they formed for Lynch syndrome. The genomic applications for Lynch syndrome and the other conditions explored are "Tier 1" techniques in that the base of collected evidence on clinical validity and utility supports implementation into practice [2]. Tiers 2 and 3 applications, such as genotyping patients to identify toxicity in irinotecan toxicity in treating metastatic colorectal cancer or genetic testing for hemochromatosis, do not meet this clinical standard of readiness for routine use.

After peering at the details of the conference and the first cancer condition to which it attended, Lynch syndrome, we will consider a model for implementing recommendations pertaining to this condition, and different categories of recommendations, from genetic testing to professional education. The chapter will conclude with a look at what is happening in the field now to support Lynch syndrome genetic testing and surveillance, and how a deliberative conference can point the way to the changes that need to take place to deliver screening to those at risk.

COLORECTAL CANCER AND LYNCH SYNDROME: EPIDEMIOLOGIC CONSIDERATIONS

The importance of Lynch syndrome (LS) lies in what could be achieved if the impact of the condition were significantly reduced. Families with members suffering from or at risk for colorectal cancer (CRC) would be the first to benefit, though Lynch syndrome is also implicated in other cancers beyond CRC. As a condition of major public health concern, colorectal cancer is the second leading cause of cancer deaths in the United States, and the third most common cancer in men and women [3]. It represents 8% of all new cancer cases in the United States [4]. In the most recent year for which compiled statistics are available, 2012, 134,784 people in the United States were diagnosed with CRC, and 51,516 persons (26, 866 men; 24,650 women) died from this cancer [3].

The lifetime risk for developing CRC has been placed at 2 to 5% for the general population, and 80% for those with LS [5, 6]. It is also the most common heritable cause of endometrial cancer (EC). One out of every 35 CRC patients and one out of every 40 EC patients have LS [7, 8]. Lynch syndrome has features that make it distinct from other non-heritable causes of CRC. Also known as hereditary nonpolyposis colorectal cancer (HNPCC), Lynch syndrome produces only a small number of polyps or none at all. It is associated with adenomas, often on the right side of the colon, that frequently progress to carcinoma. The average age of CRC diagnosis in someone with LS is 45, compared with 72 for a new diagnosis of CRC in the general population [9]. LS is a possible diagnosis when multiple family members have been diagnosed with CRC. Lynch syndrome is also associated with other cancers beyond CRC and EC, including cancer of the ovaries, stomach, small intestine, pancreas, and urinary tract. These features reflect the criteria used to identify LS in the revised Bethesda guidelines [9]:

- Developing CRC younger than age 50
- Developing CRC and other cancers associated with LS separately or simultaneously
- CRC in one or more first-degree relatives with another LS-related cancer, with one of these cancers developing before age 50
- CRC in two or more first- or second-degree relatives with another LS-related cancer

The last set of criteria resurfaces in the Healthy People 2020 recommendations:

> Family members could benefit from knowing whether the colorectal cancer in their family is a hereditary form called Lynch syndrome. Screening interventions could

potentially reduce the risk of colorectal cancer among men and women with Lynch syndrome by 60 percent [1].

The *Healthy People 2020* recommendations have been incorporated into the public health genomics education programs of several states, such as Connecticut and Michigan, and are part of the 2013 American Public Health Association policy statement *Advancing Cancer Genomics in Public Health* [10]. The APHA policy statement represents the tip of the iceberg in what is happening now in public health genomics. The *New Strategies* conference occurred at a significant point in public health's implementation of cancer genomics when possible directions had been mapped out but were yet to be crystallized into specific strategies for conditions like Lynch syndrome.

METHODOLOGY

A Consensus Building Approach to Genomics

The *New Strategies* event took place on the Centers for Disease Control and Prevention (CDC) Roybal Campus on September 7, 2012. The participants, 74 total, came from a variety of sectors: Disease Research & Advocacy (10); Governmental Agency (both CDC and non-CDC health-related) (15); Public Health (state and local public health, public health professional organizations, and university schools of public health) (19); Medicine & Nursing (medical/nursing professional organizations, and university schools of medicine and nursing) (16); Health Care Plans and Systems (8); and Industry (2). Many of the public health and medical/nursing participants had significant genetics-related responsibilities; 4 individuals worked full-time in genetics but did not fit these categories. Experts in both the clinical and public health domains were present to offer their perspectives and leadership. Industry participants from Myriad Genetics and Genzyme also took part. Members of the "Disease Research & Advocacy" group came from organizations addressing the three Tier 1 conditions – LS, HBOC, and FH – or from agencies that address cancer in general. Advocacy representation was important to assure that recommendations would reflect the consumer viewpoint. Conference goals were for participants to learn about each other's relevant efforts, foster collaborative relationships, and develop specific recommendations on the implementation of the three conditions, those for LS described herein. These conditions each hold Tier 1 status and their ethical-legal-social implications have been considered and addressed.

Continuity of the event with the preceding CDC-sponsored *Priorities for Public Health Genomics* project was emphasized. The prior project tapped professional and consumer opinion on the expanse of possible directions that public health genomics might take over the next half-decade [11]. The *New Strategies* conference was organized to develop strategies for the directions that might be taken, with a focus on validated conditions that were cited as examples but not at the center of attention in the earlier *Priorities* conference.

Decision-making in the *New Strategies* conference depended on diverse participant voices. The agenda for Lynch syndrome began with a pair of speakers, the first an expert describing the disease condition and associated screening and genetic testing, the second an expert on the public health application of Lynch syndrome genetic testing. A Patient and

Community Perspectives Panel Session followed, which led to break-out sessions yielding group recommendations for Lynch syndrome and the other two conditions. A plenary session concluded with summary reports from the break-out session facilitators on the strategies their groups developed.

Table I. Select New Strategies Report recommendations

1. Collaboration and partnership building
   - A. Build political will through the identification of effective leader(s) who will excite, connect, and convene the necessary stakeholders. The leader will need to work with different levels of state leadership. It is important and necessary to bring the state comprehensive cancer programs on board. (New Strategies Report, p. 52) [13]
   - B. Once the state comprehensive cancer program is on board, it can use its leverage to convene a meeting of state level stakeholders. (p. 52)
   - C. A toolkit for states should include a collection of evidence–based publications, a collection of narratives, and an inventory of successful programs that have been implemented in other states. (p. 56)
2. Program support
   - A. The Centers for Disease Control and Prevention (CDC) can bring groups together by creating RFPs that require groups such as public health departments and advocacy groups to work together at a state or local level. (p. 54)
   - B. Partnerships are necessary to generate buy-in, and share costs with cancer registries that may be willing to participate in surveillance efforts but lack the financial means to revise their current program or system to capture additional data. (p. 64)
   - C. Pilot programs may provide data that can be used in grant or research applications seeking additional funds. (p. 65)
3. Screening and surveillance
   - A. Successful Lynch syndrome (LS) screening programs from other states can be used as examples to convince state health departments of the potential impact of LS screening for their own state. (p. 53)
   - B. Universal cascade screening for LS in all confirmed CRC patients should be integrated into the practice of pathology. (p. 63)
   - C. The appropriate use of cancer registries, electronic medical records (EMR), and other means of data collection is important for accurate surveillance. Data should be collected through cancer registries on all measures of universal screening for Lynch syndrome, which may include immunohistochemistry (IHC), microsatellite instability (MSI), *BRAF* mutation, and methylation testing. (p. 63)
   - D. Public health departments should also investigate ways to link relatives of those with CRC to the cancer registries. (p. 55)
4. Electronic health information
   - A. EMRs can be used to track family history data and collect statewide data on the number of newly diagnosed CRC individuals who have been screened for LS. (p. 55)
   - B. Electronic versions of guidelines for clinical decision-making should be made available to physicians and should be compatible with EMRs. (p. 62)
   - C. EMR systems can implement clinical checks of data to alert clinicians to the need for LS screening. (p. 64)
   - D. Develop and use a centralized data warehouse that allows data to be shared among hospitals and is based on a health information exchange design. (p. 63)

Muin Khoury, MD, PhD, director of the CDC's Office of Public Health Genomics (CDC-OPHG), introduced an adaptation of the *Public Health in America* framework [12] that the groups could use as a conceptual template for developing an action plan for Tier 1 genetic testing implementation. Originally conceived by the Core Public Health Functions Steering Committee (1994), the adapted essential public health functions framework moves from partnership building and community mobilization to policy development, public health and health care personnel workforce training, clinical intervention, surveillance, and consumer education. Inherent in the process is an alternation between clinical and public health expertise, a balance reflected in the peopling of the conference.

As the conference unfolded, a working group might examine various policymaking strategies to cover the costs of genetic screening, incorporation into existing strategies, or coalition building to enable new program start-up. Group deliberation on clinical implementation often evoked suggestions for a unified screening protocol or set of screening criteria, optimal means of referral, and promotion of the most recent practice guidelines.

Consideration of surveillance strategies would lead groups to consider avenues for development of surveillance measures, and for patient identification and data sharing, such as using electronic medical records (EMRs) to flag at-risk patients, using state health information exchanges (HIEs), and establishing centralized disease registries. Groups could approach educational avenues through consideration of either consumer needs for basic and understandable information delivered by providers and support groups, or provider needs for information on disease diagnosis, genetic testing, and referral. Groups were to report on recommendations for strategies in these action categories and key features that might constitute a "toolkit" for their adoption by state and local public health with relevance to advocacy organizations and professional bodies. An extensive 82-page report, available on the Internet, describes group process and recommendations for the entire conference ("NSR") [13]. Here we examine those recommendations which offered a variety of solutions for Lynch syndrome genetic testing requiring group deliberation. These recommendations, summarized in Table 1, point towards optimal strategies for screening program implementation taking into account at-risk families and clinical populations.

RESULTS

Speaker Points and Group Findings on Collaboration and Partnership Building

Heather Hampel, M.S., C.G.C. of the Ohio State University Clinical Cancer Genetics Program and Comprehensive Cancer Center, a national expert on Lynch syndrome, explained that colorectal cancer risk varies with the particular mutation – from 15% for individuals with *MSH6* or *PMS2* mutations to 56% for those with *MLH1* and *MSH2* mutations. Screening of presymptomatic individuals through microsatellite instability (MSI) or immunohistochemistry staining (IHC) of tissue leads to a decision for the patient to undergo or abstain from genetic testing to identify specific LS mutations. *BRAF* testing and *MLH1* promoter methylation testing can be used to exclude the possibility of a mismatch repair gene mutation, thus obviating the need for mutation testing. Presymptomatic individuals with a high risk can be given colonoscopy starting at the recommended age and at the recommended frequency, granting the possibility of catching adenomas before they have developed into carcinoma.

The progression to cancer can occur over a span of 2-3 years, as opposed to the 8-10 year interval typical of sporadic CRC [14]. Lives can be saved by diagnosing the patient early, which in part depends on comprehensive evaluation of multigenerational cancer family history, but also on the consistent use of molecular screening. Universal screening and genetic testing for LS among newly diagnosed CRC patients has been found feasible and cost-effective [15]. The identification of an individual harboring an LS mutation can also lead to predictive genetic testing in at-risk relatives. In the United States, assuming three affected relatives per proband, testing of family members (cascade screening, moving from one family member ascertained to have a mutation to the next) has the potential to identify another 12,345 individuals at high risk who can consider earlier and more intensive screening. The Evaluation of Genomic Applications in Practice and Prevention (EGAPP) Working Group has concluded based on systematic review that sufficient evidence exists to recommend offering genetic testing to reduce morbidity and mortality in relatives with LS [16].

The optimism of identifying and monitoring families with a high risk for Lynch syndrome must be tempered, though. Debra Duquette, M.S., C.G.C. of the Michigan Department of Health and Human Services Public Health Genomics Program commented it is quite possible that the vast majority of families with a history of CRC do not know they may have LS, or even that a genetic test is available. Systemic deficiencies also exist. LS screening was performed in less than 2% of CRC cases in an audit of 2006-2010 medical records [17]. A 2010 surveillance effort by the MDHHS to explore health plan coverage for LS testing found no health plan in Michigan consistent with the EGAPP recommendation [17]. NCCN screening guidelines emphasize the revised Bethesda/Amsterdam criteria, though the current version does acknowledge the EGAPP recommendation, noting that an infrastructure needs to be in place to handle the screening results. Duquette emphasized the value of network collaboration to promote universal LS screening on all newly diagnosed colorectal and endometrial tumors. "Lynch syndrome is a genetic condition that brings clinical, public health, and advocacy groups together. [It] may be used as a model of how to build local, regional, national, and international collaboration" (New Strategies Report (NSR), p. 5).

The LS work groups also stressed the need for collaboration. Group 2 suggested the formation of expert bodies within the U.S. Department of Health and Human Services to advise on LS cascade screening. Public health and industry could partner in advocating for this need and helping with their formation. Other partnering agencies and organizations, including the Centers for Disease Control and Prevention, the National Institutes of Health, the Health Resources and Services Administration, the Personalized Medicine Coalition, and organizations representing clinical laboratories could combine efforts to press for coverage of cascade screening.

Conference Findings Addressing Opportunities and Obstacles in Genomics-Based Prevention

Collaboration to implement screening on an expanded basis would require the leadership of one or several major bodies. EGAPP efforts have catalyzed wider awareness of Lynch syndrome genetic testing. Initial and follow-up work by EGAPP examined four different clinical strategies involving microsatellite instability (MSI) screening and immunohistochemistry (IHC) staining, mismatch repair gene (MMR) gene sequencing and deletion testing for *MLH1*, *MSH2*, and *MSH6* mutations, and preliminary *BRAF* mutation testing in probands and relatives [18, 19]. EGAPP found acceptable detection rates (up to 85%) and costs (down to $18,863 per case detected) for Lynch syndrome risk assessment, at the same time leaving room for decisional trade-offs between the different strategies. The evidence review process led to the release of a recommendation statement [16], which served as the basis for actions by other bodies, such as *Healthy People 2020* and major health plans, to incorporate LS testing into their policies [20].

Proof of test validity and its dissemination are crucial. Participants in the New Strategies conference also foresaw that widespread efforts to institute Tier 1 cascade and universal screening would require sufficient leadership. Public health authorities are cognizant of the necessity for obtaining buy-in and help from stakeholders when instituting a program. A program needs to contain elements that appeal to the interests and well-being of the various stakeholder groups that will be impacted. The political will to move a program through, given that competing draws on resources exist, is also a necessity [21]. The LS Workgroups discussed how "the first and most essential step to securing buy-in from public health departments for LS screening is building political will through the identification of effective leader(s) who will excite, connect, and convene the necessary stakeholders" (NSR, p. 52). The leader may be a state level champion, such as an individual from a health department or from business or the community, or the leader may emerge from the national level, such as the Centers for Disease Control and Prevention. The program leader would need to work with different levels of state leadership, as resources already exist (e.g., CDC's Colorectal Cancer Control Program) that could be tapped into. Once a state comprehensive cancer program is on board, it can use its leverage to convene a meeting of state level stakeholders.

Public health genetics and genomics programs have in the past depended on leadership and advocacy from a variety of directions. LS Group 2 cited advocacy groups as well as the media as conduits for working with communities and publicizing programs at their start-up. Both the *New Strategies* and the *Priorities* reports suggested partnering with advocacy groups that already have large buy-in from public health departments [11, 13]. These relationships would allow the identification of at-risk families and make cascade screening more efficient and less costly.

Lynch syndrome screening initiatives must address the needs of both consumers and providers. State chronic disease directors have been involved with the maintenance and use of cancer disease registries, and could be major participants in developing informed consent protocols for individuals and families and in implementing data collection. It is conceivable that influential professional societies – the American Society of Clinical Oncology, the American Gastroenterological Association, the American College of Medical Genetics and Genomics, and the National Society of Genetic Counselors, for example – could take leading roles in administering Tier 1 programs.

The emphasis in the past, however, has been on bench to bedside translation and guidelines formation, and on management of the individual patient. Conference participants suggested it would be possible for public health professionals connected with these societies to facilitate incorporating Tier 1 genomics efforts into their existing activities, enlarging the programmatic scope to the community level.

Conference Findings on Lynch Syndrome Program Support

Participants distinguished between support for screening programs, and coverage for individualized testing. In Britain, Ireland, and Denmark, personal engagement in cascade screening is supported either by the state or the program itself if it is investigational [22].

Likewise, newborn screening in the United States is heavily subsidized, with any residual costs picked-up by the family's payer. However, the day has not yet been reached where payment for individual testing for the Tier 1 conditions is automatic. During the Patient and Community Perspectives Panel session, Cristi Radford of Lynch Syndrome International shared her success in helping hospitals to obtain reimbursement for IHC testing, though she had found that obtaining coverage for germline mutation testing and for *BRAF* mutation analysis and hypermethylation testing remain an issue. Insurance coverage of germline mutation analysis for LS varies, depending on whether the payer's guidelines stipulate the patient must be 50 years of age or younger and meets the Amsterdam II criteria or the Bethesda guidelines. In various points in the conferencing among the working groups, it was reasoned that medical payers would need to be among the partners in discussions by public health and health care providers to implement the screening programs.

In terms of the screening programs per se, LS Group 1 suggested that the CDC could bring groups together by creating requests for proposals (RFPs) which would require that public health departments and advocacy groups collaborate towards a population-based response at state or local levels. It could be that such efforts would require linkage between the two U.S. federal health agencies – the CDC and the National Institutes of Health (NIH) – to ensure adequate funding for relevant activities in numerous states. The earlier Priorities Report suggested that new or bolstered genetic screening programs could piggyback on existing funded programs, such as CDC's Colorectal Cancer Control Program [23] and its National Breast and Cervical Cancer Early Detection Program [24]. This solution parallels LS Working Group 1's suggestion that the CDC could bring on-board the state Colorectal Cancer Cancer Control programs. The piggybacking idea has the advantage of prior evidence of success and cost-effectiveness from state programs that have been up-and-running. CDC's Colorectal Cancer Control Program currently provides funding to 25 states for screening programs that promote population-based CRC screening and follow-up for underinsured or uninsured individuals ages 50-64 [23].

If a central public health-related body could bring key state examples to bear on the implementation of Tier 1 genetic screening and coordinate agencies that have been involved in the process, then such a "knowledge network" could help train other states. CDC as well as the Association of State and Territorial Health Officials (ASTHO) have published examples of states that have developed heritable cancer (Lynch syndrome, hereditary breast and ovarian cancer) surveillance programs [25, 26]. LS Group 1 members envisioned the toolkits for states including a collection of evidence–based publications, a sample of narratives, and an inventory of successful programs that have been implemented in other states. Pilot programs may provide data that can be used in grant or research applications (testing- and education-related) seeking additional funds. States with approved coverage for Tier 1 testing could create active partnerships with other states interested in engaging in Medicaid expansion or in building screening programs around tests that are already covered.

Conference Findings Addressing Conduct of Genetic Screening and Surveillance

In 2014 the National Comprehensive Cancer Network (NCCN) produced clinical practice guidelines on genetic/familial high-risk assessment of colorectal cancer under separate cover from their general guidelines for colorectal cancer screening [27]. Very much in line with *New Strategies* conference recommendations, NCCN proposed that newly diagnosed CRC patients be screened for Lynch syndrome if the colon cancer is diagnosed before age 30. Cancers of the endometrium and ovaries in relatives should also be considered, in line with Amsterdam II criteria. The EGAPP Working Group found sufficient evidence to recommend genetic testing for individuals with newly diagnosed colorectal cancer, but insufficient evidence to recommend choice of a specific molecular screening and mutation testing strategy [16]. These recommendations and the forms of genetic testing and surveillance to which they apply may be found in Table 2.

With respect to family members of affected individuals, NCCN recommended advising them about possible inherited cancer risk, options for risk assessment, and management. It recommended genetic counseling and consideration of genetic testing for relatives [27]. Statistics have been compiled on this kind of follow-through. Seventy-five % of high-risk family members in a clinical cancer LS surveillance program in Finland received counseling and ultimately were tested [30]. Sharaf has suggested that the success of involving family members in LS testing may be a function of the closeness of relatives to the proband, and whether they feel safe with how the results are used [31]. Health systems such as Kaiser Permanente Northwest have found a general level of acceptance of the possibility of undergoing LS testing among their CRC positive enrollees [32].

Duquette recommended that state health departments look for opportunities to integrate universal Lynch syndrome screening into their colorectal cancer screening and detection efforts. This advice pertains both to screening administered by public health at the clinical level, and to public health cancer surveillance efforts. LS Group 1 pointed out that for such screening to be truly "universal," new endometrial cancer cases would need to be included as well. Bellcross et al. have cautioned that universal LS screening "will require significant collaborations between healthcare systems and public health agencies, with strategies and interventions targeted at multiple levels across the healthcare continuum" [34].

This comment echoes the perceived need for partnership building and networking to make LS universal screening workable as discussed at the conference. The Lynch Syndrome Screening Network, comprised of 66 institutions, reports that the majority of its member institutions have implemented universal screening practices, suggesting the move to universal screening is feasible [35]. Speaker Heather Hampel mentioned that in a Columbus-area study of 35 CRC probands using MSI screening, 52 of 99 first degree relatives who were tested turned out to be positive. The MSI screening was quite useful. Conference participants maintained that public health professionals should set benchmarks and goals for universal LS cascade screening. Clinical algorithms are available. Steps should be taken to ensure that those who have screened positive for LS, through techniques such as IHC and MSI, receive the necessary preventive procedures such as annual colonoscopies.

Table 2. Lynch syndrome genetic testing policies and interventions

	Policy Guidelines			Cascade Screening		Universal Screening		Surveillance and Registries	
Condition	Published [Y/N]	Implemented [Y/N]	References	Achieved [Y/N][b]	References	Achieved [Y/N]	References	Achieved [Y/N]	References
Lynch Syndrome (LS)	Y	(Y)[a]	EGAPP [16]; NCCN [27]	(Y)	Dilzell et al. [28]; Hampel et al. [29]; Atkan-Collan et al. [30]; Sharaf et al. [31]	(Y)	Hunter et al. [32]; Schneider et al. [33]; Bellcross et al. [34]	Y	Mange et al. [35]

[a] "(Y)" means limited achievement of the policy or program at the current time.

[b] Cell will be marked "Y" only if program is occurring in both Europe and the U.S.A.

LS Group 2 argued that the appropriate use of cancer registries, EMR, and other means of data collection is important for accurate surveillance of Lynch syndrome cases. Members stated that data should be collected through cancer registries on all measures of universal screening for LS, including IHC, MSI, and exclusionary *BRAF* mutation and methylation testing [36]. Issues of informed consent and confidentiality may arise due to the adding of genetic testing results to registry data. The utility of such data collection would be to use state cancer registries to filter all existing diagnoses of CRC for additional LS testing and disease identification. "Analyzing cases within the state cancer registries would close the clinical feedback loop and ensure that patients are not missed" (NSR, p. 64). EMR systems could be used to communicate data to registries, and conversely, to alert clinicians to the need for LS screening in high-risk families. To be practicable, participants also suggested utilizing state level health information exchanges (HIEs) to detect at-risk individuals and monitor health outcomes. Recommendations addressed the working parts of what might be done, including linkage with clinical systems and death certificates via EMRs, and establishment of secondary data systems beyond index cases to inform providers of at-risk family members.

Conference Findings on Lynch Syndrome Genetics Education

A clear obstacle to performing the necessary screening, as commented on by speaker Duquette, is the general provider lack of knowledge regarding Lynch syndrome. A study by Tan et al. of 144 physicians in Australia, including oncologists and gastroenterologists, indicated that most of the professional respondents demonstrated suboptimal knowledge of Lynch syndrome [37]. Male general practitioners who had been practicing for at least 10 years were less likely to offer genetic referral for Lynch syndrome than specialists, with one third not feeling their role was to identify patients for referral. Many clinicians did not recognize that IHC testing is not germline testing. Knowledge deficiencies may start early. In a survey of 405 medical students from Weill Cornell Medical College, 59% of students reported they had learned about Lynch syndrome, and of those, 18% were aware of available genetic screening and 24% were aware of the criteria used to screen for the syndrome [38]. These findings suggest a general need to educate providers in the existence of genetic services for Lynch syndrome, including referral. Patient and Consumer Perspectives Panel participants also felt that as visibility for LS screening tests becomes more prominent in the public eye, both providers and patients must be educated about the benefits and limitations of IHC testing to prevent negative outcomes such as incorrect ordering of tests, misinterpretation of test results by physicians, false assurance about risk, and the election by patients of unnecessary preventive surgeries.

The LS work groups discussed different categories of activity that could be mounted to increase provider awareness. LS Group 1 suggested that medical societies incentivize best practices for Lynch syndrome genetic testing and referral by offering educational programs that meet maintenance of professional certification requirements, specifically Part IV (Practice Performance Assessment). To encourage accountability within medical organizations for the delivery of care relating to Lynch syndrome, accountable care organization accreditation could be offered as an incentive. LS Group 2 commented on the dissemination of existent guidelines. Members stressed accessibility. Electronic versions of guidelines for clinical decision-making should be made available to physicians that are compatible with electronic medical records (EMRs). EGAPP could work with the American Medical Informatics Association and the Office of the National Coordinator for Health to accomplish this type of guidelines conversion.

Debra Duquette stated that health departments can take steps to enhance public and provider awareness of and knowledge about the condition. LS Group 1 suggested that public health departments could collaborate with accreditation organizations to incentivize education for healthcare professionals. An example provided was a web-based CRC educational program for providers created by the National Coalition for Health Professional Education in Genetics (NCHPEG) and the American Medical Association. The program discusses hereditary CRC red flags and CRC family history [39]. In addition to being an educational tool, the course acts as an incentive. Physicians who complete the online course can receive 6 AMA PRA Category 1 credits, and if a performance improvement component is completed, 20 credits. Public health departments could partner with other organizations, e.g., disease advocacy, universities, to expand the array of credit-conferring educational modules touching on Lynch syndrome.

Accessibility of materials is a factor in Lynch syndrome awareness-raising. The need exists for "succinct and clear educational materials with relevant information about LS screening procedures and their availability at this time" (NSR, p. 57). One-page fact sheets would have premium value for consumers and busy providers. The LS toolkit envisioned by participants could contain such fact sheets, LS statistics, model cases, and links to professional organizations and resources.

DISCUSSION

Recent Developments: Emergent Electronic Networks and Health Care Reform

The novel concept of linking public health surveillance systems with medical systems using HIEs is coming to pass. Michigan and Minnesota now have systems that allow the sending and receiving of clinical information between providers and health care organizations, and of health information between medical systems and health departments [40, 41]. The Michigan Department of Health and Human Services is one of several health sectors in that state participating since 2012 in a coordinated, electronic health information network (MiHIN) that: (1) allows for real-time reporting by providers and hospitals of health trends and threats to state public health agencies; and (2) supports statewide and interstate electronic submission of public health data (e.g., reportable labs, disease surveillance) [40]. A 2012 Association of State and Territorial Health Officials (ASTHO) report describes other state efforts, including in New York, Rhode Island, Indiana, and Utah, to create comprehensive electronic systems that electronically link infectious disease, immunization record, newborn screening, and birth defects tracking [42].

These systems are states' electronic answers to the health care exchanges required under the Patient Protection and Affordable Care Act (ACA), building on the momentum of prior legislation such as the Health Insurance Portability and Accountability Act (HIPAA) which paved the way for secure sharing of electronic health records. The relevance of the ACA is that it mandates coverage without co-pay of adults over 50, including "surveillance screening" for those at higher risk than the general population [43]. A clarification from the Centers for Medicare and Medicaid Services allows for the attending provider to make the determination of whether the individual is part of a "high-risk population," allowing for the service, such as annual colonoscopy, to be covered without cost-sharing [44]. This progress within the U.S. system is a step in the right direction for individuals and families who might benefit from Lynch syndrome molecular screening and genetic testing, and from the vigilance of surveillance systems.

Conclusion: A Mergence of Strategies

The recommendations developed by the Lynch syndrome work groups in this conference went considerably beyond the straight mapping of directions for the future, touching on strategies that are coming to pass and yet to be realized. The toolkit concept has already actualized in the March 2014 release of a basic resource toolkit that states can adopt [45]. In the last decade public health genomics literature and developments have tended to focus on the incorporation of family history into the clinical arsenal, with the *Priorities* conference recommending cascade screening of family members. Of note, assessment of family history missed 25% of CRC patients with LS and 65% of EC patients with LS in the Columbus HNPCC study cited by conference speaker Heather Hampel. This finding underscores the importance of molecular screening of tumor samples followed by genetic testing for positive screens. Clinical protocol is thus shifted towards both cascade screening of at-risk relatives, and universal screening of individuals with CRC. This shift, and the readiness of public health practitioners and medical providers to entertain universal screening, provided the motivation for the *New Strategies* conference.

Resources are another question. Cascade genetic testing in Europe has benefited from national health system support and ongoing clinical trials, while in the United States commercial health care systems and disease advocacy-related networks have much more recently taken on this responsibility. The Lynch Syndrome Screening Network has both institutions actively performing routine tumor testing on colorectal and/or endometrial tumors, and promotional organizations such as federal/state agencies and patient support/advocacy groups among its membership. Public health can be a major player in identifying and educating individuals and families who might benefit, and in developing coalitions combining the strengths of clinical medicine, public health practice, and the community at large. The assimilation of data on at-risk individuals and its pooling into electronic systems, a goal prioritized by conference participants, is rushing forward fairly rapidly due to HIPAA and ACA requirements, and the involvement of multiple sectors. The report card on the states is currently mixed. Several states are already engaged in Lynch syndrome epidemiologic and test utilization surveillance and education. Likewise, a number of states are aiming their health information exchanges towards public health and the interchange of heritable disease information. This growth needs to continue and, in accordance with what conference participants suggested, a mergence of clinical and public health strategies needs to take place. A barbell is only as useful as the weight at both ends and the connection in between.

Genetic testing policy remains in evolution as the recent update of NCCN colorectal cancer policy indicates. This conference developed a spectrum of policies – the “broad end of the stick” – that addresses next steps. A variety of issues remain unresolved, however. One is the question of whether initial identification of Lynch syndrome should start with individuals who have just been clinically diagnosed with CRC or EC, or with high risk relatives who are as yet unassessed. Where should the resources be committed – towards cascade screening, which exists at the family level, or universal screening, which takes place clinically? Can the “toolkit” that has materialized now be utilized by states to grow their own programs? The conference outlined where actions are needed, but final choices remain, calling for further dialogue.

With any dialogic exchange, the timeliness issue acts as a barometer of the potential relevance of what is discussed. The United States has just emerged from an explosion of events in the health care arena, including the liberalization of gene patenting and an overhaul of the national health care system. The price of genetic testing is down, and new tests like Cologuard © for colon cancer screening are coming to market. Truly a new window of opportunity exists. In the colon cancer screening area, patient preference has always had a marked influence on the type of test performed. The traditional colorectal screens consumers select are a first step in diagnosis, but now the genetic tools are at hand to definitively identify cases of Lynch syndrome and curtail disease progression. Colorectal cancer is the second leading cause of death among all cancers, but Lynch syndrome need not be the topmost heritable contributor.

REFERENCES

[1] Secretary’s Advisory Committee on National Health Promotion and Disease Prevention Objectives for 2020. Healthy People 2020: genomics. http://www.healthypeople.gov/2020/about/history-development/Secretary%E2%80%99s-Advisory-Committee.

[2] Centers for Disease Control and Prevention, Office of Public Health Genomics. Genomic testing and family history by levels of evidence: tier 1. Atlanta, GA. 2015. http://www.cdc.gov/genomics/gtesting/tier.htm.

[3] Centers for Disease Control and Prevention, Division of Cancer Prevention and Control. Colorectal cancer statistics. Atlanta, GA. 2015. http://www.cdc.gov/cancer/colorectal/statistics.

[4] National Cancer Institute, Surveillance, Epidemiology, and End Results Program. SEER stat fact sheets: colon and rectum cancer. Bethesda, MD. 2015. http://seer.cancer.gov/about/contact.html.

[5] American Cancer Society. What are the key statistics about colorectal cancer? Atlanta, GA. 2015. http://www.cancer.org/cancer/colonandrectumcancer/detailedguide/colorectal-cancer-key-statistics.

[6] Strafford, J.C. Genetic testing for Lynch syndrome, an inherited cancer of the bowel, endometrium, and ovary. *Rev. Obstet. Gynecol.* 2012; 5(1): 42-49.

[7] Mulcahy, N. NCCN: test all colorectal cancers for Lynch syndrome. *Medscape Med. News.* 2014. http://www.medscape.com/viewarticle/821981.

[8] Hampel, H., Frankel, W., Panescu, J., Lockman, J., Sotamaa, K., Fix, D., Comeras, I., La Jeunessa, J., et al. Screening for Lynch syndrome (hereditary nonpolyposis colorectal cancer) among endometrial cancer patients. *Cancer Res.* 2006; 66(15): 7810-7817.

[9] American Society of Clinical Oncology. Lynch syndrome. Alexandria, VA. 2015. http://www.cancer.net/cancer-types/lynch-syndrome.

[10] American Public Health Association. Advancing cancer genomics in public health. (APHA Policy # 201317). Washington, D.C. 2013. http://www.apha.org/policies-and-advocacy/public-health-policy-statements/policy-database/2014/07/23/10/25/advancing-cancer-genomics-in-public-health.

[11] Center for Public Health and Community Genomics, Genetic Alliance. Priorities for public health genomics 2012-2017. Ann Arbor, MI. 2011. http://genomicsforum.org/files/geno_report_WEB_w_RFI_1122rev.pdf.

[12] Core Public Health Functions Steering Committee. Public health in America statement: public health core functions. Atlanta, GA. 2004. http://www.cdc.gov/nphpsp/essentialservices.html.

[13] Center for Public Health and Community Genomics, Le, L.Q.; Skiba, J., eds. New strategies in public health genomics: actions to save lives now ("NSR"). Ann Arbor, MI. 2012. http://genomicsforum.org/editoruploads/ActionstoSaveLivesNowReport.pdf.

[14] Grover, S., Syngal, S. Risk assessment, genetic testing and management of Lynch syndrome. *J. Natl. Compr. Canc. Netw.* 2010; 8(1): 98-105.

[15] Dinh, T.A., Rosner, B.I., Atwood, J.C., Boland, C.R., Syngal, S., Vasen, H.F., Gruber, S.B., Burt, R.W. Health benefits and cost-effectiveness of primary genetic screening for Lynch syndrome in the general population. *Cancer Prev. Res.* 2011; 4(1): 9-22.

[16] Evaluation of Genomic Applications in Practice and Prevention (EGAPP) Working Group. Recommendations from the EGAPP Working Group: genetic testing strategies in newly diagnosed individuals with colorectal cancer aimed at reducing morbidity and mortality from Lynch syndrome in relatives. *Genet. Med.* 2009; 11(1): 35-41.

[17] Centers for Disease Control and Prevention, Office of Public Health Genomics. Genomics translation: EGAPP: informing the effective integration of genomics into health practice – Lynch syndrome. Atlanta, GA. 2012. http://www.cdc.gov/genomics/gtesting/EGAPP/lynch_study.htm.

[18] Palomaki, G.E., McClain, M.R., Melillo, S., Hampel, H.L., Thibodeau, H.N. EGAPP supplementary evidence review: DNA testing strategies aimed at reducing morbidity and mortality from Lynch syndrome. *Genet. Med.* 2009; 11(1): 42-65.

[19] Bonis, P.A., Trikalinos, T.A., Cgung, M., Chew, P., Ip, S., DeVine, D.A., Lau, J. Hereditary nonpolyposis colorectal cancer: diagnostic strategies and their implications. *Evid. Rep. Technol. Assess.* 2007; (150): 1-180.

[20] Centers for Disease Control and Prevention, Office of Public Health Genomics. Identifying opportunities to improve health and transform healthcare. Atlanta, GA. 2015. http://www.cdc.gov/genomics/gtesting/file/print/EGAPP_factsheet.pdf.

[21] Lezine D.A., Reed, G.A. Political will: a bridge between public health knowledge and action. *Am. J. Public Health* 2007; 97(11): 2010-2013.

[22] Modell, S.M., Kardia, S.L.R., Citrin, T. Stakeholder consultation insights on the future of genomics at the clinical-public health interface. *Transl. Res.* 2014; 163(5): 466-477.

[23] Centers for Disease Control and Prevention, Division of Cancer Prevention and Control. Colorectal Cancer Control Program. Atlanta, GA. 2015. http://www.cdc.gov/cancer/crccp.

[24] Centers for Disease Control and Prevention, Division of Cancer Prevention and Control. National Breast and Cervical Cancer Early Detection Program. Atlanta, GA. 2015. http://www.cdc.gov/cancer/nbccedp.

[25] St. Pierre, J., Bach, J., Duquette, D., Oehlke, K., Nystrom, R., Silvey, K., Zlot, A., Giles, R., et al. Strategies, actions, and outcomes of pilot state programs in public health genomics, 2003-2008. *Prev. Chronic Dis.* 2014; 11: E97.

[26] Association of State and Territorial Health Officials. The 2010 state public health genomics resource guide. Arlington, VA. 2010. http://www.astho.org/Programs/Access/Genomics/The-2010-State-Public-Health-Genomics-Resource-Guide.

[27] National Comprehensive Cancer Network. NCCN guidelines: genetic/familial high-risk assessment: colorectal, Version I. Fort Washington, PA. 2015. Available online: http://www.nccn.org/professionals/physician_gls/pdf/genetics_colon.pdf.

[28] Dilzell, K., Kingham, K., Ormond, K., Ladabaum, U. Evaluating the utilization of educational materials in communicating about Lynch syndrome to at-risk relatives. *Fam. Cancer* 2014; 13(3): 381-389.

[29] Hampel, H., Frankel, W.L., Martin, E., Arnold, M., Khanduja, K., Kuebler, P., Nakagawa, H., Sotamaa, K., et al. Screening for the Lynch syndrome (hereditary nonpolyposis colorectal cancer). *N. Engl. J. Med.* 2005; 352(18): 1851-1860.

[30] ***[Editor, please apply umlaut symbols (double dots) over the indicated vowels, then remove the five "(umlaut over vowel)" comments. Thank you.] Atkan-Collan, K., Mecklin, J.-P., Ja(umlaut over a)rvinen, H., Nystro(umlaut over o)m-Lahti, M., Peltoma(umlaut over a)ki, P., So(umlaut over o)derling, I., Utela, A., de la Chapelle, A., Kaaria(umlauts over the three a's)nen, H. Predictive genetic testing for hereditary non-polyposis colorectal cancer: uptake and long-term satisfaction. *Int. J. Cancer (Pred. Oncol.)* 2000; 89(1): 44-50.

[31] Sharaf, R.N., Myer, P., Stave, C.D., Diamond, L.C., Ladabaum, U. Uptake of genetic testing by relatives of Lynch syndrome probands: a systematic review. *Clin. Gastroenterol. Hepatol.* 2013; 11(9): 1093-1100.

[32] Hunter, J.E., Zepp, J.M., Gilmore, M.J., Davis, J.V., Esterberg, E.J., Muessig, K.R., Peterson, S.K., Syngal, S., et al. Universal tumor screening for Lynch syndrome: Assessment of the perspectives of patients with colorectal cancer regarding benefits and barriers. *Cancer* 2015; 121(18): 3281-3289.

[33] Schneider, J.L., Davis, J., Kauffman, T.L., Reiss, J.A., McGinley, C., Arnold, K., Zepp, J., Gilmore, M., et al. Stakeholder perspectives on implementing a universal Lynch syndrome screening program: A qualitative study of early barriers and facilitators. *Genet. Med.* 2015, 16 April, doi: 10.1038/gim.2015.43.

[34] Bellcross, C.A., Bedrosian, S.R., Daniels, E., Duquette, D., Hampel, H., Jasperson, K., Joseph, D.A., et al. Implementing screening for Lynch syndrome among patients with newly diagnosed colorectal cancer: summary of a public health/clinical collaborative meeting. *Genet. Med.* 2012; 14(1): 152-162.

[35] Mange, S., Bellcross, C., Cragun, D., Duquette, D., Gorman, L., Hampel, H., Jasperson, K. Creation of a network to promote universal screening for Lynch syndrome: the Lynch Syndrome Screening Network. *J. Genet. Counsel.* 2015, 24, 421-427.

[36] Parsons, M.T., Buchanan, D.D., Thompson, B., Young, J.P., Spurdle, A.B. Correlation of tumour BRAF mutations and *MLH1* methylation with germline mismatch repair (MMR) gene mutation status: a literature review assessing utility of tumour features for MMR variant classification. *J. Med. Genet.* 2012; 49(3): 151-157.

[37] Tan, Y.Y., Spurdle, A.B., Obermair, A. Knowledge, attitudes, and referral patterns of Lynch syndrome: a survey of clinicians in Australia. *J. Pers. Med.* 2014; 4(2): 218-244.

[38] Frey, M.K., Biewald, M.A., Worley, M.J., Jr., Taylor, J.S., Lin, S.N., Holcomb, K. Lynch syndrome: awareness among medical students at a United States medical school. *Curr. Womens Health Rev.* 2012; 8(3): 242-247.

[39] National Coalition for Health Professional Education in Genetics. Colorectal cancer: is your patient at high risk? Lutherville, MD. 2012. http://www.nchpeg.org/index.php?option=com_content&view=article&id=382:colorectal-cancer-are-your-patients-at-high-risk&catid=35:todays-highlights%27.

[40] Michigan Health Information Network (MiHIN). Public health reporting. East Lansing, MI. 2015. http://mihin.org/services/public-health-reporting.

[41] Minnesota Department of Health, Office of Health Information Technology. Local public health: e-health capacity, capability, and challenges, 2013. 2014. St. Paul, MN. http://www.health.state.mn.us/e-health/summaries/reportlph2013.pdf.

[42] Association of State and Territorial Health Officials. State options for enhancing health information exchange for MCH systems. Arlington, VA. 2012. http://www.astho.org/Maternal-and-Child-Health/Collaborations/MCH-and-Health-Information-Exchange-Issue-Brief.

[43] U.S. Department of Health and Human Services. Preventive services covered under the Affordable Care Act. Washington, D.C. 2012. http://www.hhs.gov/healthcare/facts/factsheets/2010/07/preventive-services-list.html.

[44] Centers for Medicare and Medicaid Services. Affordable Care Act implementation FAQs – set 12. Baltimore, MD. 2013. https://www.cms.gov/CCIIO/Resources/Fact-Sheets-and-FAQs/aca_implementation_faqs12.html.

[45] Centers for Disease Control and Prevention, Office of Public Health Genomics. Genomics implementation: tier 1 genomic applications toolkit for public health departments. Atlanta, GA. 2014. http://www.cdc.gov/genomics/implementation/toolkit/index.htm.

INDEX

I

J

K

L

M

N

O

P

R

S

V